D1213112

The Holistic Rx

The Holistic Rx

Your Guide to Healing Chronic Inflammation and Disease

Madiha Saeed, MD

ROWMAN & LITTLEFIELD
Lanham • Boulder • New York • London

Published by Rowman & Littlefield
A wholly owned subsidiary of The Rowman & Littlefield Publishing Group, Inc.
4501 Forbes Boulevard, Suite 200, Lanham, Maryland 20706
www.rowman.com

Unit A, Whitacre Mews, 26-34 Stannary Street, London SE11 4AB

Graphics designed by Anna R. Cunningham

British Library Cataloguing in Publication Information Available

Library of Congress Cataloging-in-Publication Data

Names: Saeed, Madiha M., author.
Title: The holistic Rx : your guide to healing chronic inflammation and disease / Madiha M. Saeed.
Description: Lanham : Rowman & Littlefield, [2017] | Includes bibliographical references and index.
Identifiers: LCCN 2017015592 (print) | LCCN 2017019677 (ebook) | ISBN 9781442279445 (electronic) | ISBN 9781442279438 (cloth : alk. paper)
Subjects: LCSH: Inflammation—Alternative treatment. | Integrative medicine. | Alternative medicine—Popular works. | Chronic diseases—Alternative treatment.
Classification: LCC RB131 (ebook) | LCC RB131 .S24 2017 (print) | DDC 616/.0473—dc23
LC record available at https://lccn.loc.gov/2017015592

∞™ The paper used in this publication meets the minimum requirements of American National Standard for Information Sciences—Permanence of Paper for Printed Library Materials, ANSI/NISO Z39.48-1992.

Printed in the United States of America

Dedicated to my extraordinary parents and to those who spread their wings of unconditional love, support, and sacrifice to ones who need it most

Contents

Disclaimer

This book represents reference material only. It is not intended as a medical manual, and the data presented here are meant to assist the reader in making informed choices regarding wellness. This book is not a replacement for treatment(s) that the reader's personal physician may have suggested. If the reader believes he or she is experiencing a medical issue, professional medical help is recommended. Mention of particular products, companies, or authorities in this book does not entail endorsement by the publisher or author.

Acknowledgments

THE TRUE POWER OF UNCONDITIONAL LOVE AND SACRIFICE

They say in order to raise a child, it takes a village. But it can also just be a few individuals' extraordinary unconditional love equal to the love of one village that can do the trick. I am blessed to have had just that. Surrounded by unconditional love from the moment I made my entrance, my parents sacrificed everything to raise their four children to become debt-free physicians—and by everything, I really do mean EVERYTHING: their home, their friends and family, their money, their clothes, their time, basically their lives. They sacrificed it all to ensure their children had what they needed to pursue their dreams and make a difference in the world. Amidst the overwhelming unconditional love, sacrifice, and support I realized anything is possible. All that matters is love.

So for this and everything, I especially thank my extraordinary parents, Nusrat and Muhammad Saeed; my siblings, Athar, Fasiha, Sophia, and Atif Saeed—who despite their busy lives as physicians come regulary to watch the kids, even post call, so I could take a shower or eat a meal by myself; my children Abdullah, Zain, Emaad, and Qasim—who inspire me daily to prevent leptin and insulin resistance so I don't spend my entire life in the kitchen; and my husband, Omer, for being my rock. I am also blessed with the love and support from my in-laws (Mumtaz and Tahira Ansari, Muhammad, Sadaf, Sadia, and Shazia), family, and friends (too many to name, but you know who you are) who continue to motivate me to be all that I can.

I'll continue to give thanks here, because gratitude lowers my inflammation—and after writing this book, I'll need all the help I can get! First, I have a confession—I didn't even know what holistic medicine was until I was taken under wing by my attendings (Uthman and Susan Cavallo, MD) and their staff, who spent countless hours "catching me up to speed" with what I had missed out on in my official medical training. For them I am incredibly grateful for opening my eyes to the true beauty of healing and caring for the whole person. I'll continue to thank my agent, Jeff Herman, who put his belief in a newbie's idea and gave her a chance in the competitive world of publishing. I thank my editors, Jess Beebe, and Suzanne Staszak-Silva, Melissa McNitt, and all those at Roman & Littlefield for doing such an amazing job in helping my dream become a reality. Thank you, Drs. Mark Hyman, Frank Lipman, David Perlmutter, Amy Myers, Josh Axe, Tom O'Bryan, Maya Shetreat-Klein, Izabella Wentz, and so many more who have blazed this trail far before me and have dedicated their lives to others, shared their wisdom, and have inspired me. I am also thankful for the support from Erik Goldman (Holistic Primary Care) and Beth Lambert (Documenting Hope) who motivate me daily with their enthusiasm, dedication, and unconditional love to spread the message of healing far and wide, bringing hope to so many. I am grateful to Mary Agnes and Tommy Antonopoulos for supporting me with tools and guidance I needed to get off the ground.

I can't forget those who strive daily to get off the hamster wheel and take back control of their health and happiness (I know it isn't easy), especially my initial patients who helped me bloom into who I am today. For all of you who spread your wings of unconditional love, support, and sacrifice to those who need it most—for exponential inspiration, I am truly, undoubtedly thankful! I can't thank the Being Above enough. I am truly blessed! I love you all from the bottom of my heart, as the power of unconditional love and sacrifice can free us, giving us exactly what we need to fly!

Introduction

Ever feel like a hamster on a wheel—huffing and puffing, stuck in a cage, while the world around you whizzes by? Chronic symptoms and health problems can do that to you—your internal life becomes a slowly turning wheel that can inhibit you from getting anywhere. In fact, according to the Centers for Disease Control, about half of all adults in the United States have at least one uncommunicable chronic health condition, while a third have two or more, and the numbers continue to grow at an alarming rate.[1] That's a lot of aimless hamsters logging in a lot of miles! What's even scarier, the rise of chronic illness is also affecting our children.

When the dark cloud of chronic disease brings despair, most people turn to their doctor for salvation. Conventional western medicine works phenomenally well for acute care but, sadly, has its limits when it comes to chronic illnesses. Generally, instead of addressing the root causes of chronic diseases, doctors may "Band-aid" the problem by prescribing medications that come with their own sets of side effects and complications. They stamp you with a lifelong diagnosis, offering very little hope of healing or lifestyle advice. Suddenly, the life that was once yours has now been taken over by your chronic conditions, your doctor, and the pharmaceutical and insurance companies!

In your quest to take back the reins of your health, you then turn to your local bookstore/library. Sadly again to your dismay, there awaits another long and exhausting maze with aisles and aisles of books about how to overcome one chronic disease or another. Many books promise success, and many of the methods outlined actually do have the power to improve your health. While you're running on the hamster wheel, it's overwhelming to try to find the energy and time to research what methods will actually work for your individual conditions. This can lead to frustration and confusion, and it can discourage you from finding the real solution to your problem. Are you truly stuck in life defined by your chronic conditions? Will you just have to live with the idea that your life is no longer in your control?

No! With every dark cloud, there is a silver lining (I know it sounds cliché, but it's so true). There is hope: it is possible to take back the wheel of your health! You are so worth it. I have escaped that hamster wheel, and I have helped thousands of patients do the same. The fact that you're reading this means you're ready to escape too. In this book, I'll show you how.

But why should you trust me? Before becoming a board-certified integrative holistic family physician and health coach, I was like most Americans—unhealthy and overweight. I had many of the same bad habits that have led half of all Americans down the road toward chronic disease. When I joined a holistic practice, I quickly realized that medical school and residency hadn't taught me what I really needed to know about how to keep people healthy and happy. I was taught not one class on nutrition and very little on stress management, and, surprisingly, my colleagues in pediatrics, internal medicine, and psychiatry were in the same boat. We'd spend only fifteen minutes on each patient, and were taught to address one condition at each visit—nothing more, nothing less. We were penalized if we spent too much time with a patient and frowned upon if we didn't see an average of twenty-five patients every workday. In those fifteen-minute visits, we discussed symptoms and treatment options, which more often than not consisted of a prescription for medication.

This didn't feel right to me. How could I truly help someone heal if I focused on only one aspect of the person's life and just treated them with pharmaceuticals? Wasn't there another way? Why was this person sick, anyway? These questions burned in my mind, day in and day out.

I knew I needed to find answers, but I was also suffering with my own chronic conditions: thyroid disease, acne, seborrheic dermatitis, weight and hormonal problems, digestive issues, fatigue and joint/muscle aches. I felt as if every year another problem was around the corner. As both doctor and patient, I was tired of a methodology that covered up symptoms and never got to the root cause of problems. I knew I had the potential to fly but was tired of being weighed down by my chronic illnesses. I needed to find another way!

On my quest for true healing, I came to understand that inflammation is an underlying cause of most chronic health conditions. Healing this inflammation is the key to renewed health, yet it is often overlooked. I discovered that the solution lies in the fields of holistic and functional medicine, which gets to the fundamental reasons of *why* you're feeling the way you're feeling. It uses all the effective tools available—complementary, alternative, and integrative medicine, combined with conventional treatments and unconditional love—to help get your body back into balance.

Years of study in holistic and functional medicine, and applying everything I learned on myself as well as my patients, has transformed my life as a doctor and coach to people with chronic conditions. I now know how to help my patients overcome inflammation and radically improve their health. Everything I prescribe, I have painstakingly researched and lived myself. With the help of *The Holistic Rx*, these simple lifestyle changes have allowed me to alleviate my symptoms from within, get rid of medications for good, and take back the reins of my health.

Every day, my patients inspire me and my passion to guide as many people as possible on the path toward true healing and real living. Two patients are particularly inspirational. The first is a twenty-one-year-old woman who had suffered from severe eczema for as long as she could remember. Her skin burned from head to toe, and she would sit in a bath eight hours a day to try to get some relief. The pain became so unbearable that she tried to commit suicide three times. She saw physician after physician before coming to me, distraught, as a last resort. After just one week of applying the strategies I will teach you in this book, the burning that had plagued her for years was gone. Tears flowed down her face as she asked, "Why hadn't I heard about this treatment earlier?" She had suffered hopelessly for years when the answer lay in the one thing that she could control: her lifestyle.

My second inspirational patient is a thirty-one-year-old woman who had been diagnosed with several autoimmune diseases, including myasthenia gravis, Hashimoto's disease, lichen planus, psoriasis, eczema, and suspected Sjogren's syndrome, along with other chronic conditions. She came to me on seven medications and because of uncontrolled symptoms was being advised to start an eighth. She reflected, "After just six months on the healing diet, I was completely off medication, I had lost weight, and my depression and anxiety had completely disappeared. I felt more like myself than I had in a very long time." She continues to do well, exercising and generally living her life without those health problems, achieving her lifelong dream of becoming a scuba instructor—a dream others had told her to abandon! Her recovery wasn't rocket science, and it didn't cost her a fortune; it was just a matter of making simple, inexpensive changes that improved the quality of her life. Even more amazing is that once you target the root cause, you can heal not just one chronic condition, but all of them simultaneously!

These stories are among thousands of examples that add fuel to my fire to help spread the word of true healing and real living. Patients like you are recovering from autoimmune diseases, skin problems, mood disorders, and digestive issues, along with a very wide range of nonspecific symptoms, without medication, simply by implementing evidence-based, cost-effective lifestyle changes. They inspire me to continue my work, even when I sometimes feel overwhelmed by my own busy and demanding life. I had to get this secret of healing out to the world!

HOW TO NAVIGATE THIS BOOK—TIME TO GET BACK IN CONTROL!

The Holistic Rx approaches healing in two parts. The first part addresses the root causes of chronic health conditions and lays the foundations of good health. It offers a simple, easy-to-follow prescription for healing inflammation and achieving lasting optimal health and happiness. I have conducted extensive and exhaustive research, converting evidence-based information straight from the experts into easy-to-follow advice accompanied with pictures, providing you with all the information you need to take charge of your health.

Chronic disease is basically your body out of balance. *The Holistic Rx* briefly examines the components of every chronic disease—which involve Digestive health and Detoxification, including what to eat—so that you will be empowered to handle the Four Big S's: stress, sleep, social health, and spirituality. This book will hold your hand, taking you step by step, at your own pace, helping to bring yourself back into balance. It will empower you to understand your body and treatment options and to take the next step on your personal healing journey. I will be cheerleading you every step of the way: You can do this!

The second part will take your healing power to the next level with comprehensive, condition-specific recommendations about additional integrative approaches that can be added to the foundations of good health for close to 30 conditions. You'll learn how to tailor your healing program to you, and then accelerate your healing with the use of various integrative modalities that are most effective for your condition. This book offers you a complete guide to self-directed, holistic, functional, and integrative treatment options for common symptoms and ailments for the whole family, empowering you to optimize your own healing and wellness.

I've made *The Holistic Rx* easy to follow, enabling you to see benefits right away, and what's even more exciting—it's cost-effective too! I'll tell you what works, so you can put your time, energy, and money where they'll do the most good.

I can confidently say that healing and preventing disease has never been easier. Even while juggling four young boys (five if you count my husband), cooking, cleaning, zumba, a busy medical practice, and my work in writing, education, and public speaking, I was able to heal and prevent my own chronic diseases and those of my patients, while staying on budget. If I can do it, so can you!

You are a gem, inside and out, no matter your age or demographics! You are a beacon of inspiration to those around you. Look at all you have accomplished despite being less than 100 percent! When you're in good health, you're free to get off the hamster wheel and actually live your life the way you were meant to. Imagine everything you'll be able to accomplish when you're feeling your best. There's no limit to what you can do.

Let's start this healing journey together—at your pace, one step at a time. You are worth it! Did I mention how excited how I am? So excited! Let's do this! Get ready to feel great! Now let the fun begin!

Part 1

THE FOUNDATIONS OF GOOD HEALTH

• *1* •

Understanding the Silent Fire Within

The Role of Inflammation in Chronic Illness

Yay, you've made it to the first chapter (I like to celebrate small successes)! I know what you're thinking: what does inflammation have to do with my symptoms? Well, have no fear because there is just one simple answer—EVERYTHING! Before you start looking the other way, let me explain. The first step of your healing journey is to understand what's fueling your symptoms—that is, why you're feeling the way you do. In order to allow your body to get on the path to recovery, we'll need to help your body get back into balance by targeting the root cause. This effort is key to your recovery; it is the very foundation of good health.

You may have struggled for quite some time with conditions like depression/mood disorders, thyroid disease, autoimmune disorders, digestive issues, skin disorders, or more general symptoms like pain and fatigue. These seem like different problems, but they actually have one thing in common: inflammation—the root of most chronic diseases.

WHAT IS INFLAMMATION ANYWAY?

Run! There's a fire! Don't look behind you, look within (great, now where are you going to run?). *Inflammation* actually means "fire inside," and it's something we're all familiar with—a hot, fierce, lifesaving reaction that occurs when your body's immune system tries to fight off infections, help heal injuries, or protect you from disease. Without inflammation, we would be in danger in a hostile world. We would have no way to fight microbial invaders or repair the damage constantly inflicted on us.

There are two forms of inflammation: acute and chronic.

Acute Inflammation—A Good Thing

Acute inflammation (or good inflammation) lasts for a short time, from a few seconds to several days. It serves a healthy purpose and is beneficial. Almost immediately after tissue damage or stimulated by infections, your immune system (specifically called your innate immunity) sends white blood cells and other hormone-like substances to help start the healing process. An inflamed part of the body is red, hot, swollen, and painful, and it actually indicates an attempt to heal infection—a good sign that your body's defenses are working properly. The innate immune system only knows one order, that an intruder equals inflammation. Thank you, acute inflammation!

Chronic Inflammation—Too Much of a Good Thing

Chronic inflammation (or bad inflammation, sometimes referred to as systemic inflammation), on the other hand, gradually destroys the magnificent masterpiece that we were born with. It is a hidden, smoldering, painless fire created by your immune system as it tries to fight off modern life's daily exposures to triggers like unhealthy food, stress, toxins, allergens, an overgrowth of bad "bugs," and even low-grade infections driving obesity and chronic disease.

The adaptive immune system, responsible for chronic inflammation, takes a little longer to kick in, developing over time. After gathering all the information about the intruder and how to attack that specific threat, it develops a plan. These triggers all cause an increase in the release of inflammatory molecules of your immune system called *cytokines*. Cytokines are important in fighting off infection and cancer, and they help your body distinguish between friend and foe. When properly functioning, the fire can remain contained; however, with constant exposure to triggers, the inflammatory cytokines and their reponses get out of control and go into overdrive—going out of control and destroying everything in its path, leading to chronic diseases of every stripe and causing damage not only in vascular tissues and organs but throughout all body tissues.[1] This self-perpetuating cycle is the common denominator of most chronic diseases and difficult-to-explain symptoms.

At this point, it may rise to the level of a chronic disorder. When this happens, many doctors prescribe pharmaceuticals to address the symptoms until they are manageable. Typically, neither they nor their patients know how to identify the cause and eliminate the inflammation. Standard medicine holds that such diseases can be managed but rarely cured. In contrast, the holistic, functional, and integrative approach recommended in this book is effective in treating all your chronic conditions, because it addresses the underlying cause: chronic inflammation. So cool!

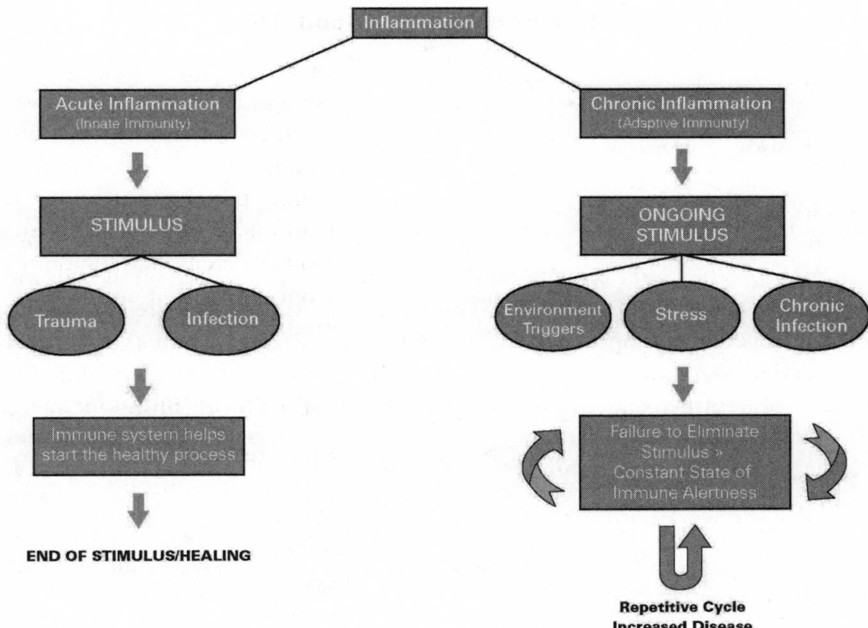

Figure 1.1. Acute vs Chronic Inflammation

OH NO! IS THERE A FIRE WITHIN ME?

You are unique, and so are your chronic conditions with their own unique symptoms. However, some symptoms are characteristic of inflammation in general:

- body aches and pains
- fever
- congestion
- frequent infections
- stiffness
- dry eyes
- digestive symptoms
- shortness of breath
- fatigue
- allergies
- mood disorders

- light-headedness and brain fog
- memory and concentration issues
- weight gain or inability to lose weight
- headaches
- and many more!

Sound familiar? If you have a chronic health condition, likely driven by inflammation, chances are good that you're struggling with one or more of these symptoms. When your body is chronically inflamed, depending on the specific body part, disease can result. For example, if your skin or lungs are chronically inflamed, you are at high risk for developing acne, eczema, asthma, or chronic obstructive pulmonary disorder (COPD). If your brain/nerves or joints are inflamed, attention-deficit/hyperactivity disorder (ADHD), depression/mood disorders, arthritis, and other degenerative diseases can result. Inflamed arteries can lead to heart attacks and strokes. Inflammation can even lead to obesity, as inflammation interferes with the job of the mitochondria (powerhouse of the cell) to burn fat and makes fat loss very difficult. It can affect every part of your body, and overall inflammation can lead to autoimmunity and cancer. Unfortunately, we are seeing more and more of it, every corner we turn!

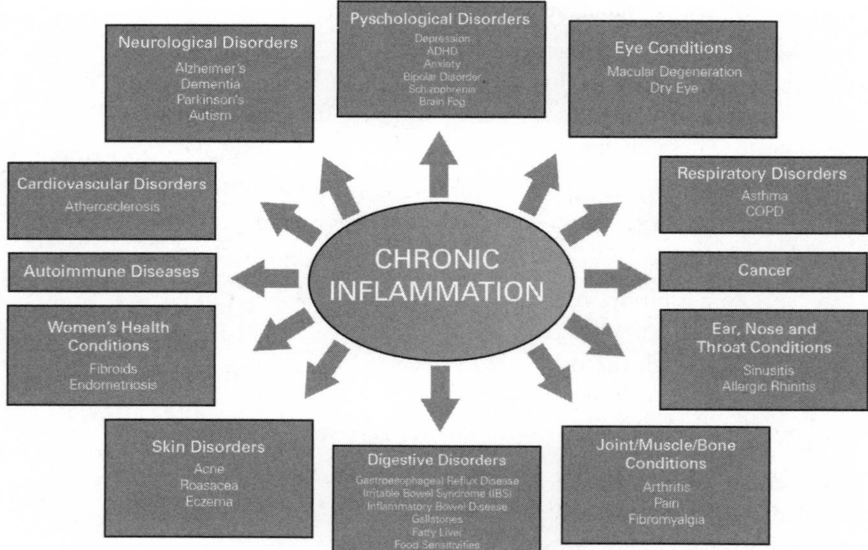

Figure 1.2. Chronic Inflammation

WHY IS CHRONIC DISEASE ON THE RISE?

If you recognize your symptoms in the description of chronic inflammation, you're not alone. The number of people with chronic conditions is rapidly increasing. The CDC states that chronic diseases are the leading causes of death and disability in the United States and are responsible for seven out of ten deaths every year.[2] Chronic disease also accounts for 86 percent of our nation's health care costs.[3] Forty-six million more Americans are projected to have at least one chronic condition in 2030 than in 2000.[4] Given current trends, one in every three children born in 2000 will develop diabetes over the course of a lifetime.[5]

This increase in the rates of chronic illness is a direct outcome of an increase in inflammation. The following factors are thought to explain why inflammation—and thus chronic disease—is on the rise.[6]

Genes in Your Control

Epigenetics is the study of change in our gene functions without physical mutations to the DNA structure. Genes may load the gun, but the environment pulls the trigger. Our diseases, medications, our internal and external environment and lifestyle, digestive health including our microbiome (our gut's bacteria), nutrition, toxins, stressors, exercise, sleep, optimism, and spiritual health, can alter how our genes are expressed. These factors have the ability to turn genes on and off, influencing the release of pro-inflammatory cytokines and thereby potentially increasing the likelihood that we will develop chronic conditions. These changes can then be passed on to our offspring. It is always important to weigh the risk over the benefits before starting on an antibiotic.

Antibiotics

Exposure to antibiotics harms the population of bacteria in our gut (microbiome), triggering a process that can lead to increased inflammation. It is always important to weigh the risk over the benefits before starting on an antibiotic.

Altered Nutrition

More than 80 percent of food in North America contains genetically modified organisms (GMOs)! A 2014 study from MIT researchers correlated the precipitous increase in chronic conditions with increased use of glyphosate (an herbicide most commonly found in GMO seed) as it impairs detoxification.[7, 8] When foods are genetically modified or full of chemicals and artificial flavors and colorings, our immune system views them as foreign invaders instead of food, and inflammation is triggered.

Excessive Hygiene

The hygiene hypothesis suggests that germs actually help build the immune system. Keeping our families in an overly clean and sheltered environment can limit their exposure to germs, restricting the growth of their immune system. The hygiene hypothesis suggests that germs actually help build the immune system. When the immune system doesn't have significant germs to work with, it overreacts to less important triggers, and inflammation may result.

Environmental Toxins

Toxins that surround us can damage the body's own detoxification mechanisms, making it harder for our bodies to get rid of them.

Regular accumulated exposure to toxins can shift our immune system, increase inflammation, and make the body more prone to developing allergies and chronic conditions.

Toxins also damage the body's own detoxification mechanisms, making it harder for our bodies to get rid of the toxins.

Methylation Defects

Methylation is a key biochemical and cellular process that affects genes and is a key element of detoxification. If methylation improves, our body systems function properly. When there is a problem with the methylation process, we can have trouble with detoxification, immune function, mood balance, DNA repair and maintenance, energy production, and inflammation control.

THE PIECES TO THE INFLAMMATION PUZZLE

Inflammation is a complex process, and there are a number of things that can trigger it or make it worse. A deficit in any of the areas discussed below can cause or worsen inflammation.[9] Remember, each individual is different. You may be eating well but dealing with a huge relationship problem. You're in a different situation than someone who is not exercising but has a great social group. Each of you has a unique story with particular implications for your health. Improving your physical, mental/emotional, social, and spiritual health is critical in healing and preventing chronic conditions. When I discuss the factors that contribute to inflammation, begin to think about where your own deficiencies might be—it may be the most productive place for you to start with your own healing.

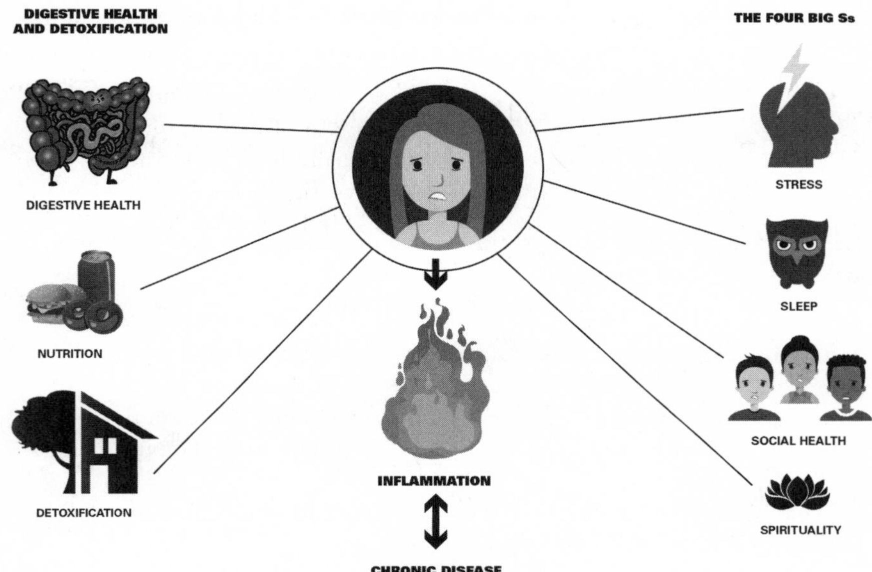

Figure 1.3. The Holistic Rx: Factors of Inflammation

Digestive Health and Detoxification

We are only as well as the way we treat our body, and the activities and choices we make daily can affect our internal world. Imbalanced digestive health, poor nutrition, and environmental toxins can impede our recovery. Let's look at the aspects of physical well-being one by one.

Digestive Health

The gut is the largest gate between the outside environment and our internal environment, playing an integral role in healing and disease prevention. About 70 to 80 percent of the immune system is located in the digestive system. When immune cells are activated through the gut, they release inflammatory molecules that travel throughout the body and cause inflammation in our joints, skin, blood vessels, brain—everywhere! So what we put in our mouths can either help us or harm us, improving or activating our immune system.

Nutrition

Proper nutrition, with an anti-inflammatory diet, not only keeps our digestive system happy but also regulates our glucose and stabilizing insulin (a storage hormone secreted by the pancreas to help regulate the levels of glucose [sugar] in the bloodstream)—managing our insulin resistance. To put it simply, insulin resistance refers to the body's diminished ability to respond to insulin and can result in rapid and premature aging and can cause strokes, dementia, heart disease, and cancer. Anything that causes insulin resistance will also cause inflammation, and vice versa. Nutritional deficiencies often interfere with the healing process, so adding certain supplements to the diet can expedite healing by supporting the immune system and restoring the body to health and balance.

Detoxification

We live in a world full of toxins, most invisible. With regular exposure, toxins can slowly accumulate in our bodies, placing a heavy burden on the liver, the organ that is responsible for removing them. When it is overwhelmed and can't eliminate the toxins, the liver tends to store them, unable to do its job in helping to decrease inflammation and thus further increasing it.

THE FOUR BIG S's: STRESS, SLEEP, SOCIAL HEALTH, AND SPIRITUALITY

Stress

Stress is the cause of more than 80 percent of complaints presented to a doctor. Your physical health affects your spiritual, emotional, and overall psychological well-being. Stress contributes significantly to inflammation. In particular, stress taxes the immune system[10] and chronically increases the levels of cortisol, a hormone that is released to prepare us to respond to threatening situations. This leads to inflammation and its accompanying diseases and ailments. Managing stress is essential in healing and preventing diseases.

Sleep

While we sleep, our body doesn't consume much energy, leaving more energy for the body to remove toxins, make hormones, and fight infections. If we fail to get enough rest, our bodies cannot complete these important tasks. This can increase the chance of developing problems due to excess toxins, inflammation, and hormone imbalances. Improving your sleep is a powerful way to boost your health.

Social Health

Your social environment is so important for healing and preventing chronic inflammation. Loneliness and negative social relationships increase cortisol levels and depress immune function—again, worsening inflammation.[11] Having positive social relationships that leave you feeling loved releases hormones into the bloodstream, strengthens your immune system, and improves your overall health and healing.

Spirituality

Negative spiritual energy is related to increased stress, more depression, and a weakened immune system, increasing inflammation.[12] Healing the soul and cultivating positivity are important aspects in preventing and healing chronic conditions.

STOP RUNNING—LET'S FINALLY PUT OUT THE FIRE!

To be truly effective at managing and/or overcoming a chronic condition or symptom, we need to address these processes at every level. Inflammation burns in the body, slowly destroying it the way fire destroys a building. Unless you put out the fire (that is, calm the inflammation in the body), you're simply allowing the building to smolder, compromising your body further. Conventional medicine doesn't put out the fire for chronic illnesses but simply Band-aids the blaze without turning off the ignition. This approach will only work superficially to keep symptoms at bay but will rarely address the root cause of the blaze. In order to effectively manage the symptoms—and, better yet, overcome the condition—we need to put out the fire once and for all and get your body and it's hormones back into balance, allow your body to stop fighting an uphill battle, and set yourself on the path to recovery. Addressing the root causes of inflammation will help you overcome not one but multiple chronic conditions and balance your hormones all at the same time. Once you have healed the root cause, you can optimize healing by using the additional healing modalities. This gives you all the tools you'll need to get you back in the driver's seat of your own health and help heal and prevent chronic illnesses. That is the power of *The Holistic Rx*.

I will take you through this entire process, step by step, day by day, with laughter and love. Join me on the road to recovery. You deserve health and happiness—let's nip chronic disease in the bud by putting out the fire of inflammation! You can do it! Watch out inflammation, here we come!

• 2 •

Digestive Health and Detoxification

PUTTING OUT THE FIRE AT THE GATE: RESTORING DIGESTIVE HEALTH

When we talk chronic disease, we have to talk about the gut. Don't look down at your belly! I'm not talking about that kind of gut—at least, not yet. I'm talking about your digestive health. Now don't go shying away to the next chapter, because your overall well-being and the health of your digestive tract are intimately integrated, such that problems with the gut are the starting point or the gateway of chronic disease. Healing chronic disease begins in the digestive system.

Ever wonder what the difference is between somebody with a health condition and somebody without? I know it may not seem like it, but we are all the same on the inside. Yes, our genetics may differ, but more and more research is pointing to how our genetics can be influenced by our environment, making a huge impact on how our insides function. Our gut and digestive system make up the largest gate between the outside environment and our internal environment. This gate plays an integral role in healing and disease prevention as the integrity of the intestinal barrier is an important component of inflammation.[1]

Being the gateway to health, your gut is the first to come into contact with the universe and the first line of defense between you and the universe, deciding between the good guys and the bad guys as it houses about 70 to 80 percent of the immune system.[2] To keep us in good health, our gut relies on carefully maintaining a symbiotic relationship with trillions of microorganisms. Your body's defenses are constantly fighting to get rid of inflammation, and this battle results in the symptoms that keep you feeling sick. Improving your digestive health is an essential way to overcome inflammation and chronic disease, so this is the foundation of *The Holistic Rx*. Let's get started! Time to give the "poop maker" the recognition it needs—let's honor thy gut!

The Ride Down

Our human digestive system plays several vital roles.

First, it processes the foods we eat, digesting the food and converting vitamins after absorption of the nutrients regulating our metabolism. The bacteria help to extract energy from undigested food products as they pass through the digestive system.

The digestive system is integral to our immune system. It prevents toxins and pathogens from entering the body. It also repairs any damage caused by foreign substances and the reactions they have caused in the body, such as inflammation and infection.

The digestive tract is also one of the key organs in detoxification, removing toxins from the body (among others that include the liver, kidney, skin, and lungs).

Finally, the digestive system is the body's neurotransmitter factory, as every class of brain neurotransmitters, about three-fourths of the body's neurotransmitters, has been found in the gut, including about 90 percent of the body's serotonin and 50 percent of the body's dopamine.

Knowledge is power, so let us briefly go through what is happening at each point in the digestive system, demonstrated in the accompanying picture.

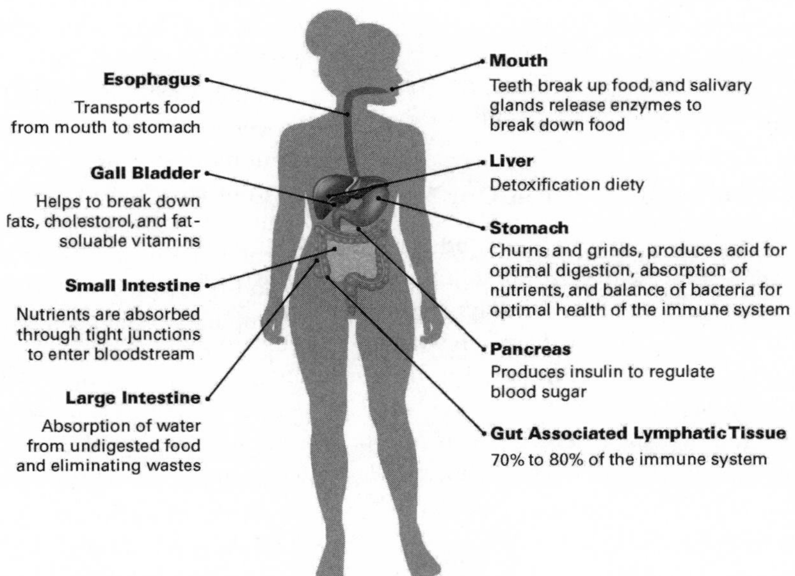

Figure 2.1. The Digestive System

The Secret Organ Within: Our Intestinal Bacteria

Shh. I have a secret: humans are actually superorganisms; we are made up of our own cells plus a huge number of microbes that live on and inside us. In fact, our human cells are outnumbered by one hundred trillion microbes, with about 3.5 to 4.5 pounds of bacteria just in our digestive system.[3] We are a complex blend of genetic traits from human and microbial cells. This gives new meaning to the phrase "you are not alone"!

Microbial balance and biodiversity are key to optimal health and well-being.[4] The unique composition of good bugs (mutualists), bad bugs (pathogens), and neutral bugs (commensals) that contain viruses, bacteria, protozoa, helminths (multicellular parasitic organisms), and microfungi are involved in most, if not all, biological processes that constitute human health and disease by directly affecting our epigenetics and our immune system.[5] To keep everything running smoothly and the immune system on its toes against bad guys, most experts believe that a ratio of about 85 percent good/neutral and 15 percent bad is key in maintaining optimal health.[6] Lowering the bacterial richness leads to higher weight, fat, high cholesterol, triglycerides, insulin resistance, and more pronounced inflammatory markers and a higher likelihood of a leaky gut as compared to those with higher bacterial richness.[7] A study of an Amazonian indigenous tribe free of chronic illness revealed the most diverse number of microbes ever documented in humans.[8] This *microbiome* can be viewed as a "new organ" that plays a vital role in the development and balance of the immune system and alterations to this new organ, either from lifestyle or various infectious triggers responsible for inflammation leading to chronic disease.[9]

The Connection between Our Mothers and Our Gut

Our health is as good as our mother's gut/vaginal bacteria. Sounds appetizing, right? I know the last thing in the world you want to think about is your mother's "hooha," but seriously, we acquire our "bugs" from our environment as we are delivered into the world. Starting from conception, via the placenta, our babies are exposed to beneficial microbes.[10] The particular microorganisms we obtain depend also on mode of delivery. For example, babies born vaginally are colonized with lactobacillus and other "good" bacteria, similar to that in a mother's vagina, while babies born via C-section tend to have more "bad" bacteria, like staphyloccous, predominant species similar to skin flora and the surrounding area, which is associated with an increased chance of developing illnesses like asthma, allergic rhinitis, dermatitis, and autoimmune diseases.

We also acquire some of our microorganisms through the way we feed. Formula feeding provides a different microbiome than breast-feeding, influencing gene transcription differently and creating permanent metabolic changes. As we grow, our microbiome also grows with us, continuously being exposed to trillions of bacteria daily, adding further gut diversity, constantly changing, determined by our environment.[11] It is so amazing that these tiny organisms will lay the foundation for our health and immune system for years to come.

The Bugs and Their Secret Agenda

A healthier microbiome means a healthier you! Taking care of our little friends is incredibly important as they have many functions. Let's take a closer look at what the microbiome does.

Digestion

The bacteria in our gut help digest multiple nutrients, balance intestinal pH, synthesize hormones and vitamins, protect the gut, and regulate peristalsis (the wavelike contractions that keep the contents of the intestines moving through).

The Immunity Ninja

The gut—more specifically, the gut associated lymphatic tissue (GALT)—is the first line of defense between the world you live in and your internal world (even communicating with your nervous system, including your brain). A healthy relationship with beneficial bacteria is required for a healthy immune system to maintain the function of the small intestinal lining protecting you from unwanted foreign proteins/toxins and infectious agents seeping into your bloodstream. The good bacteria interact with both innate and adaptive immune systems, influence the T cells (a critical part of the immune system), help fight off colds and infections, and break down bacterial toxins, helping to organize the right level of response to any invader.[12] And if all of that isn't enough, a healthy microbiome has an added bonus of possessing antitumor and anticancer effects. Yay, immune ninja!

Energy Reaper

Intestinal bacteria help extract energy and harvest calories from undigested food as it passes through the digestive system.

Metabolism Regulation

Bacteria produce vitamins and folic acid, increase the absorption of minerals, and manufacture short-chain and essential fatty acids. They break down, rebuild hormones, promote optimal growth, and help you maintain a healthy metabolism and weight.

Gene Expression

Our DNA isn't our destiny—we have the power to change our genes. With twenty-three thousand human genes and eight million microbial ones, our environment, particularly our microbiome, can influence the expression of our genetic code. The absence of healthy gut bacteria alters genes and signaling pathways involved in learning, motor control, and memory. Your microbiome influences your cellular functions—for instance, by telling your genes whether to burn fat or store fat (FYI, whispering to your microbiome in an effort to brainwash it to burn fat doesn't work . . . I've tried).

Mood and Behavior—The Neurotransmitter Factory

We've all heard the phrase "The way to a man's heart is through his stomach," but now science is concluding that it's also the way to his brain. Your microbiome helps shape your brain, your mood, and your behavior. The gut contains all the same neurotransmitters found in the brain, including most of the body's serotonin. Changes in microbial composition can cause either a stress response or a calming response, in part by way of the vagus nerve. Negatively altering the microbiome can also lead to cytokine release, increasing stress and inflammation and leading to mood disturbances. So the key to keeping someone happy is to keep their gut bacteria happy.

With trillions of tiny organisms inhabiting our bodies and influencing everything down to the expression of our genetic code, it is empowering to think that every bite of food, every interaction with our environment, and every lifestyle choice creates a ripple effect that reaches into the microbiome. The next time you look in the mirror, remember: you are really never alone—then thank your mom's gut bacteria.

When Things Go Wrong, Things Get Leaky

Now that I have completely grossed you out, but most importantly informed you, let's talk about what happens when things start to go wrong. Your gut is naturally permeable to allow vital nutrients, like properly digested fats, proteins, and starches, to pass through the tight junctions and enter the bloodstream.[13] Normally, the cells that line your intestine stick together very tightly to form a protective barrier that is hard to penetrate, keeping out bigger particles that can damage your system.

If an imbalanced gut microbiome, or dysbiosis, goes on for a while, pathogenic microbes or improperly digested proteins may activate the immune system, creating a fire or war in the gut as they trigger an inflammatory response from immune cells. This inflammation then damages the gut wall epithelial cells and the junctions become leaky and increasingly permeable,[14] over time leading to increased intestinal permeability, or leaky gut syndrome.[15]

When your gut becomes leaky, the intestinal barrier becomes weak and compromised, allowing things to pass through the membrane into the bloodstream that normally would not, such as gluten, undigested food particles, viruses, yeast, bad bacteria, and toxins that trigger the immune system[16] and unbalance your gut microbiome further. What is bad for your gut is also bad for your microbiome, and vice versa. Biodiversity is key to keeping the immune system happy.

In acute inflammation, this isn't a bad thing, but when the immune system is constantly in the "on" position for months, over time the immune system becomes highly reactive, responding to stimuli that it would have previously ignored, like zonulin and other foreign substances, and keeping the gates open. When this continues for months and becomes chronic, it can lead to translocation of bacteria, and bacterial products like lipopolysaccharides (LPS), also known as an endotoxin, penetrate the bloodstream, activating the immune system and releasing cytokines that instigate inflammation through the body and central nervous system (CNS). This can lead to impaired glucose metabolism; insulin resistance; obesity; metabolic syndrome; type 2 diabetes; food sensitivities; nutrient deficiencies like that of B12, magnesium, and iron; neurotransmitter deficiencies; allergies; chronic intestinal disease like inflammatory bowel disease; autoimmunity; and carcinogenesis, at the very least.[17,18] This process can even begin in utero if a mother has an infection or chronic inflammation herself.[19,20]

How Did Your Gut Get Out of Whack?

There are a number of possible reasons why your gut got out of whack, and *The Holistic Rx* is specifically designed to address them. Regaining good health by reducing this exposure to triggers can help put out the fire and lead to optimal health and healing for years to come.

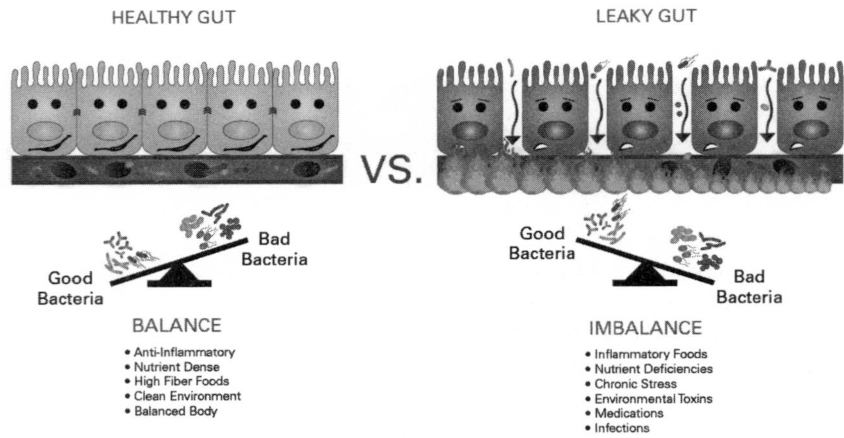

Figure 2.2. Healthy Gut vs. Leaky Gut

Nutrition

What we eat and drink can either help us or hurt us, because it directly affects the composition and metabolism of our microbiome. Our health is largely determined by whether we're feeding the "good" bugs or the "bad" bugs. (See Figure 2.2.) A high-fiber, nutrient-rich, anti-inflammatory diet promotes the beneficial bacteria, enriching the microbiome and helping it do its good work for you. Eating the wrong foods—with limited or no nutritional value, processed, an excess of sugars, including alcohol, unhealthy fats, unsprouted hybridized grains, and especially foods that one becomes sensitive to, along with nutritional deficiencies—can throw off the bacterial balance and create an inflammatory effect, leading to chronic disease.

The body undergoes an inflammatory response specifically when gluten is consumed. In 2000, Dr. Alessio Fasano at the University of Maryland isolated a physiological substance that directly controls the tight junctions in the gut wall, a substance he called "zonulin" that leads to leaky gut.[21, 22] Two things can trigger the release of zonulin in the small intestine—exposure to bacteria and exposure to gluten.[23] We are now exposed to more zonulin than ever before, leaving our immune system in the "on" position and our bodies vulnerable to becoming chronically inflamed.

Chronic Stress

Emotional and social stress can increase levels of stress hormones that negatively affect the microbiome. Studies have shown that stressful experiences have decreased probiotic diversity, causing overgrowth of yeast in the gut. This alters gut permeability, and also influences our epigenetics, leading to inflammation. This connection also works in reverse: the wrong microbes can create more inflammation and stress.

Environmental Contaminants

Daily exposure to hundreds of household and environmental chemicals is hard on the microbiome. All these chemicals put a stress on our immune defenses, straining the body's ability to repair itself and leading to chronic delay of necessary routine repairs. We have now made it routine to oversanitize our bodies and our homes, killing off many beneficial strains and microbes. Spending too much time indoors can limit diversity in the gut.

America represents less than 2 percent of the world's population, but we use 24 percent of its pesticides.[24] A diet of genetically modified crops and food additives, which are made with the widespread use of pesticides, creates a dangerous toxic load in our bodies and has degraded our gut health over time.

Medications

Seven out of ten Americans are on at least one prescription medication, and NSAIDs and other painkillers are consumed at record levels. Many medications can affect the microbiome and lead to dysbiosis. Such medications include:

- NSAIDs (nonsteroidal anti-inflammatory drugs, such as ibuprofen)
- birth control pills
- steroids
- chemotherapy drugs
- sleep medications
- acid-blocking medications/antacids
- opiates

Antibiotics deserve special mention when it comes to the microbiome. The purpose of an antibiotic medication is to kill off some populations of bacteria, but in doing so it also kills off beneficial bacteria, negatively affecting the diversity of the microbiome and damaging our intestinal villi. Antibiotics can be lifesaving in certain situations, but they are often used when they aren't truly necessary. The overuse of antibiotics has fueled the dramatic increase in conditions such as obesity, type 1 diabetes, inflammatory bowel disease, allergies, and asthma; what is sad is that antibiotics can even kill off good bacteria in kids permanently.[25] The increased use of antibiotics and environmental toxins creates imbalances in our microbiome, leading to leaky gut.

Overly Strenuous Exercise

Overly strenuous exercise may increase pro-inflammatory cytokines in the bloodstream and harm the lining of the intestine. Probiotic treatment may help protect the gut from increased permeability caused by strenuous exercise.[26]

Genetics

Many of the autoimmune conditions linked to leaky gut have a genetic component, yet researchers have determined that less than 10 percent of those with the genes for an autoimmune disease will actually develop it. We have control over our epigenetics.

Infections

Infections or exposures that were never resolved—either bacteria, viruses, fungi, or parasite—all affect the microbiome.

Do I Have a Leak?

According to research published in journals like *Clinical Gastroenterology* and *Hepatology and Gut,* there are a number of health conditions that cause leaky gut or can be caused by it, including the following:

- Autoimmune diseases[27, 28] like Hashimoto's,[29] celiac disease and non-celiac gluten sensitivity,[30] lupus,[31] multiple sclerosis,[32] and rheumatoid arthritis.[33]
- Blood vessel problems like hypertension,[34] hyperlipidemia, and CVD.[35]
- Skin inflammation (eczema, psoriasis, rosacea, dermatitis, and acne).[36]
- ENT problems like allergies[37]and sinus problems.
- Endocrine issues like metabolic syndrome[38] and diabetes 1[39, 40] and 2.[41]
- Gastrointestinal problems like Crohn's disease,[42] ulcerative colitis,[43] gas, bloating, and digestive pain,[44] irritable bowel syndrome,[45] ulcers, non-alcoholic stertic hepatitis,[46] Non alcoholic fatty liver disease (NAFLD) and other liver issues,[47] pancreatic disease,[48] and other digestive symptoms like belching, bloating, and bad breath.
- Gynecological problems like yeast overgrowth[49] PCOS (polycystic ovarian syndrome)[50] and other hormonal chaos. Damage to the microbiome can lead to estrogen dominance that can lead to painful breasts, lumps, heavy periods, infertility, increased risk of miscarriages, and lowered libido and even can increase the risk of estrogen dependent cancers (breast, endometrial, and ovarian).

- Neurological problems like ALS,[51] Alzheimer's,[52] migraines,[53] and Parkinsonism.[54]
- Cancer[55] and anemia.
- Eye problems.
- Psychological disturbances like alcoholism,[56] anxiety and depression,[57] ADHD,[58] schizophrenia, bipolar disorder, and sleep disturbances.
- Pulmonary disorders like asthma.
- Rheumatological problems like arthritis[59] and other degenerative diseases, chronic fatigue syndrome,[60] fibromyalgia,[61] and restless leg syndrome (RLS).[62]
- Pediatric issues like autism.[63]
- Urological problems like interstitial cystitis.
- General problems like malnutrition and nutrient deficiencies, infections, and even acute inflammation like sepsis.[64]
- Food sensitivities.[65]
- AIDS.[66]
- Weight gain/obesity.

As you can see, leaky gut can cause a vast number of symptoms and disorders, as it starts off as general inflammation but then over time advances to nutrient malabsorption and then food and other chemical insensitivities. For this reason, healing the intestinal lining is the foundation of *The Holistic Rx*.

Foods That May Be Doing More Harm Than Good

Food is a critical factor in causing or exacerbating chronic disease or chronic symptoms. The foods you eat always influence your health—the effects can be either dramatic and immediate or subtle and gradual. Certain foods can contribute to leaky gut syndrome or worsen their symptoms, which in turn increases your risks of developing food sensitivities and together amplify one another.

For instance, in a leaky gut, food is improperly digested. Particles of it then leak through a weak intestinal barrier. The immune cells read the "name tags" on the food particles, telling your body how it should respond. If the immune cells label the particles as invaders, they can make antibodies against the specific food. When this happens, you develop a food allergy that can in turn lead to the symptoms that we described above, including heart palpitations, postnasal drip, cough, congestion, digestive issues like cramping, fatigue, and brain fog. Because the reactions can be outside the realm of the digestive tract, and often are delayed, it can be hard to connect a particular food to how you feel.

There's a subtle but important difference between a food allergy and a sensitivity or intolerance to a food. When you eat the food that you're allergic to, you experience an immediate response like hives, swelling, or difficulty breathing, as you have developed IgE antibodies to it, and are allergic to the exposure.

If the food causes other symptoms of inflammation, we would say that you have an intolerance or sensitivity to it. Food sensitivity involves IgG antibodies. Although the symptoms are usually less severe, food sensitivities play an integral part in causing immune-mediated conditions. If you suspect you have food allergies or sensitivities, you may find it helpful to consult with an allergist or functional integrative physician, who can check for IgE and IgG antibodies.

The following foods are the major common culprits in allergies or sensitivities, inflammation, and chronic disease. Removing these foods from your diet can greatly improve your health, so it's a great place to start.

Noooo, Not the Bread, Anything but the Bread!

We have all heard of this new fad called gluten. But what is it, and why are people trying to avoid it if they don't have celiac disease? Gluten (the word comes from the latin word for "glue") is a protein found in grains such as wheat, barley, rye, kamut, and spelt—so basically all the delicious stuff that you crave. About twenty-one million Americans are thought to have non-celiac gluten sensitivity, which causes inflammation, including mental illnesses[67] like depression and schizophrenia,[68] autism,[69] dementia,[70] obesity, heart disease, and even cancer.[71] Simply removing gluten from the diet can help improve symptoms drastically.

Why does gluten cause such problems? People all over the world eat wheat for breakfast, lunch, and dinner, so in order to increase the yield, in the last fifty years modern wheat has been hybridized, genetically manipulated, and sprayed with massive amounts of chemical fertilizer and pesticides.[72] This high-yielding dwarf wheat has a much higher amount of gluten, more phytic acid and amylopectin, but fewer nutrients. So this new gluten protein molecule is large, and we lack the specific enzymes to fully break it down. When the partially digested molecules come in contact with the small intestine, they spark your immune system and create inflammation. Gluten can cause the gut cells to release zonulin, the protein that can loosen tight junctions in the intestinal lining, creating a permeable barrier and leading to—you guessed it—leaky gut syndrome.

Not only can gluten lead to leaky gut syndrome and food sensitivities, but it also causes large spikes in blood sugar (as two slices of whole wheat bread raises your blood sugar more than two tablespoons of table sugar), contributing to blood sugar deregulation, insulin resistance, and obesity, leading to further inflammation. Gluten binds to opioid receptors in the gut, the same receptors that morphine and heroin bind to. This makes the body crave it and even creates a withdrawal effect when you stop eating gluten. Wheat has been genetically modified in such a way that we are exposed to more gluten today than ever before, making non-celiac gluten sensitivity a widespread problem. One study reported that an inflammatory gut response was noted in the intestinal cells of healthy volunteers, suggesting that gluten may cause reactions in almost everyone.[73]

To throw you another caveat—there are certain foods that the body (your adaptive immune system) might confuse with gluten—for example, corn, dairy, millet, oats, rice, and yeast. These can cause similar reactions or cross-reactivity and can also increase chronic inflammation by triggering leaky gut, according to a 2013 European study.[74]

My goal is to reduce all your inflammation, so I will ask you to eliminate all grains to optimize and expedite healing—in other words, remove all the potential igniter fluids and put out all the fire. Once you've put out the fire in the gut, and let your body heal, you might be able to introduce some grains, including gluten foods, back into your diet in moderate amounts, depending on what your body can tolerate.[75] But again, if this is too overwhelming, start with removing all gluten from your diet.

No, Not the Sugar Either!!

We are a culture literally surrounded in sugar, as it permeates our daily lives—every holiday, every treat, every celebration, every trip to the doctor and every sadness, disappointment, and time of stress. It is found in 74 percent of packaged foods. Sugar stimulates the brain reward centers[76] via neurotransmitters, and when you stop eating sugar, especially suddenly, you experience withdrawal symptoms, just like when you withdraw from dopamine and other addictive drugs.[77] Unfortunately, sugar can be directly related to all chronic diseases, like heart disease, cancer, stroke, and diabetes, and it has no redeeming nutritional value. A major study from the Harvard School of Public Health published in the *Journal of the American Medical Association* found that those who took 25 percent or more of daily calories as sugar were twice as likely to die from heart disease than those who consumed less than 10 percent.[78]

Bad bacteria thrive on sugar, leading to bad bacterial overgrowth of pathogenic bacteria and yeast species like fungi, which then increases more cravings for more sugar, creating a vicious cycle. This imbalance in the microbiome leads to inflammation, as it interferes with the ability of your white blood cells to destroy toxins and fight infection, making you sick—all this within minutes after eating sugar, and it can last for several hours!

Sugar disrupts your blood sugar balance, with insulin spikes that can be dangerous and can lead to fatigue and brain fog, anxiety, and mood swings; reduces HDL ("good" cholesterol) and raises LDL ("bad" cholesterol); causes weight gain and accumulation of belly fat; increases your appetite and sugar cravings; and also leads to fatty liver.

Sugar also increases oxidative stress, leading to inflammation. So basically, sugar makes you obese, old, and ill. It's scary that we feed this regularly to our children! As you get off sugar, you can relax cravings by drinking calming teas, increasing vitamin C, sleeping more, and engaging in other activities that relieve stress and increase happiness.

Artificial Sweeteners—the Cold (Not So Sweet) Truth

Artificial sweeteners are synthetic chemicals and have been shown to cause allergic reactions and various physical ailments leading to gut irritation, insulin resistance, and inflammation. They cause hunger (leading to leptin resistance, which prevents you from knowing when you're full), gas and bloating, headaches and migraines, CVD, and type 2 DM according to a 2013 study in *Trends in Endocrinology and Metabolism*.[79] Sucralose especially has a detrimental effect on gut bacteria.[80] Researchers at Duke University Medical Center also discovered that Splenda significantly reduces beneficial bacteria in the gut and increases fecal pH, which decreases the amount of nutrients you can absorb.[81]

Studies have found that people who use artificial sweeteners actually gain weight and increase waist circumference instead of losing it, increasing the chance of developing type 2 diabetes (by 67 percent)[82] and metabolic syndrome, worsening the obesity epidemic.[83]

Lettin' Go of the Booze

Alcohol provokes a leaky gut, increases intestinal permeability, opens up junctions between enterocytes, and inflames the liver.[84] It impairs your impulse control, so you're more likely to eat more—and to do so mindlessly. In addition, it is simply sugar in another form, meaning that it causes spikes in blood sugar levels, contributing to insulin resistance and increased anxiety, fatigue, and brain fog. It can also trigger the release of histamine, which causes gastric juices to flow, constricts lung tissue, and plays a major role in many allergic reactions in the body. If you are suffering from chronic issues, alcoholic beverages are more likely doing more harm than good, despite the benefits shown with moderate consumption.

Got Milk? . . . Actually, Keep It

Dairy products can trigger an inflammatory response capable of attacking the body's own tissues. After the age of five, the body stops producing the enzymes that break down the macromolecules in milk (lactose and milk proteins). Commercial cow's milk contains growth hormones and chemicals—pasteurized to kill the bad bacteria.[85] Normally, milk should separate easily for easy digestion, but now it's been modified by pasteurization and homogenization, which destroys healthy probiotics, vitamins, minerals, enzymes, and nutritious proteins, makes lactose difficult to digest, creates free radicals, and alters the casein protein, creating a molecule that resembles gluten. The undigested molecules lead to leaky gut syndrome, causing an inflammatory response. Dairy also contains a protein called A1 beta-casein that releases beta casomorphine-7, an opioid that can create a shortage of antioxidants in the brain and has been linked to autism and schizophrenia.[86] Another concern pertains to the natural estrogens from pregnant cows that can increase the risk of hormonal sensitive cancers and early puberty. For someone with sensitivity to dairy, even cultured products like yogurt can cause problems.

If you are worried about calcium, be assured that there are plenty of good calcium sources besides dairy products. I'll discuss alternatives later in this chapter.

Stay Away From the Frankenfoods

Processed foods, also referred to as frankenfoods, contain a lot of ingredients, like hydrogenated oils (canola, soybean, corn, and other vegetable oils) that damage the gut flora and give rise to intestinal inflammation, leading to chronic illnesses like leaky gut.

Processed foods also contain genetically modified plants like corn, soybeans, and more than 750 different products that contain high levels of glyphosate, an active ingredient in the weed killer Roundup. As it turns out, this chemical is very active in disrupting beneficial bacteria,[87] leading to leaky gut, imbalanced gut bacteria, and damage to the intestinal wall. Even vitamin D3 activation in the liver may be affected negatively by glyphosate's effect on liver enzymes, potentially explaining epidemic levels of vitamin D deficiency. It is best to avoid glyphosate, as we simply just don't know enough.

There IS Hope!

Now that you've absorbed the information in this chapter and I have completely overwhelmed you, pause and take a deep breath and put that ice cream back in the freezer as you sulk in the depths of your despair. I know I just took off everything from your "happy food" list. But there IS hope!!! These are the foods that may be leading to your pain, agony, and multiple trips to the doctor. Removing them for a short time will allow you to see what foods are actually bothering you. Once you have extinguished the fire and healed your gut, adding healthy alternatives back in is very much possible! Now guess who's back in charge? You are now empowered to use what you've learned to improve your health. So exciting!

Getting a Clear Picture

The only way to properly treat dysbiosis is to first remove problematic food, bad bacteria, and infections that elude the radar of conventional medical tests, but that doesn't mean you must fly completely blind or rely totally on guesswork. There are a number of testing methods—some of which have been around for decades, others of which are very new—to help guide treatment. I always start out with the cheapest option—listening to your body. If your symptoms sound like leaky gut, trust your gut. A comprehensive stool test is a noninvasive test that gives a picture of some of the organisms present in a patient's GI tract, as well as some sense of bacterial balance and presence of yeast. IgG and IgE tests can check for food sensitivities. A lactose breath test or hydrogen or methane breath test can check for SIBO (which I'll discuss in detail later), and the leaky gut and organic acids test reveals vitamin and mineral deficiencies.

Putting Out the Fire in the Gut

Now I will guide you through the process of putting out the fire in your gut and giving your body a fighting chance to heal. With diet, lifestyle changes, and occasionally supplements—here's to a happy and healthy gut!

There are so many gut-healing diets out there, it can get confusing as to where to go and what is right for you. Again, my approach is focused on what is the easiest, most cost- and time-effective way to heal. Everyone is different, but starting with the key basics and then adjusting as you need to is the best way to go.

What all the gut-healing plans have in common is the importance of changing your diet. To heal your digestive system, putting out the fire in the gut is the critical first step. You will need to first stop putting gasoline on the fire by avoiding all the foods that are likely to be causing problems. You'll then take steps to restore a healthy balance of bacteria, replenish nutrients, repair the lining of the gut, and generally rebalance your system. Once a minimum of three or four weeks have passed, or your symptoms have improved/resolved, you'll be ready to take the next step—reintroducing foods one at a time and carefully noticing which, if any, cause problems so that you can exclude them from your diet. A short-term gut healing diet is better than a lifetime of pain and suffering! Let's do this! You deserve it!

THE GUT Rx

Through diligent attention to changing your lifestyle and diversifying your foods you can start diversifying your microbiome for the better. The idea of making a major change in your diet can be scary, but think about it: right now, every other doctor is probably telling you that you are going to have to live with these symptoms and possible medication forever. I am telling you that it doesn't have to be forever, and three to four weeks of a different diet is not going to hurt you; it will only help you. Instead of focusing on the foods you can't eat, focus on the foods you *can* eat and start repairing in less than twenty-four hours.

Plan ahead and set a date. Find a four-week stretch of time that you can dedicate to yourself, when you will be able to spend some time preparing for and adapting to a different way of eating. The first week is usually the hardest, since you will be adjusting to new foods and possibly going through withdrawals. You may also experience a die-off reaction (discussed below), which can make you feel worse before you feel better. Just be patient and take it one day at a time. There is a light at the end of the tunnel. We can do this together!

Remove

In order to put out the fire in the gut, we first need to remove all the possible offending triggers.[88] Remove all of the following:

- Grains (amaranth, barley, brown rice, buckwheat, bulgur, corn, farro/emmer, grano, kamut, millet, oats, oatmeal, popcorn, muesli, rolled oats, quinoa, rye, sorghum, spelt, teff, triticale, wheat, and wild rice; quinoa and corn are technically not grains, but they contain proteins similar to grains)
- Dairy
- Sugar
- Alcohol
- Starchy vegetables

- Nutrient-depleted foods, processed foods (full of poor-quality fats and oils [commercial liquid vegetable oils, hydrogenated oils, and trans fats] and GMOs)

You will also need to remove infections that will increase intestinal inflammation and stop bacterial overgrowth—like viruses, parasites, yeast, and small intestinal bacterial overgrowth (SIBO: good bacteria in the wrong place). Use a combination of berberine (active against candida albicans and staphylococcus aureas), wormwood, caprillic acid, grapefruit seed extract (antimicrobial and antifungal), garlic (active against bacteria, fungi, viruses, and parasites), oregano oil, and peppermint oil (will discuss specific treatments for each infection later in the autoimmune and digestive chapters).

Most people start to see improvement of symptoms when they remove these foods; if after a couple of weeks you're still not seeing any improvement despite *The Holistic Rx*, you may also want to consider eliminating other problematic foods like beans/legumes (some people do okay with lentils and navy beans), soy, eggs, nightshades, and nuts. Also remove any foods that you think (or know) you are allergic or sensitive to.

You may be tempted to remove just one food at a time, but I recommend taking out *all* the foods that may bother you. Taking out one at a time may not help you feel better and can actually be more discouraging. Removing the foods all at once will help you feel better faster, and once you feel better, you'll be ready to reintroduce each food one at a time to see how you are affected.

That said, if removing all the foods is too overwhelming, then don't. Stress causes more problems and inflammation, and I don't want you to stress out. I suggest you start with eliminating gluten and dairy.

Replenish Food and the Ability to Digest

Now it's time to restore and replenish the vitamins, minerals, nutrients, and essential ingredients for proper digestion and absorption that might have been depleted by diet, medication, disease, or aging. To do this, incorporate power foods into your diet by getting back to the earth and replacing any deficiencies necessary for digestion.

First let's replenish with nourishing food, so instead of focusing on what you can't eat, let's focus on what you can eat. The following need to part of every meal (discussed in more detail in the following section):

1. **Vegetables**: Nonstarchy vegetables are easy to digest and packed with vitamins, antioxidants, minerals, and fiber.

2. **Protein**: Choose grass-fed beef, pastured chicken, eggs from pasture-raised hens, wild-caught seafood, and hemp seeds.
3. **Fat**: Get your fats from coconut oil, avocados, olive oil, nuts (if you aren't sensitive to them), and seeds.
4. **Water**: Drink filtered water when possible.

It is important to increase the biodiversity of the microbiome by exposing yourself to the external world around you and being cautious about the soil the foods you intake grows in.

Other foods for healing the gut include the following:

- **Bone broth and collagen**. Have at least one cup a day of bone broth. Bone broth and collagen are rich in amino acids like L-glutamine (energy source for your intestinal cells), glucosamine, chondroitin, collagen gelatin, proline, and glycine, all of which help repair, seal, soothe, and restore gut mucosal lining and lower inflammation. These are also full of bioavailable, easily absorbed minerals like calcium, magnesium, phosphorus, silicon, and sulfur,[89, 90] and these nutrients are necessary to support the immune system. I recommend cooking with meat, collagen, fat, and bones in a crock pot for at least eight hours.
- **Herbs that reduce inflammation**: black seeds, turmeric, rosemary, and ginger are a few examples that can be added to your dishes.
- **Fermented foods** should be added if tolerated. Fermented foods can actually feed the good guys and the bad guys, so it is best to add fermented foods as you continue to heal your gut.

Optimize the Ability to Digest

If you're putting in the effort to eat healing foods, also make sure you're actually digesting the foods you're eating. Keeping your stomach at an appropriate pH is key in optimal digestion. Too much stomach acid can cause reflux and other symptoms, but too little can cause bloating, an inability to break down food or activate digestive enzymes, and an overgrowth of yeast and bacteria. Causes of a decrease in stomach acid include alcohol, antibiotics, caffeine, hypothyroidism, imbalanced microbiome, nicotine, and stress—especially chronic stress.

You can easily check your acid level with a baking soda test:

1. First thing in the morning, before eating or drinking anything, mix ¼ teaspoon of baking soda in 4–6 oz. of cold water.
2. Drink the baking soda solution.
3. Time how long it takes you to belch, up to five minutes.

Any belching after three minutes indicates a low acid level. Betaine hydrochloric acid supplements can be helpful while your gut is healing if you carefully follow these guidelines: Start with one capsule or tablet at the beginning of each meal. Increase the dose by one capsule per meal until you have a warm feeling in your stomach. Then drop back down to the dose just before the warm feeling occurred. Stay on it for one to two months, then stop and see how you feel.

I also recommend starting the day off with a glass of water with lemon. With each meal, drink half a cup of water with half a teaspoon of raw apple cider vinegar. Digestive bitters can also help to boost stomach acid.

If your symptoms don't improve within four weeks, you might need digestive enzymes to help break up macronutrients and absorb the nutrients you need from food. I recommend a plant-based enzyme formula along with an enzyme blend, especially one with protease, amylase, and lipase.

Repopulate

Restoring the balance of good bacteria in your gut is absolutely crucial to overall health. You can accomplish this by using probiotics (helpful bacteria) and prebiotic, fiber-rich foods.

Probiotics

Probiotics are found in fermented foods such as unpasteurized natural sauerkraut. (They're also found in yogurt and kefir, but these are dairy products, so you won't be eating them during this phase.) You can also take probiotics in the form of supplement capsules or powders. Take a probiotic supplement with or after food, as it binds to food particles to make sure it survives the stomach acid.[91] Probiotics are safe for the general population, but there's a small risk for people who are immunocompromised.

What should you look for in a probiotic supplement?

1. **Strains Diversity.** The human gut contains hundreds of known species of different bacteria, and it should be our goal to mimic that environment as best as we can. Different species of probiotic bacteria have different strengths and weaknesses. To gain maximum benefit, a probiotic should have a mixture of at least ten or more strains. Look for lactobacilli (especially plantarum and brevis), bifidobacteria (longem and lactis), and soil-based organisms, such as endospore probiotics like bacillus subtilis and bacillus coagulans.

Soil bacteria have a number of added benefits. Along with supporting your gut, they also improve nutrient absorption, reduce inflammation, nourish the cells in the colon and liver, create new compounds like B vitamins, vitamin K2, antioxidants, and enzymes, and lower the amount of harmful pathogens like candida, fungi, and parasites.[92]

Added bonuses:

Bacteriophages. Phages are viruses that specialize in breaking open and killing certain kinds of bacteria. Taking supplemental phages could be helpful in improving inflammation, specifically ear infections, yeast infections, cystic fibrosis, and other lung diseases (swimming in the ocean will also get you the phages you need).[93]

Mushroom mycelia and *Saccaromyces boulardii* are good yeasts that fight the bad yeast and restore normal flora in the intestinal tract. These help lower inflammation by having an antitoxin and antimicrobial effect, destroying pathogenic yeast like *Candida albicans.*[94, 95, 96] Yeast-based probiotics may improve SIBO, while spore-based can increase lactobacillius, improving gut diversity. All the different strains will make sure they colonize in the gut.

Choose a product that is condition appropriate when it's available—for example, add l. rhamnosus, l. gasseri, b. lactis for weight loss;[77] for IBS, use bacillus infantus, b. animalis, b. lactis, l. plantarium; for IBD use l. plantarium 299v; for vaginal and urinary health, use l. rhamnosis, l. reuteri, l. plantarium, l. crispatus; and for elevated cholesterol and blood sugars, use l. acidophilus, l. ramnosis, b. lactis, and b. longus. If taking an antibiotic, make sure your probiotic includes l. brevis.

There are now supplements that are specific for lactose intolerance, sugar malabsorption, IBS, and diarrhea. Make sure to avoid supplements that contain soy, dairy, gluten, grains, or artificial ingredients.

2. **Strength.** You need to provide probiotic bacteria in large enough dosage to see an improvement. A good probiotic supplement should have a concentrated amount of bacteria: at least eight billion bacteria cells per gram.

   Start slow at one billion organisms daily and gradually go up to twenty billion organisms daily, or until you are rebalanced and feeling well; everyone is different, as it can range anywhere from fifteen billion to one hundred billion CFU.

   When you introduce the probiotic into your digestive system, it begins to destroy the pathogenic bacteria and viruses, which release toxins. You may experience worsening of your symptoms. We call this a *die-off reaction*. Fatigue, digestive reactions, low-grade nausea, mild headaches, and emotional irritability are quite common. The specific reaction depends on the individual. It usually lasts from a few days to a few weeks.

To help manage this, I recommend that you start at a low dosage and watch for die-off symptoms. If no symptoms occur, then gradually increase the dose. If you see a die-off reaction, stay on that dosage until the symptoms disappear. If symptoms are hard to deal with, you can space out the doses (that is, take the supplements less often) to help relieve some of the symptoms. Once the symptoms resolve, gradually increase the dosage. Continue this process until you reach twenty billion organisms daily or whatever dosage keeps you feeling well.

Epsom salt baths, sea salt, seaweed, and sodium bicarbonate (baking soda) can help with the die-off reaction and speed up recovery. Take an Epsom salts bath one day, then a sea salt bath the next day, then a seaweed bath the next day, then a baking soda bath the next day, then start again with Epsom salts. Half a cup in the bath water for thirty minutes is best. Again, do what you can do easily; if daily is too much, start with whatever you feel comfortable with.

3. **Duration.** Once you've reached the dosage of probiotic supplements that's right for you (typically twenty billion organisms daily), I recommend that you keep taking the supplements for about six months in order to reestablish normal gut flora. You may then be able to reduce the dosage somewhat, as long as you still feel well. You can even change them every three to six months, but remember that the probiotic foods are extra important in maintaining gut health.

   It's important to continue eating healthily even when you're using probiotics. For now, keep following the gut-healing diet. When you're finished with that, you'll switch to an everyday healthy diet—a topic I'll cover in the next section.

Prebiotics

Prebiotics play an important role in healing the gut to decrease inflammation.[98] Prebiotics are "food" for probiotics. They nourish and stimulate the growth of "good" bacteria while promoting the reduction in disease-causing bacteria such as clostridia, klebsiella, and enterobacter. They work with the probiotics; together, they optimize gut healing.

I would recommend eating your prebiotics—as the supplement form can create a lot of gas and bloating. This can be confusing if you're trying to get to the root of your digestive issues. If you eat vegetables and fruit every day, you're consuming sufficient quantities of prebiotics to feed your hungry bacteria. Green leafy vegetables and other high-fiber foods are especially good at promoting growth of good bacteria, along with asparagus, carrots, garlic, leeks, raw onions, radishes, and tomatoes.

Repair

After you have removed the offending foods from your diet (that is, stopped adding fuel to the fire), supplemented the digestive process as needed, and restored the normal bacterial balance, the gut wall needs to be healed. Repairing the gut lining is important to ensure proper absorption of nutrients.

I recommend that you continue drinking bone broth, one cup per day minimum. Bone broth is powerful in regenerating the gut wall lining.

It's also helpful to eat foods that are rich in zinc (lean beef and poultry, nuts such as cashews and almonds) and vitamins A (carrots, dark leafy greens, winter squash, lettuce, dried apricots, cantaloupe, bell peppers, fish, liver, tropical fruits), C (bell peppers, dark leafy greens, kiwi, broccoli, berries, citrus fruits), and D (tuna canned in water, sardines canned in oil, beef or calf liver, egg yolks or cod liver oil) and omega 3, which improves inflammation and heals the gut lining, along with vitamin E and selenium.

In addition, I recommend taking the following supplements. These will soothe inflammation and continue healing the gut:

- Probiotics are the most important part of resealing.
- L-glutamine, 5 g twice daily, with meals.[99] L-glutamine can be found in the bone broth, also in animal proteins and raw spinach, red cabbage, and parsley. It helps to rejuvenate and preserve the gut lining and prevent worsening of leaky gut, as it is a fuel source for the cells in the small intestine that help moderate the body's IgA immune response, which is associated with food sensitivities and allergies.[100]
- Omega 3 (2–4 g per day with meals) overall improves inflammation and heals the gut lining.
- Digestive enzymes are nutrients that completely break down what you eat; these include proteins, fats, complex sugars, and starches, which can reduce intestinal inflammation. Look for ones with protease (breaks down proteins including gluten), amylase (breaks down starches), lipase (breaks down fats), lactase (breaks down lactose in dairy) and DDP IV.
- Others can be zinc carnosine (30 mg per day), turmeric, slippery elm (200 mg per day), aloe vera (100 mg per day), licorice root, DGL (500 mg per day specifically for leaky gut exacerbated by emotional stress), frankincense (an essential oil that helps heal leaky gut and lower

inflammation),[101] quercetin (500 mg three times per day with meals), colostrum powder, chamomile, organic sulfur compounds, methylsulfonylmethane (MSM), boswellia powder, marshmallow root (100 mg per day), butyric acid or butyrate, and plantain.

Special Consideration—Children

Probiotics can be given to babies born with C-section and/or had history of yeast, antibiotics, or steroids during pregnancy, labor, or while nursing. Probiotics can also be considered if there is a family history of increased intestinal permeability issues, like autoimmunity or metabolic syndrome. Look for lactobacillus acidophilus and bifidobacterium infantis. Dosage depends on age. Infant up to twelve months: 1–2 billion of bacterial cells per day; one to two years of age: 2–4 billion per day; two to four years: 4–8 billion per day; four to ten years: 8–12 billion per day; and twelve to sixteen years: 12–15 billion per day.

Digestive enzymes: younger than five years old: pinch of digestive enzyme powder with each meals; older than five: ½ teaspoon with each meal.

Glutamine powder: Give your child 1.5 g of glutamine powder twice daily if your child is over four years old.

Rebalance

Rebalancing is key to lower inflammation overall and is what *The Holistic Rx* is all about. Focusing on activities that will add diversity of microbes from the soil will help to balance the microbiome and help lower stress. Remember this is your time to prioritize taking care of you. Add activities like gardening, spending time walking barefoot outside (will help improve sleep, raise energy, and lower inflammation by stabilizing your internal bioelectrical environment), shopping at local farmers markets for fresh produce, swimming in the ocean and fresh water lakes (decreases skin inflammation, RA, and psoriasis).[102] Getting a pet will also diversify the microbes in your home.[103]

Reintroducing Foods, Step by Step . . . Yay!

Once you've been on the gut healing diet for a minimum of three to four weeks, you should be feeling better. You will know if your gut is healed once you feel as if you can start weaning off your medications (only under doctor's supervision) and your symptoms have improved or have resolved. If you aren't, I recommend that you stay on the healing diet and consult with a holistic or functional health care practitioner, as it may take time to heal, depending

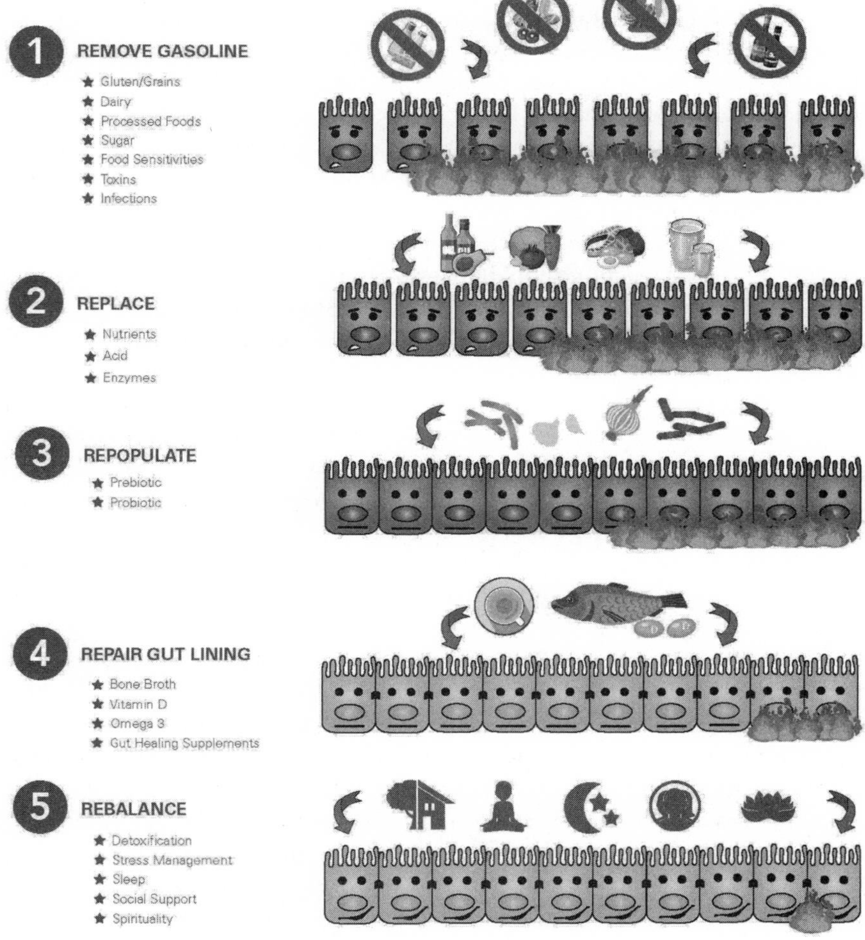

Figure 2.3. The Gut Rx

on your condition and how long you have been dealing with your condition. Remember, if you have been dealing with chronic inflammation for a long time, then any improvement is better than no improvement—patience is key.

When your symptoms are where you want them, you can begin reintroducing foods. It's very important to reintroduce one food at a time and to pay careful attention to whether your symptoms return. That way, if you do have symptoms, you'll know exactly what food caused them, and you can choose to give up that food, until you heal more completely. If you have no reaction to the food, then you can move on to the next food.

Start with the food that you miss the most. Eat that food in the most pure form for a couple of days and notice how you feel. On day three, don't eat that food but continue to observe how you feel. Because sensitivities can take up to seventy-two hours to manifest, it is important to wait and see if symptoms develop. Use a food reintroduction log to keep track of this process.

Symptoms to look for are digestive symptoms, headaches, joint pain, abdominal pain, fatigue, mood swings, congestion, or rashes. If you experience any of these symptoms, other symptoms you've had before, or new symptoms, it is an indication that you have sensitivity to the reintroduced food, so remove it again. The food reaction should go away within a day or two, but for some people it can take longer.

Once a reaction goes away, then it's time to try reintroducing the next food.

Repeat this process with the next food. Following this schedule, you will be trying a new food every four days. When the reintroduction phase is complete, you'll know exactly which foods you can eat and which cause problems.

What to Do If You Relapse

It's possible that you will eventually experience a relapse, meaning that your symptoms might return. This may happen because you've eaten a food to which you're sensitive, or it may happen despite your being on a good diet, as deficits in any of the other processes we talked about in the first chapter may induce relapse. Antibiotic therapy is another common reason for relapse. If you are prescribed an antibiotic and want to avoid relapse, take a probiotic with 50–100 billion CFUs in between the antibiotic doses and stay on the probiotic for three times the length of the antibiotic course.

Here's what to do if you have a relapse:

- Make sure you're implementing the entire Holistic Rx, as increased stress, infections, toxins, or insulin resistance can lead to inflammation.
- Trim back consumption of suspicious foods. You are likely overconsuming some food that is bothering you.
- Begin to take two capsules of digestive enzymes with food, if needed.
- Continue with a maintenance dose of probiotics.
- Monitor symptoms for one to two weeks.

If your symptoms are not improving, then you may need to start back at the beginning of the Gut Rx or start a stricter and more structured gut healing approach.

Gut Healing Diets

Multiple gut healing diets exist. What I have done is simplified it for you. But for those with serious issues, you may need to follow a more structured approach. I recommend diets like the Gut and Psychology Syndrome (GAPS) diet, keeping in mind your sensitivities and balancing glucose; it is helpful for patients as it offers a stagewise approach to healing. See appendix for further details. Others include the Specific Carbohydrate Diet, FODMAPS, Autoimmune Protocol, Paleo, and so many more. Everyone is different, so use what works best for you.

Congratulate yourself! Healing your digestive system is the hardest step of *The Holistic Rx* to go through, but it's also the most powerful. By rebalancing the bacteria in your gut and healing the intestinal lining, you have reduced inflammation throughout your body and taken a huge step toward improving your overall health. Your body is now in good shape to get the most from the foods you eat. In the next section, I'll lay out an everyday approach to eating for optimal health.

EAT TO HEAL, TRIUMPH, AND THRIVE

Hooray! Cue the trumpets! You've made it this far! In the last section, we talked about the importance of gut health in inflammation. Now let's talk about everyone's favorite topic and an integral part of our lives—FOOD! We have all been there, running through our lives, flying through one meal on to the next, grabbing anything we find to put in our mouths. With each meal comes frustration, about what to cook that is cost-effective, is healing, and will "tame the inner beast." Most of us raise the white flag when it comes to mealtime, giving in to inner desire or the bad bacteria in our gut.

But have no fear—I have come to your rescue! Food is power, and it's information that influences the expression of your genes, it literally talks to your genes! Healing food gives us the ability to take back control of our health. We touched on food in the last chapter; let's dive in a little deeper now. We all eat. Food can either hurt you or help you to prevent and heal from the inside out. So if you think about it that way, let's focus on foods that will help you feel more energetic, help you lose weight, and heal chronic disease! Now what's better than that?! Actually, it's going to get better . . . keep reading.

Anti-Inflammatory Food Lifestyle—Why?

Everyone is different; some things that work for some don't work for others, but all have this in common—inflammation is the driver of chronic disease. So with that in mind, it makes sense to eat more of the foods that decrease inflammation, eliminating/limiting the foods that increase it, whether you have a diagnosed illness or want to prevent one. I recommend adopting an anti-inflammatory approach to eating. This is not a meal plan but a way of life.

This anti-inflammatory diet/lifestyle enhances your metabolism to help your body function optimally—eating a plant-based, antioxidant-rich diet and minimizing toxic exposures all can lower inflammation. No more counting calories, just choosing the right foods in the right balance. Good healthy food is the biggest investment you can make for you and your family, for now and the future. I promise you: your future self will thank you.

Healing food not only communicates with your genes, but whenever you put a bite in your mouth, it also:

1. **Keeps your gut happy.** Paying extra attention to your diet is crucial to stopping the inflammation where it starts and gets to the root of your problem (as discussed in the previous chapter).
2. **Regulates glucose, decreases insulin resistance, and balances hormones.** Anything that causes insulin resistance will also cause inflammation, and vice versa. Insulin resistance leads to rapid and premature aging, and causes stroke, dementia, heart disease, cancer, hormonal imbalances, and so much more.[1]
3. **Provides dense nutrients.** Focusing on foods that are nutrient dense provides your body with the strength it needs to heal inside and out. Nutrient density creates resilience.

What Is Insulin Resistance?

What is insulin resistance, and why does it matter? Well it all starts when we take that bite of food. As discussed in the previous chapter, it enters our bloodstream after being absorbed by our digestive system. The glucose in our body is needed for the cells for energy and fuel. But glucose can only enter the cells with a key—insulin. Insulin is a storage hormone produced by the pancreas; it is responsible for controlling blood sugar levels and determines our metabolism.

Over time, the flood of inflammatory signals starts to wear down this key as the body stops listening to the insulin that is always present, until it stops working and the cells stop opening their doors to insulin, unable to absorb glucose adequately, leading to insulin resistance. In order to keep the glucose levels in a healthy range, the pancreatic beta cells start producing even more insulin. Over time the beta cells can't keep up with the body's increased demand for insulin, leading to excess glucose in the bloodstream, a state that makes the body uncomfortable. Prolonged states of insulin resistance can result in increased insulin levels that can lead to fat storage, obesity, metabolic syndrome, prediabetes, diabetes, premature aging, and inflammation, aggravating many other serious disorders. Managing insulin resistance is critical to heal balance hormones, and prevent chronic disease.

What Causes It Anyway?

Diet

As discussed in the last chapter, dietary sugars and refined flours are the biggest triggers of inflammation and cause insulin spikes. Artificial sweeteners have been linked to weight gain and diabetes. The lack of fiber can lead to increased visceral fat, and an increased amount of omega 6 and a deficiency of omega 3 can contribute to system inflammation, leading to worsening insulin resistance.

Stress

Increased cortisol increases insulin levels, which in turn worsen insulin resistance.[2]

Dysbioisis and Leaky Gut Syndrome

The bad bacteria increases inflammation and worsens insulin resistance, causing obesity and belly weight.

Deficiencies

Vitamin D deficiency contributes to insulin resistance due to the role it plays in glucose tolerance through its effects on insulin secretion and insulin sensitivity. The lower the vitamin D, the higher the insulin resistance. Magnesium deficiency has also been linked to developing insulin resistance.[3]

Medications

Medications like steroids and hydrochlorothiazide, a first-line medication for blood pressure, can actually cause hyperglycemia, leading to insulin resistance. Check with your doctor and read the side effects to know which ones can increase your blood glucose levels, and ask for an alternative if available.

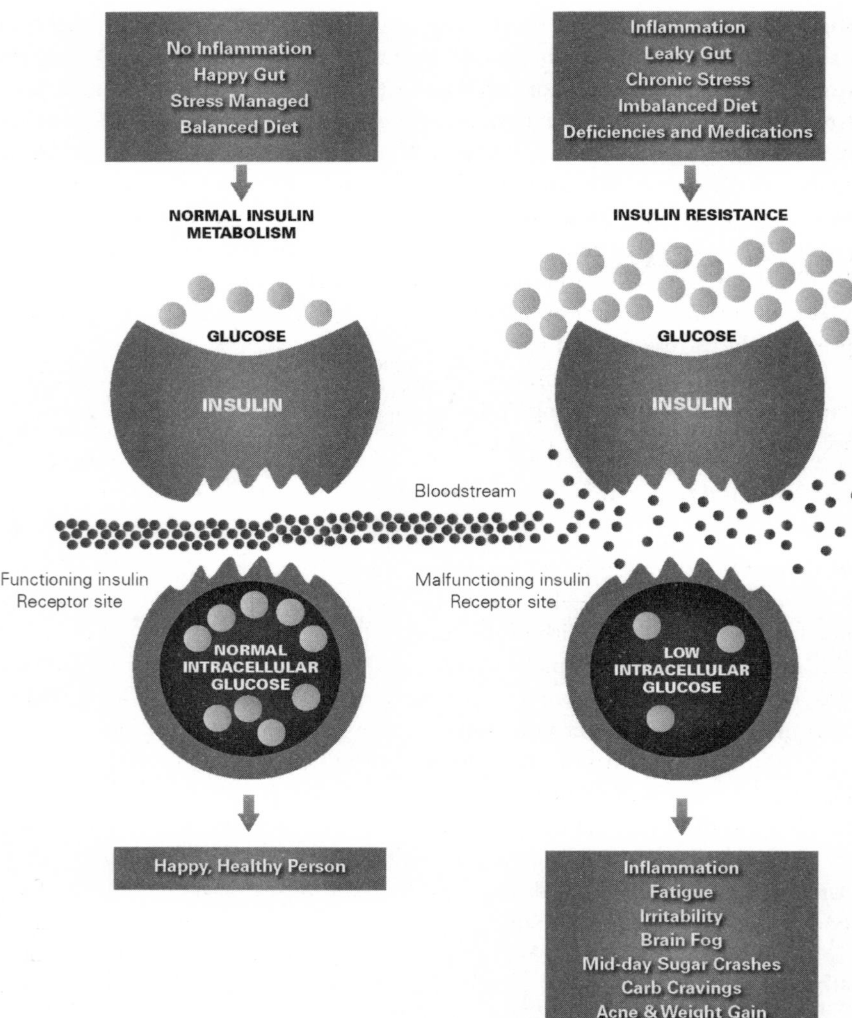

Figure 2.4. Insulin Resistance

Could I Be Insulin Resistant?

Ok, before you go down through this list, be forewarned, as according to the CDC, one out of every third American has prediabetes, and nine out of ten don't know they have it.[4] Unspecific symptoms are fatigue, irritability, brain fog/memory and concentration issues, weight gain around the midsection, sugar crashes in the middle of the day, carbohydrate craving, and inability to lose weight; missing a meal can lead to being cranky and irritable, weak, and tired. After meals one feels drugged and sleepy; you feel that you are addicted to carbohydrates; you have hypoglycemic attacks, poor sex drive, acne, increased hair growth, acanthosis nigricans (skin becomes dark and thick, in the folds and the creases like back of the neck, groin, and armpits), infertility, and cysts; you have difficulty losing weight, and you gain weight easily and aggressively. If you are experiencing irregular menstrual periods or have a history of PCOS or infertility, you could be insulin resistant. Also be more cautious if you have a family history of diabetes, hypoglycemia or alcoholism, high blood pressure, heart disease, and type two diabetes.

Any of these sound familiar? What's even scarier is that these symptoms can be present in very young children and are constantly overlooked, and we are seeing more and more of it daily.

Recipe for Success

Now that you know why it's important to fill your belly with foods that will heal you, not hurt you—let's talk about specifics. So whenever we eat, we need to eat for success. With hundreds of diets out there leaving you confused, I'm going to make it simple. Focusing on nutrient-dense foods, in the right proportions, that keep your gut happy, your glucose regulated, and balance hormones will help lower your inflammation and optimize healing!

When hunger strikes, don't focus on the foods you can't have (because believe me, you will want them even more) and don't listen to your pesky bad bugs as they will manipulate your mind and your cravings, as they work by changing neural signals along the vagus nerve, altering your taste receptors to make you crave foods that will help them thrive.[6] Focus on the foods you CAN have. I ask my patients (and children) to go down a checklist of foods that need to be on their plate, before they consider eating anything else. If we eat the starchy carbohydrate first, we deprive our body the nutrient-dense foods it really needs to functional optimally. Each meal should contain a balance of vegetables, fats, and protein with adequate hydration (if you notice, it is very similar to the gut healing diet, I described previously).

1. **Vegetables:** half your plate
2. **Protein:** about 4–6 oz. (15 grams)
3. **Healthy fats:** one to two teaspoons of oils, nuts, seeds (if tolerated) or avocados.

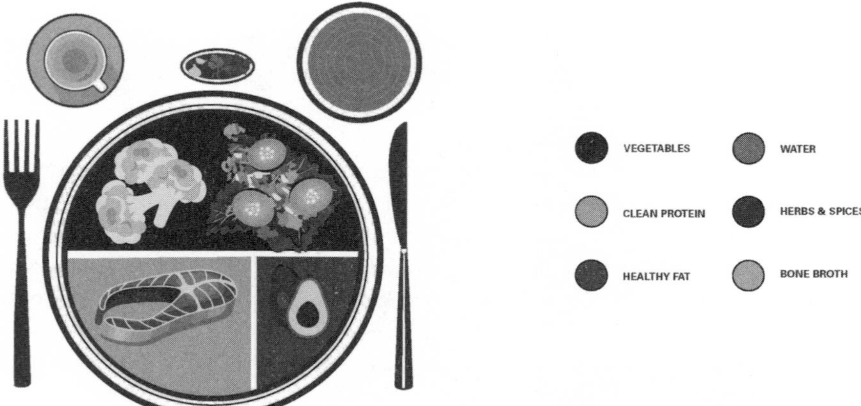

Figure 2.5. The Healing Plate

If you remain hungry, then you can either have a fruit or a healthy grain-free or gluten-free carbohydrate (depending on your individual body's need). It is very important to always combine protein and fat with all carbohydrates (and remember veggies are carbohydrates).

All these meals quickly satiate and optimize gut health and decreases insulin resistance,[5] thereby improving the immune system—healing and preventing chronic disease. So where do we begin? In order to eat for success you need to prepare for success.

Let's focus on what you and your family CAN eat (demonstrated by the healing food pyramid below)! There is so much variety, and the combinations of mouth-watering healing foods are endless—you can never get bored. Let's get started!

Basic Healing Foods for Every Plate

Start with the Colors of the Rainbow

No, I'm not talking about Lucky Charms, so put that box away, but the hidden gems of the grocery store . . . vegetables! Sadly, during 2007–2010, half of the total U.S. population consumed less than 1 cup of fruit and less than 1.5 cups of vegetables daily; 76 percent did not meet fruit intake recommendations, and 87 percent did not meet vegetable intake recommendations.[7] This needs to change, as vegetables help to keep your body alkaline, optimize detoxification, and reduce inflammation.[8] Anytime you feel hungry, they should consist of the majority or half of your plate, leaving room for clean protein and healthy fats. This dynamic combination will reduce your risk of chronic illness.

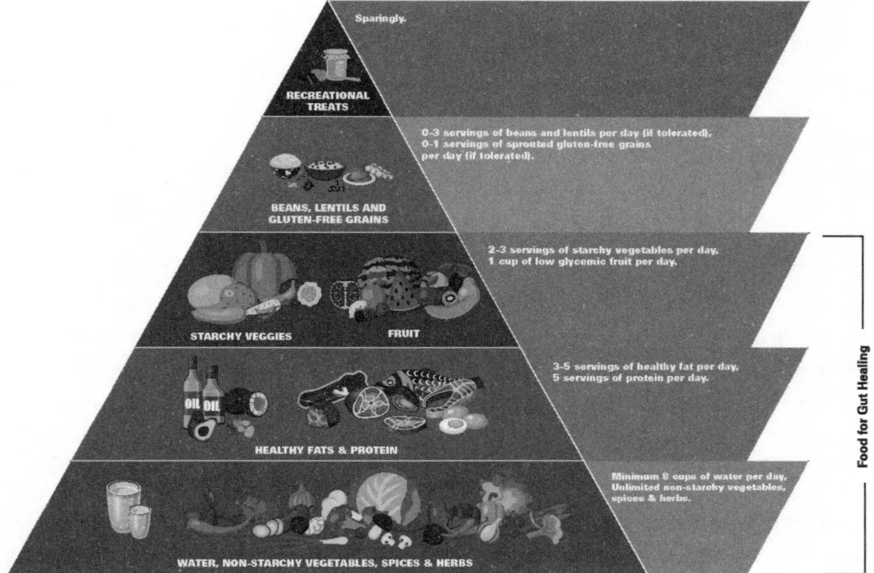

Figure 2.6. The Healing Pyramid

Eat local, whole organic vegetables when possible—the whole plant is full of vital nutrients. These can be eaten raw, cooked, cultured, juiced, or in soups and stews. Make sure not to power wash your veggies; it's fine to rinse, but the tiny bit of soil is good for you as it will also add diversity to your microbiome, lowering inflammation. Keep skin and peels of fruits and vegetables on, as they are a great source of bitters. Bitters are highly nutritious; they regulate your appetite and affect fat storage[9] and insulin release,[10] control blood sugar levels (even in diabetes),[11] optimize wound healing, improve detoxification, and overall improve inflammation.

Examples: Artichoke, asparagus, bamboo shoots, beets, bok choy, broccoflower, broccoli, broccolini, Brussels sprouts, cabbage, carrots, cauliflower, celery, chives, cucumbers, kale, leeks, lettuce, mushrooms, okra, olives, onions, parsnips, sea veggies, spinach, squash (acorn, yellow and butternut, spaghetti) sweet potatoes, turnips, zucchini, and bitters like arugula, bitter melon, kale, and other leafy greens.

Veggie Spotlight

Prebiotic foods: Chicory root, dandelion greens, eggplant, garlic, Jerusalem artichokes, Jicama, kefir, leaks, onions, peas, asparagus, burdock root. Prebiotic foods help heal the gut lining by providing food for the probiotics, optimizing detoxification, soothing inflamed tissues, and protecting against further inflammation.

Fermented foods: If your gut is healing, adding fermented foods to your diet will optimize health and healing by supporting digestion, detoxifying your liver, and strengthening your immune system. Foods like sauerkraut and kimchi help regulate glucose levels and decrease total cholesterol and LDL just after one week of eating them.[12] They are also rich in glutamine, key in improving inflammation, and rich in lactic acid to help balance production of stomach acid. Natto is made from fermented soybeans (if you can tolerate soy); it has been shown to enhance vitamin K2 (will discuss later in this chapter), boost immune system, support cardiovascular health, and contains bacillus subtilis.[13] Other fermented foods to try are miso, kombucha, kvass, pickles, apple cider vinegar, pickled ginger, and homemade ketchup.

Mushrooms: Mushrooms have great benefits as they contain beta-glucans that keep the immune cells alert and antioxidants that lower inflammation. The part incredibly healing is the part of the mushroom that is called the mycelia (part below the ground) and has been shown to balance the microbiome, help detoxification, destroy cancer cells, protect the heart, lower blood sugar, provide antifungal and antiviral benefits, and has liver-protecting properties that also balance cortisol and other stress hormones.[14] Types include cordyceps, reishi, shiitake, lion's mane, and turkey tail.

Sea vegetables: Sea vegetables are excellent sources of iodine, vitamins, and minerals like iron, calcium, and iodine, along with vitamin K2, folate, and magnesium, just to name a few. They help to alkalinize the body and improve detoxification, lowering inflammation, supporting thyroid function, improving blood pressure, and relieving asthma. Examples include kelp, kombu, nori, arame, and wakame; they are great for soups, salads, and snacks.

Protein Power

Your body needs protein to heal and is crucial for the immune system, appetite control, and muscle synthesis. Protein ensures that your gut lining will be appropriately constructed and that there will be enough building materials for enzymes. Studies show that inflammation went down when people added lean meats instead of carbohydrates in their diets.[15]

Your body needs about 80 to 120 g of clean protein per day (depending on your age, body composition, and activity level), and it is essential to get protein at every meal and snack—whether it is from a vegetarian or animal source. Eating protein increases your metabolic fire and ability to burn calories while reducing your appetite, helping you feel full. After the vegetables, make room for about 4–6 oz. of protein per meal, but everyone is different. If you feel fatigued or are exercising, you may need to eat more protein.

Protein Spotlight

The quality of the protein is more important than the quantity—choose clean protein.

Fish: Small wild-caught fish are highly nutrient dense and are great sources of omega 3s, vitamin D, and vitamin B12.[16] Consume smallish fish, wild or sustainably raised cold-water fish, including wild salmon, mackerel, sardines, herring, small halibut, anchovies, and sable (black cod). Look for sustainable organic fisheries, and when purchasing farmed fish, look for farms with high environmental welfare standards; organic standards are best in closed systems.

Poultry and eggs: Look for animal products that are pastured raised, eating nonGMO feed and antibiotic, hormone, and pesticide free. Pastured poultry have more EFAs. Eggs are an excellent source of choline that is needed for brain health and detoxification. They are also full of antioxidants, minerals, and vitamins, especially vitamin D. Eggs protect against heart disease.[17] They are prepared best poached, soft boiled, or cooked on low temperature.

Meat: Meat has always been a gray area, with research on both sides of the spectrum. But one thing is for certain, we need to focus on the quality. Grain-fed animals are more inflammatory to humans. Meat from grass-fed animals is full of micronutrients.[18] It is full of beneficial fats and omega 3s with an optimal ratio between omega 6 and omega 3, lower overall fat content, higher absorbable form of vitamin E content,[19] higher conjugated linolenic acid and vaccenic acid; it lowers inflammation and rebuilds healthy cells.[20] Switching from grain-fed to grass-fed meat and dairy products has lowered women's risk of breast cancer by 60 percent compared to those with the lowest levels of CLA.[21] So make sure the meat that you are eating is grass-fed and grass-finished. (I use the term *grass-fed* not only for meat but also for dairy and other items, as it has come from grass-fed cows.)

Vegetarian option: Hemp seed protein and chia protein power. Pea protein powder, lentils, and beans are also great if you can tolerate them.

Protein powders: There are numerous protein powders on the market. Opt for the least ingredients as possible. Beside the ones I listed above, egg protein powder, collagen or beef gelatin powder, and hydrolyzed beef protein are great sources and will help heal gut lining. Rotate protein sources, to avoid developing sensitivities.

If you can't eat clean, eat lean protein like beef sirloin, turkey or chicken breast, avoiding the cuts of meat with lots of fat and ground beef. Avoid pork as it harbors viruses and parasites, and processed meat like ham, bacon, and sausage can lead to increased risk of cancer.

Healthy Fats

Yes, that wasn't a misprint, fats can be healthy. Fats have gotten bad press, but they are actually key in lowering inflammation [22] and helping people to lose weight.[23] Over the last couple of years, the truth is finally coming to the surface. Fat is essential for your body to work optimally and the key ingredient for cellular function. We have all heard about the effects fat has on heart disease, but now studies have shown no link between cholesterol, saturated fats, and heart disease.[24]

Fats help with weight loss (especially compared to low-fat diets), give us energy, are vital for brain and nerve function keeping it sharp, balance mood, aid in preventing dementia, are required to make hormones like testosterone and estrogen and to metabolize vitamin D,[25] and actually are key in reversing every single indicator of heart disease risk, including cholesterol, hypertension, diabetes, inflammation, and more.[26] Fat is required to make cholesterol, found in every single cell in the human body, needed for cell structure, aids in the body's important metabolic and hormonal functions, helps absorption and use of fat-soluble nutrients, and optimizes digestive health and bone health. A low cholesterol diet just forces your body to work harder to make its own, revs up its own production, causing higher cholesterol levels.

Fat satiates us by turning on leptin, the hormone that regulates feelings of fullness, which is often disrupted by eating too many processed refined carbohydrates and bad fat.

There are different types of fats: Saturated (butter and coconut oil), monounsaturated (olive, avocado, and many nuts), polyunsaturated (omega 3 and 6), and trans fats.

Saturated fat is what we have known till now as the "forbidden fat." Saturated fat is essential for fat-soluble vitamins and nutrients, and is actually beneficial as it can actually lower triglycerides, raise HDL and the less harmful (fluffy) type of LDL, lower inflammation by turning off the genes that produce cytokines, and prevent leaky gut. Fats like coconut oil and butter don't raise saturated fats,[28] but it is actually the carbohydrates you eat that force your liver to make fat, leading to high cholesterol, especially the bad type of LDL, triglycerides, lowering HDL.[29]. Saturated fats reduce inflammation and chronic disease, like heart disease, cancer, diabetes, depression, and others. Adding fats to your diet can also reduce overall calorie intake.[30] It is important to be careful with saturated fats in the presence of a high refined carbohydrate diet[27]and low omega 3 intake as it may lead to inflammation. Healthy fat sources are great snacks for in between meals to balance your blood sugar and immediately satiate. A typical serving of fat is about a tablespoon of oil, handful of nuts, or 4 oz. of fish or other animal protein. Your goal should be between four and five servings of fat a day.

Examples of good fats: fatty fish and fish oils, flaxseed oil (full of essential fatty acids, improves constipation, reduces risk of heart disease, and optimizes cellular function),[31] avocado, nuts, seeds, olives, olive oil, coconut oil, medium chain triglycerides (MCT oil), butter (organic pasteurized raw), ghee (clarified butter, free of A1-beta casein), and palm oil. Animal fat can be your friend, like tallow, lard, and schmaltz.

Fat Spotlight

Avocado: Full of nutrients, fiber, antioxidants, and minerals to help reduce inflammation, prevent cancer, and satiate. It is full of protein, compared to any fruit, and helps to build lean muscle mass; detoxify; build healthy skin, hair and eyes, brain, digestion; protect against insulin resistance; and help burn fat! Pass the guacamole!!!

Coconut oil: Contains anti-inflammatory fats like lauric acid, increasing metabolism and promoting weight loss. Coconut oil fights off fungus[32] and bad bacteria,[33] improves digestion, metabolism, blood lipids, sugars; acts as an antioxidant; improves memory for those with Alzheimer's disease; improves cholesterol;[34] lowers insulin levels;[35] and improves sport performance. It contains conjugated linolic acid, which strengthens the immune system and helps cells communicate better, protecting you from cancer. Actually, coconut oil is not associated with an increased risk of heart attack and stroke.[36] Coconut oil remains stable with heat up to 400 degrees F, so it can be used for cooking. Look for virgin, organic, expeller cold pressed, unrefined, and unbleached.

Medium chain triglycerides: Coconut oil is about two-thirds MCT oil, but other more concentrated ones are present in the market. These are also great sources for fat with great antioxidant and antimicrobial properties, supporting your immune system. They actually promote weight loss, heal obesity-related fatty liver, and reduce the ratio of total cholesterol to HDL.

Palm oil: Has been shown to protect blood vessels,[37] reduce blood pressure, improve cholesterol profiles,[38] and reduce heart disease risk.[39] Look for sustainable oil with the label CSPO.

Olive oil: Is great for your brain and lowering inflammation,[40] hsCRP, and even cancers.[41] Just a few tablespoons will do the trick, lowering blood pressure,[42] preventing heart attacks[43] and cholesterol panels.[44] Olive oil is also great for optimizing gut health[45] by lowering bad bugs like H pylori. Purchase extra virgin olive oil as it possesses more anti-inflammatory properties[46] (in dark tinted glass bottles to prevent oxidation). Olive oil is best as it contains polyphenols that are powerful antioxidant compounds, reducing the risk of heart disease.

Butter: Science has now concluded that butter is instrumental in heart disease prevention[47] and reducing inflammation. Choose grass-fed butter, which is full of choline and vitamin A[48] and has three to five times more CLA than grain-fed butter.[49]

Ghee: Ghee has the same anti-inflammatory properties as butter, so you can also look for grass-fed ghee. Grass-fed ghee is full of vitamin D, A, omega 3s, CLA, and butyrate, which promotes intestinal health. In ghee, the milk solids have been removed so it can easily be tolerated by those with dairy allergies.

Nuts and seeds: Nuts are a great source of proteins, minerals, fiber, and essential fatty acids. Studies[50] have proven that nuts lower the incidence of cardiovascular disease,[51] improve cholesterol,[52] prevent blood glucose from spiking,[53] lower risk of type 2 diabetes,[54] reverse brain dysfunction,[55] and even lower the risk of death.[56] Nuts should ideally be purchased raw, soaked (overnight for up to twenty-four hours), sprouted then roasted, to be stored in closed, tight, and dark containers in a cool location that helps to reduce the lectins and phytates content. You can freeze nuts and seeds for up to three months. A handful or two a day of nuts like almonds, pecans, walnuts, hazel, macadamia, and pistachio and seeds like chia, flax, and pumpkin is enough to gain all the benefits.

Respect the oil: Oils begin to get damaged at certain temperatures, destroying valuable nutrients (smoke point), and even good oils can start to go bad if not treated properly. Below I have listed the oils that can be used at what temperatures. Let's respect the oil, for them to respect us!

High heat: coconut oil and ghee.

Med/low heat/no heat: extra virgin olive oil, and unrefined coconut oil, walnut oil, macadamia oil, sesame oil, avocado oil, walnut oil, almond oil, and butter.

Water, Water Everywhere . . . But What Else Can I Drink?

Optimal hydration is key in decreasing inflammation. Being well hydrated flushes out toxins through your kidney, promotes weight loss, increases energy, and promotes healthy bowel movements. To optimize healing, drink at least eight glasses of water each day. Remember not to drink after a meal, as it may hamper digestion.

Filtered water is best. Other options are carbonated water, fresh raw veggie juice, spring water and chilled drinking tea, and organic tea (black, white, green, herbal, or yerba mate). Green tea is anti-inflammatory and has antioxidants, phytonutirents, and detoxifying properties. Try adding slices or wedges of orange, lemon, or lime to water. Throw in a mint leaf for an extra refreshing flavor along with stevia. Some people can tolerate coffee (black or with coconut milk). Remember to drink about a minimum of a cup of bone broth per day. Smoothies are also a great option for a fast meal; add all the key nutrients: a fruit; veggies; nondairy milk or water; smart fat like chia, flax, or coconut oil or MCT oil; and a protein powder.

Nature's Candy—Fruit!

The health benefits of fruit are endless. If after the veggie, protein, and good fat source, you're still hungry, I recommend going to dessert by eating a small amount of low-glycemic fruit. If you are doing fruit as a snack, always balance it with some sort of protein and fat source, to keep inflammation at bay. You can include ½ cup to 1 cup per day of the low-glycemic fruits like berries, oranges, cantaloupe, apples, peaches, plums, pomegranate, kiwi, and even watermelon, as it is mostly water.

Berries are rich in antioxidants, which prevent toxins from damaging the body; they are also rich in pranthocyanidins, which have been shown to reverse inflammation, and they have gallic acid, which protects our brains from inflammation, oxidative stress, and cancer,[57] supports heart health and digestion, and controls appetite, promoting weight loss. Pomegranate seeds, as an antioxidant, also heal from the inside out, as they are anitcarcinogenic,[58,59] reduce arthritis and joint pain,[60] and are cardioprotective, lowering blood pressure.[61]

Finally, Give Me My Carbohydrates!

Yes, finally down to everyone's favorite part of the meal, and guess what? Most of the meal should be carbs! Shocked? Vegetables are carbohydrates, and you're allowed unlimited refills. Other great carbs are nuts and seeds, lentils, and even fruit.

So listen to your body!

I bake with nut, seed almond flour or coconut flour, which are great for anyone healing from leaky gut. Once you have healed your gut some, you can occasionally add back in rice, quinoa, or other forms of gluten-free grains and even sourdough bread, as tolerated. Avoid high-glycemic carbohydrates, as best as you can.

Fiber

Fiber suppresses appetite, helps you feel full, controls craving, stabilizes the rise in your blood sugar and insulin levels after a meal, decreases inflammation and lowers blood pressure, improves cholesterol and memory, helps fight chronic disease like cancer, and helps to remove toxins from your system, feeding the healthy bacteria. Fiber should be part of every meal and can be found in nuts, seeds, and fresh produce like avocados, broccoli, asparagus, kale, green beans, artichoke, sweet potato, okra, tomatoes, and butternut squash. Fruit sources include apples, pears, blueberries, oranges, raspberries, strawberries, peaches, and pineapple. Beans and lentils are also great sources, if tolerated. Aim for about 25–30 g or about ten servings of fiber per day.

Sweeteners

Most of us have a sweet tooth, and as an occasional treat, we can still enjoy sweet things (cue happy dance now). Sugars like refined sugar, corn syrup, and agave nectar (very high in fructose, worsening insulin resistance) should be avoided, but raw honey, evaporated cane sugar, date sugar, maple syrup, and black strap molasses are all high in phenols and antioxidants.[62]

Honey is a natural, least-processed sweetener and is full of antioxidants, vitamins, and minerals. It helps to lower inflammation, aiding the gut by acting like a prebiotic and neutralizing free radicals. It also helps in improving conditions like allergies, coughs, and asthma.[63] It is best to choose cold expressed raw organic honey, or manuka honey, but again sparingly to keep glucose levels under control. Maple syrup also contains lots of beneficial antioxidants,[64] decreasing the plasma glucose, protecting the microbiome, and protecting against cancer.[65, 66, 68] Other sweeteners that are full of antioxidants are molasses from raw cane sugar[69] and date sugar. Organic stevia whole plant extract can also be used, as it doesn't raise your glucose levels. Dark chocolate, higher than 70 percent cocoa is best, with numerous health benefits.

Herbs and Spices

Herbs and spices are powerful antioxidants, anti-inflammatories, and detoxifiers. Garlic decreases blood pressure, prevents clots, and improves cholesterol (crush and chop to release its secret power: allicin); cardamom stimulates bile and optimizes liver health and fat metabolism; cinnamon helps to stabilize blood sugar and blood pressure and lowers bad cholesterol; turmeric is a powerful anti-inflammatory and optimizes detoxification; and ginger lowers inflammation and atherosclerosis. Green herbs like thyme have powerful antiseptic, antioxidant, and anti-inflammatory properties, aiding in digestion; sage lowers blood sugar and blood pressure; oregano has antifungal, antibacterial, antiparasitic, and antioxidant properties; and others like mint, basil, dill, chives, paprika, rosemary, and parsley are also beneficial. Add the powerful effects of black seeds with antioxidant, antimicrobial, anticancer properties, preventing insulin resistance and optimizing hair, skin, and liver function. Adding these nutritious herbs and spices is the best way to battle inflammation with every morsel you eat. So awesome!

Salt

Salt is another one that has been shined the caution spotlight. But table salt is different than sea salt. Table salt has been overly processed, its chemical composition altered and stripped of its nutritional benefits, causing fluid retention; and, it's toxic. Now sea salt, Celtic salt, and Himalayan salt are the real deal. These are full of trace minerals that keep you hydrated, essential minerals like magnesium and calcium, and so many more that are all needed for the body to function optimally. I usually recommend about 1–2 tsp a day of sea salt, but use with caution if you have a health condition that is sensitive to your salt intake.

To Go Organic or Not to Go Organic—That Is the Question

This question crosses our mind every time we step into the grocery store: Is the price markup worth the benefits? Well the difference between the two is how the crops are grown. For organic foods, with the USDA label, the guidelines prohibit the use of pesticides or herbicides, hormones, genetic engineering, and antibiotics, while the conventional produce doesn't have to follow any of these restrictions.

In a study published in the *Journal of Applied Nutrition*, organically and conventionally grown apples, pears, potatoes, wheat, and sweet corn were compared and analyzed for their mineral content over a two-year period; organic produce was found to be incredibly more nutrient dense.[70] So choosing from organics is best, but if you can't, take a look at the Environmental Working Group, which has a list of the "dirty dozen" and the "clean fifteen" (foods with and without pesticides) and stick to organic with those foods on the dirty dozen list.

Foods to Avoid/Limit

Gluten

Examples of foods that have obvious or hidden gluten are barley, rye, wheat, durum, graham, kamut, semolina, spelt, oats, and soy sauce and other condiments like ketchup. Avoid foods that are packaged, processed, and canned with "natural flavors." Also, beer and seitan can often have gluten, unless it is marked gluten free. Gluten can be hiding in anything, so always make sure it is marked gluten free—even your body products.

Sugar

Avoid sugar and all its other code names: agave, barley malt, brown rice syrup, bran sugar, dextrose, glucose, dextran, lactose, disaccharides, fructose, high-fructose corn syrup (HFCS), hydrogenated starch, maltodextrin, maltose, monosaccharides, sorghum, sucrose. and xylose.

Fructose, like in agave and HFCS, has been shown to be associated with insulin resistance, hypertension, and impaired glucose tolerance. A diet full of processed sugar leads to obesity and inflammation and is responsible for the obesity, diabetes, heart disease, and dementia epidemic, leading to premature death.[71]

Processed/Junk/Fast Foods

Here is where you will need to watch out for all the white stuff, like white flour, bread, cakes, cookies, and other baked goods. They have a very high glycemic index, full of partially hydrogenated oils and GMOs.

Soy

Soy, as most is genetically modified, is not recognized by the digestive system. Its molecules remain unbroken, leading to leaky gut syndrome as it stimulates the immune system to produce antibodies, food sensitivities, and inflammation.[72] It also contains inhibitors that shut down the digestion of proteins, causing gastric discomfort and reducing the absorption of amino acids and minerals such as calcium, iron, magnesium, and zinc. Soy disrupts the endocrine system, especially disregulating thyroid and estrogen, and interferes with leptin, leading to leptin resistance, making you overeat.

Soy is found in tempeh, tofu, edamame, soy sauce, and tamari and can be found in meat substitutes and protein shakes, bars, and powders. If you're going to eat soy, make sure it's fermented, as in tempeh. The fermentation process breaks down indigestible carbohydrates and dissolves the protein-digestion inhibitors.

Corn

Corn can be equally as dangerous as gluten; it can also contribute to leaky gut.[73] When you digest corn, your body can react to it as if it were gluten. In this program, we will eliminate all grains, because of the potential for cross-reactivity of gluten. Corn is also one of the most commonly genetically engineered foods, with about 90 percent of corn being genetically modified. It is present in many products—such as high-fructose corn syrup, corn oil, and cornstarch—and is even being fed to our livestock and poultry, leading to inflammatory saturated fats.

Alcohol

As discussed in the gut section, alcohol is basically just another code name for sugar.

Food Additives, Artificial Colors, Flavors, or Preservatives, and GMO Foods

Anything artificial causes inflammation. Food additives cause uncontrollable hunger and binge eating. MSG (causes headaches and allergies and damages your gut), artificial sweeteners and flavors, soy protein isolate (processed soy extract, causes cancer in animals), sodium and calcium caseinate (toxic dairy extract), phosphoric acid, dipotassium phosphate, tricalcium phosphates, carrageenan (causes leaky gut and inflammation), sulfides (cause allergies and inflammation), nitrates and nitrites in processed deli meats (cause cancer),[74] microwave popcorn (contains PFOA, a synthetic chemical linked to cancer and hormone disruption),[75] and industrial food additives like emulsifiers such as polysorbate 80 or lecithin (commonly found in vitamins, chewing gum, and ice cream) are all linked to autoimmunity.[76]

In 2015, glyphoside was linked to cancer by the World Health Organization and the International Agency for Research on Cancer (IARC).[77] Pesticides were engineered to contain Bt toxins, which kill insects by destroying their digestive lining, and glyphosate doubles as an antibiotic, disrupting our guts also. The pesticide disrupts the microbiome, compromises the ability to detoxify toxins, depletes vitamin D and other key nutrients, and can mimic hormones like estrogen, which can lead to cancers. The pesticide can be linked to a fourfold increase of celiac disease and other autoimmune conditions, according to 270 studies compiled by MIT in 2013.

Refined Oils, Hydrogenated Oils, and Trans Fats

Avoid trans fats, as they lead to inflammation and immune dysfunction. They also increase bad cholesterol and lower good cholesterol, raising the risk of heart attack.[78] They promote obesity, insulin resistance, prediabetes and diabetes type 2,[79] cancer,[80,81] and dementia. Trans fats include shortening, margarine, spreads, anything that is hydrogenated and are commonly found in refined baked goods.

Avoid vegetable oils like corn, soybean, canola, safflower, and sunflower, as these vegetable oils are partially hydrogenated oils, and 90 percent of canola oil is from genetically modified plants. These oils also contain pro-inflammatory omega-6 fats and lead to gut dysfunction/leaky gut, interfering with normal cell metabolism, and are hazardous to health, increasing our chances of heart disease.[82] The imbalance between omega 6 and omega 3 has been shown to depress the immune system function, contribute to weight gain, and lead to chronic disease[83] and inflammation.[84] Omega 3 should be eaten in the correct ratio to omega 6; ideally, the omega 6 to omega 3 ratio should be from 4:1 to 1:1 to optimize health, fight disease, and stop premature aging.

Dairy

Most people can't tolerate dairy, especially those with a leaky gut as it triggers their immune system leading to inflammation, weight gain, and chronic disease.[85] But once you have healed, you can gradually add dairy back in. Ideally, full fat, raw sheep and goat's milk, organic and pastured, hard cheese, and homemade yogurt are best, and these are lower in lactose, so the nutrients are easily digested, like vitamin B12, magnesium, calcium, folate, enzymes, and probiotics. One can also make goat's milk kefir to boost healthy fats and improve gut flora.[86] Raw milk (best from Jersey or Guernsey cows or from source-certified cows) modulates epigenetics, increasing microbial diversity and lowering allergies. Grass-fed dairy also contains the ideal ratio of omega 6 and omega 3 needed to optimize health and healing.[87] Low-heat boiling preserves the milk benefits better than high-heat boiling.

Alternatives include: coconut milk kefir, with its wonderful antifungal, antiviral properties to help heal leaky gut; and almond milk, which can help to lower bad LDL cholesterol and support cardiovascular health, as it is high in monounsaturated fats, high in omega 3 fats and amino acid L-arginine, great for healing leaky gut.

Most people can tolerate grass-fed butter and ghee, as these have great antioxidants and good fats like CLA, which boosts metabolism, but avoid if you have serious dairy sensitivity.

For calcium necessary for optimal bone health and good general health focus on these foods: flaxseeds, spinach, sardines, walnuts, Brazil nuts, greens (e.g., mustard and collard), sesame seeds, wild salmon, broccoli, and kale.

Drinks

Drinks to avoid are soda, diet soda, sports drinks, fruit juice, and other sweetened beverages like iced tea and lemonade that is full of sugar; these all have limited nutritional value.

Grains

Grains have been a key part of the current food pyramid. Grains are the edible part of the plant, the seed with the embryo. The plant produces natural insecticide to help it pass undigested through the animal system. The truth is that all grains are anti-nutrients (as they contain phytates), preventing your body from absorbing the nutrients and minerals (like calcium, magnesium, iron, zinc, and potassium) and decreasing the digestion of fats, protein, and starches, which leads to deficiencies of key nutrients the body needs. Grains can promote leaky gut, feed unfriendly bacteria, and damage the intestinal cells.

Grains can be problematic for most because they contain amylopectin, causing blood sugar spikes that lead to insulin resistance, increasing belly fat and inflammation,[88] and lectins (like agglutinins, a natural insecticide, and prolamines), specifically in oats, corn, or quinoa, which can cause leaky gut and dysbiosis by stimulating the immune system, interfering with cell function, and making it hard to digest. Some may even contain toxins from molds, called mycotoxins, increasing weight gain and irritability. Seeds and seed-bearing plants like grains and legumes contain amylase inhibitors, which block the enzymes your body uses to break down carbohydrates, and protease inhibitors, which block the enzymes your body uses to break down proteins. These enzyme inhibitors even survive cooking, providing a meal for unhealthy bacteria promoting SIBO and yeast overgrowth; they contain saponins, which occur in legumes, pseudo grains, and nightshades, which potentially destroy red blood cells, threatening your gut integrity and leading to leaky gut. Grains are not needed to sustain a healthy existence free of disease, as they offer very little nutritional value compared to all the other categories.

So eliminating these is critical in *The Holistic Rx*, even amaranth, barley, buckwheat, corn, millet, oats, quinoa, rice, sorghum, spelt, and teff. Coconut, nut and seed flours are great alternatives, as both are highly nutrient dense and are high in protein, fiber, and minerals. Coconut flour even lowers bad LDL[89] and is easier to digest than almond flour for some people.

Once you have healed, as tolerated, adding some occasional grains back into your diet can be accomplished. Sprouting the grains makes them easier to digest and the nutrients easier to absorb, deactivates the phytic acid, and increases dietary fiber by 50 percent.[90] Examples that can be added include organic sprouted grain flours like buckwheat, sorghum, quinoa, millet, amaranth, corn, oats, rice, and even sourdough.

Other Possible Inflammatory Foods for Chronic Disease

If you're still not improving after four weeks (despite optimizing *The Holistic Rx* and fixing deficiencies), here are other common food allergens that you can focus on eliminating, as patients can also be sensitive to the following:

Eggs

Eggs are a great source of proteins, especially if organic and pasture raised. But for those who are susceptible, they can be allergenic. They contain lysozyme, a protective enzyme that breaks down the cell membrane of gram-negative bacteria, leading to leaky gut.

Legumes

Beans can be great sources of minerals, proteins, and fiber. Some people can also have problems with beans and legumes as they contain lectins,[91] phytates,[92] and saponins, as they are difficult to digest and can worsen digestive function by irritating the lining of the small intestine, which in turn creates inflammation, impairs the absorption of nutrients and minerals, and spikes blood sugars.

For those with sensitivity to legumes and beans, presoaking, sprouting, or fermenting these foods can improve digestion and absorption. Legumes to restrict are black beans, garbanzo beans, lentils, lima beans, soybeans, and white beans.

Nightshades

Vegetables in the nightshade family like tomatoes, white potatoes, bell peppers, eggplant, and spices like cayenne pepper, paprika, and red pepper flakes are to be avoided if you still continue to have problems. They contain a variety of compounds like solanine, chaconine, and lectins, which can worsen leaky gut.

Caffeine

Though some may be able to tolerate caffeine in the right amounts, caffeine can cause problems especially in patients with insomnia and mood disorders, as it stimulates the release of stress neurotransmitters like adrenaline and excess estrogen and can make you anxious and irritable, impacting sleep. If you're going to drink caffeine, don't consume it after 1 pm. Getting off of caffeine can release you from cravings and normalize your brain chemistry, only helping your adrenals.

So if you feel like caffeine is holding you back, here's how you can slowly wean off. Starting on a weekend, slowly cut your dose in half every day until you're down to a little bit, and then stop. Make sure to drink lots of water during this time, and if you get a headache, go to bed. Taking vitamin C (1,000 mg) can help to decrease the withdrawal effects and headaches.

So overall, grains, legumes, seeds, caffeine, and nightshades can contribute to leaky gut by damaging intestinal cells, opening tight junctions, and feeding unfriendly bacteria to create gut dysbiosis; these should be avoided if you have serious inflammation.

Other Sensitivities to Consider

One can also be sensitive to certain foods that may contain histamine, sulfates, salicylate, and oxalate.

Listen to Your Body

I know you hate me right now, but in about two weeks, you might change your mind once you discover the real you! I'm going to say this again, you are taking the problematic foods away for a short time, and once you heal, those can be added back as tolerated. So listen to your body!

NOW WHAT DO I EAT?! Go Down the List

Now that I've confused you once again, let me clarify. Whenever you get hungry, focus on foods that will lower inflammation, not add fuel to the fire that is already burning within. Again, whenever you're hungry, ask yourself: what is my veggie, my clean protein source, and my healthy fat, and make sure you're optimally hydrated, as dehydration can lead to cravings.

Example meals include:

Breakfast: veggies, clean protein and healthy fat. Examples include foods made with coconut, nut and seed flours like pancakes, waffles, muffins, banana bread/zucchini bread, eggs, quiche, no-nitrate sausages (chicken, beef, and turkey) or kabobs, no-grain cereal in almond milk with fresh or frozen berries, smoothies, greens, fruit or nut or seed butter, fresh fruit, chia pudding.

Snacks: veggies, clean protein, and healthy fat and fruit. Examples include sugar snap peas and guacamole, nuts with blueberries, veggie and protein rollups.

Lunch and dinner: veggies, clean protein and healthy fat. Examples include soups, egg/chicken/tuna salad, veggie and protein rollups, zucchini pasta with meat sauce, lettuce wrap, stir fry, no-grain tortilla/naan, cauliflower rice.

Grocery Shopping Tip: Go Down the List

Grocery shopping can be so confusing with so many options! When going grocery shopping, remember not to go when you're hungry, and choosing whole, one-ingredient food is the key to your success. Going down the list, again, makes it easy. Choose veggies, clean protein, and healthy fat and fruit. Remember to read labels, avoiding the list we just talked about. Stick to the basics, and you won't go hungry!

Out and About: Go Down the List

I love the quote by Ghandi, "Be the change you wish to see in the world," and I take that everywhere I go. Leading by example is key and something I stress to my kids all the time. Going to parties and restaurants is going to take more will power, but by using these simple tips, you can be empowered and not fall victim to the foods that will hurt you. Being prepared by doing your homework before going out can help you prepare for success. Researching the menu or taking your own food to parties can help you. Communicate with your server and be clear about what you're trying to avoid. Avoid the bread and appetizers at the table (remember, they give that stuff out for free, so it is literally worthless to you and your body) and ask for a gluten-free menu. Replace the grains with extra vegetables and ask for very simple food preparations, choosing foods that are roasted, broiled, baked, grilled, seared, steamed, or sautéed. Stay away from foods that are glazed, fried, crispy, breaded, and creamy. Ask to replace salad dressing, dips, and sauces with olive oil, salt, and pepper. Fill up beforehand and drink one to two glasses of water before the meal to reduce your appetite. Remember to continue to follow the list. Focus on veggies, clean protein, and healthy fat, and ask for fruit for dessert.

Travel: Go Down the List!

Take the crazy out of the fun and always be prepared! Plan ahead for traveling, do advanced research, pack your own food, bring ice packs and insulated bags, ask for a fridge, or bring a cooler. Examples of what you could take with you are wild canned salmon, all natural mayo, natural no-nitrate grass- or pasture-raised jerkey/kabobs, nut and seed butters, coconut butter, almond flour or flaxseed crackers, whole food protein bars, water, grain-free baked goods, hard boiled eggs, olives, broccoli slaw, sweet potato or veggies chips (fried in coconut oil), and all the veggies and low-glycemic foods.

The options are endless!!!! So exciting!!!

Special Note for Vegans

A vegan diet can be healthy as long as you're eating mainly vegetables and getting good sources of vitamin B12, B2, taurine, vitamin D3, iron, DHA, and minerals like magnesium, copper, and zinc. Remember to continue to balance and go down the list, choosing healthy protein and fat options. It might be a little difficult to heal the gut being vegan, but adding in vegetable broth with lots of healthy fat can help.

Pregnant or Breast-feeding

Pregnancy and breast-feeding are critical moments that will determine your and your child's health. Continue to follow the list, cutting back on fish consumption to once or twice a week, but add back in DHA (900–1,000 mg per day). The health of your gut determines your child's health, so eat to keep your gut happy. Continue prenatals and probiotics.

Other Tips for Health and Improving Insulin Resistance

- Begin your morning with water and lemon.
- Eat and drink until you're two-thirds full.
- Breathe, really enjoy your meal, and chew every bite well.
- Fast three to four hours in between meals (and up to two snacks per day).
- Stop eating and drinking at least three hours before you go to bed; intermittent fasting can help to break the cycle of elevated insulin levels.
- Cut out foods with a glycemic index above 55.
- Always combine carbohydrates with clean protein and healthy fats.

I Need Help!

Consider going to a functional medicine or holistic practitioner, nutritionist, or health coach to help you figure out the right food plan for you. Sometimes even the best intentions aren't enough, and finding the right person to help guide you and help you get organized will help you get and stay on that path toward healing! It never hurts to have an extra cheerleader on your side. Sometimes checking your specific genetic profile, with the help of a practitioner, will help tailor your specific plan that will work the best for you.[93]

SUPPLEMENTS

Living healthy and boosting immunity always starts with diet and can't be replaced. Supplements can give you the extra push in the right direction toward healing, supporting the immune system, allowing it to be healthy and balanced. Nutritional deficiencies can interfere with you getting better, so supplementing can give you the extra boost you need to expedite healing.

Why Are We Deficient?

What with our conventional and commercial farming practices, the standard American diet is full of processed foods and low on microbial diversity; increased stress and toxins can decrease nutrient absorption and increase inflammation. Also, the older you get, the harder it becomes for your body to absorb nutrients.

Medications can also lead to deficiencies; examples include the following:

- Proton pump inhibitors and H2 receptor antagonists cause depletions of beneficial flora; calcium; digestive enzymes; folic acid; B12; vitamin C, D, E, K; biotin; chromium; and zinc. If you are taking calcium, use calcium citrate. Vitamin C can increase the absorption of aluminum and antacids.
- Anti-anxiety drugs diminish melatonin.
- Antidepressant medications like SSRIs diminish melatonin, iodine, selenium, and folate. Do not take St. John's wort, 5-HTP, or SAMe without talking to your healthcare provider first. Others diminish B2 and CoQ10.
- Oral contraceptive pills diminish vitamin B2, B5, B6, folate, B12, magnesium, zinc, vitamin C. Do not drink grapefruit juice as it can increase estrogen levels up to 30 percent.
- Bisphosphonates can diminish calcium.
- Albuterol can diminish magnesium and potassium.
- Inhaled corticosteroids can diminish vitamin A, calcium, magnesium, melatonin, selenium, zinc, B6, folate, B12.
- Antibiotics deplete good bacteria; vitamins B1, B2, B6, B3, B12, vitamin K (if antibiotic is taken for more than ten days); calcium; magnesium; and potassium.
- Antidiabetic drugs diminish coenzyme Q10, vitamin B12; metformin can deplete B9, B12, and possibly CoQ 10; insulin can deplete magnesium.
- Hormone/estrogen therapy can deplete vitamin A, B1, B2, B6, B12, C, magnesium, and zinc.
- Anti-inflammatory drugs diminish iron, vitamin C and potassium, folate, melatonin, and zinc.
- Aspirin diminishes vitamin B1, biotin, folate, C, iron, and zinc. Take aspirin before taking niacin.
- Stronger anti-inflammatory drugs like steroids diminish potassium, vitamin C, zinc, vitamin D, selenium, calcium, folic acid, and magnesium.
- Blood pressure lowering medication diminishes calcium, vitamin B6, B1, vitamin C, zinc, sodium, potassium, and magnesium.
- Ace inhibitors deplete zinc, CoQ10 magnesium, potassium.
- Beta blockers deplete CoQ10, choline, melatonin, vitamin B1, vitamin D. Do not eat oranges within two hours of taking atenolol as they reduce its effectiveness. Vitamin D supplementation may interfere with

the absorption of these drugs, take four hours apart, do not exceed the daily recommended amount of calcium if taking more than 50 mg of B6 to monitor blood pressure.
- Thiazide diuretics can deplete vitamin B1, B2, folate, CoQ10, magnesium, potassium, sodium, zinc.
- Calcium channel blockers deplete melatonin and vitamin D.
- Cholesterol lowering medications diminish CoQ 10; do not drink grapefruit juice. High doses of vitamin D may reduce the effectiveness of atorvastatin.
- Hormone replacement therapy diminishes magnesium, vitamin B6, folic acid, zinc, and vitamin C.
- Oral contraceptive pills diminish zinc, vitamin B2, vitamin B3, B6, B12, folic acid, magnesium, vitamin C, and tyrosine.
- Thyroid replacements like Synthroid diminish calcium.
- Tranquilizers diminish CoQ10 and vitamin B2.

How to Choose a Supplement?

If you decide to supplement, remember that the supplement industry is largely unregulated, so be sure you're using products made with integrity, and always read labels. You want to make sure the brand is known for quality; look for large reputable brands and FDA approval. Make sure it is third-party tested and follows good manufacturing practices. Check for the initials USP, GMP, or NSF, to make sure the product doesn't contain additives, synthetic ingredients, and colorings. Purchasing from supplement companies that use organic ingredients is an added bonus. Check the expiration date and make sure the product is fresh. Your best insurance is to purchase supplements from natural health stores or through a healthcare provider properly educated in quality professional supplements. You can also get affordable quality supplements from online nutritional stores. Always check with your licensed primary care practitioner before starting a supplement. More is not better—do not exceed the recommended dosage.

Let's start with the key four supplements that will benefit you in boosting your immunity. (As always, before beginning any new supplement program check with your healthcare practitioner.)

Vitamin D

Vitamin D is an interesting vitamin or prehormone that is an essential precursor to hundreds of disease-preventing proteins and enzymes, binding to many receptors causing changes to cell function. We make D3 as the sunlight hits our skin. When this happens, the liver and kidneys transform the vitamin D into a more active form, allowing our cells to read DNA instructions more effectively, important for our genetic code. Vitamin D regulates vital components of hormones and neurotransmitters like serotonin, helps control cell growth, is a cancer fighter, is essential in mineral metabolism, is a major player in bone strength, and regulates absorption and transport of calcium, magnesium, and phosphorus for bone mineralization and growth. Vitamin D is a disease preventer and vital in decreasing inflammation and lowering insulin resistance. Its deficiency is strongly linked to autoimmune disease.[94]

Most patients are deficient in vitamin D because of the lack of sun exposure and sunblock that blocks the ultraviolet B rays needed to convert the vitamin D to its active form. We look for a range of about 50–80 mg/ml to optimize health. It is best to have your physician check your vitamin D 25OH lab value. If you work closely with a professional, they can prescribe the appropriate dose to quickly increase your vitamin D level. Always make sure you're taking D3, as D2 isn't metabolized by the body. Once it is optimized, continuing on a dosage about twenty times your weight in pounds daily or 2,000–4,000 IU per day is appropriate. A vitamin D overdose is rare but possible as a high vitamin D level (greater than 150 ng/ml) leads to excessively high calcium in your bloodstream, kidney damage, even psychosis. Remember to take vitamin D and other fat-soluble vitamins with meals containing fats.

Be cautious with vitamin D if you have hyperparathyroidism, Hodgkin's or non-Hodgkin's lymphoma, granulomatous disease, like sarcoidosis and tuberculosis, kidney stones, kidney disease, or liver disease.

If looking for a natural way to optimize vitamin D, you'll need exposure of at least 40 percent of your skin to the sun, just until it turns pink or one shade darker, sunbathing at close to noon to 1 pm, using mineral-based sunscreens to help optimize vitamin D conversion. Foods that are also rich in vitamin D include sea vegetables, fish (especially sardines, salmons, and mackerel), beef liver, some cheeses, mushrooms like portabellas, eggs, raw milk, and cod liver oil yolks.

Cod Liver Oil

Cod liver oil provides DHA, vitamin A, and D3 and to a lesser extent vitamins K and E, which help in the absorption and utilization of minerals and nutrients and helps to fight inflammation, as it is fermented, preserving the essential oils in the fish. Some don't tolerate vitamin D supplementation and do better with cod liver oil. Since fermented cod liver oil has twice the vitamin A and D3 of regular cod liver oil, only half the amount is needed. If you're not using fermented, I recommend butter oil in conjunction with a high-vitamin cod liver oil. About 1 tsp high-quality cod liver oil is usually recommended.

Vitamin K

Vitamin K, another nutrient we don't get enough of, is necessary to prevent calcification and clotting and is essential in bone, brain, and immune health. There are two forms: K1 and K2. Vitamin K1, important for blood clotting, is easier to get as it is found in most green vegetables like lettuce, broccoli, and spinach. K2, important for cardiovascular protection, cancer, and strong bone, is found in dietary sources like fermented foods and is produced by bacteria in your gut. Its job is to tell the calcium where to go, so in doing so it helps to reduce calcification in the arteries and improve the calcium intake into bones and helps to restore cancer cells' ability to die.

When we increase our vitamin D intake through supplement use, we can create a relative insufficiency of vitamins K, A, and E. Vitamin K2 or MK-7 is needed for vitamin D to work effectively. A dose of 100–250 μg K2 daily or 50 μg for every 5,000 IU of D3 is beneficial. So when you are taking your vitamin D or calcium supplement, make sure you are meeting your vitamin K needs, by eating enough greens, fermented foods, nuts, cod liver oil, liver, and organ meats. Don't mix vitamin K1 with warfarin.

Magnesium

Magnesium is an essential mineral especially for your nerve cells, muscles and bones and has a major role in immunity.[95] About 75–80 percent of the population are deficient in magnesium because of our acidic diet and constant fluoride exposure.[96] Your cells need magnesium to work, including more than three hundred enzymes and hundreds of body processes that use or synthesize ATP, DNA and RNA, cofactors in methylation and detoxification; vital in muscular contractions and in the production of testosterone and progesterone; production and utilization of fat, protein; and carbohydrates; metabolism of calcium, sodium, and potassium; and is a constituent of bone and teeth. Magnesium can help to reduce spasticity in muscles; improve chronic pain; improve digestion, mood, and sleep; helps you relax; widens blood vessels; lowers blood pressure; increases HDL; lowers TG; lowers hsCRP; improves cardiovascular health, arrhythmias, and blood sugar.[97] Deficiencies are linked to heart disease.[98]

When one is deficient in magnesium, one can feel fatigued, anxious, experience chronic pain or cramps, have difficulty sleeping, feel numbness and tingling in extremities, feel heart racing or abnormal heart rhythms, and have carbohydrate cravings, loss of appetite, and problems in blood sugar regulation, leading to chronic illness.[97]

Ideally, taking about 350–400 mg of elemental magnesium by mouth every day will help fix the deficiency. Even though magnesium glycinate, chelate and maleate are the best absorbed, magnesium citrate is great for constipation and sleep issues. Avoid magnesium supplementation if you have poor kidney function; and if you are constipated, avoid magnesium oxide. Take the magnesium and calcium at least two hours apart from your multivitamin/mineral supplement. Sources of magnesium are green leaves, like frozen spinach, Swiss chard, avocados, dark chocolate, artichoke hearts, almonds, cashews, pumpkin and squash seeds, salmon, halibut, and meat.

Fish Oil

Fish oils are rich in essential fatty acids, like omega 3 and omega 6 fatty acids, which are needed for our cell membranes to work, and can't be produced by our body so they need to be consumed. Their use has been beneficial for a wide array of medical conditions. Essential fatty acid, specifically omega 3, helps to improve your immune system; improves blood chemistry; promotes brain and heart health; lowers triglycerides and increases HDL;[99] improves insulin sensitivity; protects against depression, digestive disorders, arthritis, asthma, and Alzheimer's; improves skin, nail, and hair strength; increases nutrient absorption; improves fertility; and prevents and heals chronic disease by lowering inflammation.[100] Studies suggest that patients with breast, prostate, and non-small cell lung cancer may derive benefit from supplementation.[101] Sixty percent of your brain weight is made up of fat, and 25 percent of that fat is DHA. Omega 3s are predominantly anti-inflammatory as they reduce the expression of inflammatory genes and molecules in the body, while omega 6 promotes the expression and release of pro-inflammatory prostaglandins and interleukins.

Omega 3 foods are coldwater fatty fish like sardines, herring, sardines, wild caught salmon, lake trout, mackerel, shellfish, clams, oysters, mussels, pasture-raised chickens, grass-fed meat (grass-fed beef has fewer omega 6s compared with soybean- or corn-fed cattle), antelope, shrimp, squid, organic, eggs, walnuts, and flax and chia seeds. DHA is found in algae. If you are a vegetarian, eating a seaweed salad several days a week or taking a seaweed supplement with DHA is an effective way to benefit from omega 3s. Your body needs docosahexaenoic acid (DHA) to make myelin, and eicosapentaenoic acid (EPA), deficient in the most of us, is very helpful in lowering inflammation. Omega 3 acid supplementation has been found to be helpful in a variety of autoimmune conditions. Doses of 1–4 grams are recommended when taking fish oil supplements. For rheumatoid or other arthritis, I suggest 3,000 mg per day of EPA plus DHA. For general support of your immune system try

1,000–2,000 mg per day. If you are a vegetarian, you can take 1,000–3,000 mg of flaxseed oil, but it isn't as potent as taking fish oil. Always be sure to get fish oil that's clear of heavy metals, PCBs, and pesticides.

Omega 3 causes platelet inhibition, so common side effects can be belching, halitosis, heartburn, nausea, loose stools, rash, increased bleeding, and bruising (mostly seen with 3 g or more a day). Bleeding risk in patients on blood thinners shouldn't be a concern, because of the low dosage. Make sure to check with your physician first, as INRs should be carefully monitored in patients initiating omega 3.

Remember, everyone is different, and you know yourself better than anyone else. Find a practitioner who will work with you to explore what works for you and what doesn't.

DETOXIFYING YOUR BODY

The Constant Attack

TAKE COVER!!! Your body is constantly being bombarded in all directions, trying to defend its borders and all the communities that live within. Everything passes through security—the liver, your body's main detoxifying organ. With toxins here, there, and everywhere, and more and more bad guys trying to pass security, this forces your liver to work extra hard to remove them. Toxins and your body work the same way. A high body burden of toxins can make it especially difficult to lose weight, damages metabolism, and disrupts the liver's ability to detoxify, worsening inflammation.

We are exposed to more and more chemicals, pesticides, pharmaceutical drugs, and radiation than ever before—with more than one hundred thousand new chemicals in the past few years slowly penetrating our everyday lives. Our bodies are not meant to handle the enormous amount of artificial pollutants we are exposed to daily inside and out. In order to deal with the toxic overload, you must avoid toxic exposures, support your body's natural ability to detoxify, and lowering inflammation, helping you become more resilient to the world around you.

Agitating Toxins

A toxin is a substance that when eaten, swallowed, breathed in, or in contact with your skin can illicit an inflammatory response as your body sees it as foreign or dangerous.

The liver is an integral component in detoxifying the body; it changes nutrients into a more usable form that can be utilized by your cells, filters out and removes cholesterol and lipoproteins, metabolizes (breaks down and builds) many biological molecules, stores vitamins and iron, excretes or detoxifies the compounds and toxins it comes across, destroys old blood cells, produces bile, and removes spent hormones, shipping them off to the large intestine, kidney, skin, and lungs in order to leave the body. If the liver does not have the ability to detoxify or metabolize a particular compound, it will store it locally, holding on to the toxic material the body should be eliminating.

In small amounts, toxins are harmless, as your body can take care of the threat easily. But the slow, hidden, cumulative overload from food or chemicals can directly damage your cells down to the mitochondria (the energy maker of the cell that produces fuel for all our cellular functions). Depending on your particular weakness and what you're exposed to, this puts a huge strain on your liver and the mitochondria. When they are happy, we are happy and feel fantastic. But when its functions are disrupted, the body starts to malfunction, leading to inflammation and chronic disease.[1] Toxins lower immunity, increasing the vulnerability to autoimmunity, cancer, and blood sugar issues; they make the body numb to insulin and leptin, increasing insulin resistance, preventing one from losing weight, and leading to heart disease, diabetes, and strokes. Toxins also affect our epigenetics, and inflame the gut, leading to leaky gut.[2] So the cumulative effect of all the bad guys trying to get past security and then the imbalance with increased stress and lack of sleep and exercise is that the immune system is weakened, further causing worsening inflammation.

Am I Toxic?

Signs of detoxification are very similar to feeling off balance. Symptoms include rashes, flushing, and sweating, dark circles under your eyes, red palms and soles, yellow-coated tongue, brown spots on skin, offensive body odor, mood and sleep issues, chronic pain, digestive issues (e.g., gas, diarrhea, or constipation), trouble digesting fats, chemical sensitivities, allergies, congestion, and frequent infections. Other general symptoms include fatigue, feeling puffy all the time, brain fog, and the inability to lose weight.

Did I scare you yet? I would rather use the term *empowered*. So let's now get you back in control and detoxify to heal and prevent chronic conditions!

Steps to Resilience . . . Let's Detoxify!

Begin by taking these simple steps:

1. Identify your toxins.
2. Keep fluids moving.

3. Eat to detoxify.
4. Swap out toxic for clean.

Just to scare you a little further (or empower you), let's identify these toxins and examine some in a little detail (warning: adult diapers [preferably made with organic cotton] may be worn to protect you from any mishap that may result from the terror).

Step 1: Identify Your Toxins

Heavy Metals

Mercury can be found in silver filings, cosmetics, pesticides, and some vaccines. It is a common pollutant released into the air from many factories, especially those that burn coal. When it settles in the soil and the bottom of our waters, it accumulates in our fish, highest in the tuna and swordfish. The health impacts are highly dependent on the form of mercury that you are exposed to. Exposure in adults can lead to dementia, while one of the types of mercury exposure can cross the placenta and impair cognitive function in children. High levels cause developmental problems that include mental retardation, cerebellar ataxia, limb deformities, altered physical growth, sensory impairments, and cerebral palsy.[3]

Arsenic is commonly found in drinking water. It is also found in insecticides' residues on fruit, vegetables, chicken, rice; in household detergents, colored chalk, wine, rat poison, and automobile exhaust. The animals eat the arsenic, and we eat the animals; our exposure to arsenic can lead to diabetes and gout and makes it harder to remove any mercury from your body, which will increase your risk of autoimmune diseases and cancer.[4]

Lead is a severe neurotoxin that accumulates in the bone, where it can be stored for years. Lead can still be present in older homes, paint, older water pipes, and occasionally in certain cosmetics and pottery from China. Exposure may lead to cardiovascular disease and IQ problems.

Hormone-Disrupting Chemicals

Hormone-disrupting chemicals are readily absorbed and mimic the effects of our hormones. They can send mixed messages to the endocrine system disrupting the hormones' natural actions. Following are examples of hormone disruptors:

Xenoestrogens are endocrine-disrupting chemicals that mimic the effects of estrogen. They build up in fatty tissues of animals and can cause effects like early puberty, difficult and early periods, male infertility, obesity, cancer, and increased inflammation. If you are a man, you might notice more breast tissue or a low sex drive. The estrogen disrupters BPA and phthalates and parabens (described next) are examples of xenoestrogens.

BPA (bisphenol-A) is found in plastics such as containers and baby formula cans. It coats store register receipts. It can cause problems in hormonal signaling, disrupting estrogen, thyroid, leptin, and androgen functions in the body. This promotes weight gain, insulin resistance, and diabetes, impairs brain development in newborn babies; stimulates autoantibody production; and causes problems in the small intestine.[5]

Phthalates and parabens are added to many personal-care and hygiene products like hair spray, perfumes, body washes, shampoos, lotions, fast food, food packaging, plastics with the #3, and detergents. They may be listed on the packaging of products (such as diethyl phthalate), or they may be disguised under the word "fragrance." Phthalates have been implicated in cancers, endocrine disruption, ADHD, diabetes, and obesity. Parabens are easily absorbed, and both phthalates and parabens disrupt hormonal balance, leading to obesity, insulin resistance, and diabetes.[6]

Triclosan is an antimicrobial agent often added to antibacterial soaps, body washes, deodorants, hairsprays, and toothpastes, along with some findings in kitchenware, toys, clothing, and furniture. Frequent exposure of triclosan has been correlated with increased levels of allergies in children, development of antibiotic-resistant superbugs, and is being studied as a potential cancer-causing agent. The Environmental Protection Agency has labeled this as a pesticide and is no more effective than plain soap.[7]

Perfluorooctainoic Acid (PFOA) is a chemical released when nonstick pans that contain Teflon or polytetrafluoroethylene (PTFE) are scratched and/or heated. Nonstick pans can release this chemical called perfluorooctanoic acid (PFOA). Our bodies have difficulty detoxing these chemicals out, so they accumulate over time adding to our overall toxic load, disrupting our hormonal and immune systems. PFOA has been shown to cause liver damage and developmental problems in animals, is a known carcinogen, and decreases energy and mental concentration.

Pesticides are used in agriculture to kill insects. Small amounts, obtained through our food, over time can disrupt our hormones and the microbiome, stimulating autoantibody production leading to weight gain, insulin resistance and diabetes; causing fatigue, irritability, depression, and forgetfulness; and leading to overall inflammation.

Dioxins and polychlorinated biphenyls (PCBs) belong to a family of very toxic chemicals which were banned in the 1970s, but they still persist in the environment and in our bodies. PCBs increase TSH and thyroid antibodies, by displacing iodine, promoting the onset of Hashimoto's thyroidits and other autoimmune diseases, like rheumatoid arthritis. They can also lead to cancers, diabetes, and myocardial infarction. Dioxins are found in meat, dairy, and fish. Chlorine is found in industrial products, lubricants, coolants, industrial chemicals, pools, plastics, pesticides, paper products, and cleaning products. Chlorine has also been shown to not only increase the prevalence of antibiotic resistance but also increase the number of genes of new antibiotic-resistant strains.

Bromide (polybrominated diphenylethers [PBDEs]), another iodine look-like, is found in flame retardants in furniture and upholstery and in our mattresses (making the mattress inflammable), baked foods, plastics used in computers/appliances, and other electronics, tea, citrus-flavored drinks, and gluten free productions. It has been shown to increase the risk of Hashimoto's, ADHD, and diabetes.

Fluoride is an industrial waste by-product added to water supplies to attempt to minimize dental decay and is classified as a drug, administered without a specific dose for all to consume.[8] As of 2010, 41 percent of kids ages twelve to fifteen had some sort of dental fluorosis, according to the CDC.[9] Flouride disrupts the endocrine system, blocks iodine absorption, increases the likelihood of thyroid issues and cancers, increases oxidative stress, and interferes with cell signaling from neurotransmitters, growth factors, and hormones. All fluoride toothpastes have a warning to call Poison Control if swallowed. In 2014, *Lancet Neurology* classified Fluoride is a neurotoxin[10] that damages more than two hundred enzymes and causes developmental neurotoxicity that persists over generations. Sadly, it can also be found in supplements, medications, toothpaste, black tea, red tea, and canned food items. Any cavity prevention can be accomplished via topical fluoride and optimal nutrition [11].

Others

DEA (diethanolamine) is used in foaming agents, shampoos and bubble baths, and toothpastes. In lab animals it is linked to esophageal and stomach cancer. It is banned in many countries but still blesses the United States with its presence.

Volatile organic compounds or VOCs are found in perfumes, air fresheners, household cleaners, and shampoos. They are neurotoxic.

Perchlorate is used to make fertilizers and can be found in our water supply, fruits, veggies, and fireworks.

Surfactants are found in 90% of all shampoos, toothpastes, hair conditioners, soaps and laundry detergent to help break up dirt. Sodium lauryl sulfate (SLS), Sodium laureth sulfate (SLES) and dextran sodium sulfate (DSS) are notoriously toxic for the gastrointestinal system, increasing permeability. They create irritation, inflammation, disrupts hormone function damaging healthy skin.

Now that I have likely scared you from ever coming out into the world again (and likely made you soil your diapers), I want to tell you that there is hope. So again, come out from under your covers, clean up, and let's talk about how we can optimize the security from any bad guy invaders. Let's give your body the fighting chance it deserves!

Step 2: Keep Fluids Moving

Keep the water flowin'. The skin is a major elimination organ for toxins, and sweating helps to eliminate what the body does not need. So get up and exercise or spend some time in a sauna, brushing/exfoliating your skin. Taking a bath with epsom salt, sodium bicarbonate, seaweed, or sea salt (preferably alternating them) may all be helpful to eliminate toxins and is great to lower any die-off reactions. Oil-pulling and infrared saunas can also be helpful to pull out the toxins. Drinking more water helps to increase urination, which will rid toxic waste, especially with hot lemon water in the morning.

Keep the caboose going and the snakes pilin'. Make sure your bowels are eliminating appropriately. Enemas and colon cleansers may be helpful with elimination of toxins and especially important for those who are not having regular bowel movements.

Rub a Rub Rub. Massage turns the extracellular matrix from a jelly-like substance into a more liquid state, improving elimination through the lymphatic system and helping to relax. Yay! More massages!

Step 3: Eat to Detoxify

Pass Me Some Alkalinity, With a Side of Sulfur and Fiber . . . Please.

The ability to create a more alkaline environment in the body with an acidic pH in the stomach may help with the detoxification process. Raw fruits, vegetables, herbs, and spices have the most potent detoxifying effects, so get as many servings in as possible. These not only help with alkalinity, but are rich in sulfur and fiber, which helps bind toxins and eliminates them through stool. Aim for about 30–40 g of fiber per day. Acidic foods consist of dairy, processed foods, sugar, flour and meat. To maintain a balance, aim for a ratio of 80 percent alkaline and 20 percent acidic foods; but this can vary depending on how much more cleaning your body needs, so listen to your body.

Focus on asparagus, bok choy, celery, citrus, green apples, kiefer, kimchi, sauerkraut, olives, plums, cruciferous vegetables such as broccoli, Brussels sprouts, beets, cauliflower, watercress, cabbage, kale, swiss chard, and collard greens (raw are more alkaline when cooked). An easy way to do this is to start your morning with a hot cup of water with lemon, followed by a green shake for breakfast or vegetable juices made with cucumbers, carrots, celery, and wheatgrass, providing antioxidants, B vitamins, and minerals. These are full of enzymes that support your liver and gallbladder. Other foods that are great for liver support are salmon, berries, pumpkin seeds, olive oil, lentils, brazil nuts, wheatgrass, and grapes. Top beverages are apple cider vinegar, dandelion tea, milk thistle tea, and chamomile tea as they all cleanse the liver and gallbladder. Herbs that can help in detoxification include caraway, dill seeds, curcumin (turmeric), rosemary, thyme, cumin, basil, poppy seeds, oregano, black pepper, and cilantro (a natural chelator). Raw fruits and vegetables are more alkaline when they are cooked.

Get Your Glutathione On!

Glutathione is the most important antioxidant and is found in every cell in your body, but its highest concentration is in your liver. It helps to mop up heavy metals like arsenic, cadmiumm, mercury, and end products and anything that can damage cells by binding to free radicals and carrying them out of the body. Lots of environmental exposure can cause the glutathione to get used up leading to damaged tissues and leading to inflammation. Glutathione also helps with DNA protection, mitochondrial and immune support; it protects against heart disease, cancer, dementia, and other chronic illnesses. Some patients have handicapped enzymes, but genetics aren't your destiny, and eating the right foods can help give you the raw materials required for making it. Help your body make its own glutathione by eating plenty of garlic, onions, cilantro, and cruciferous veggies like broccoli, kale, cauliflower, and cabbage. N-acetyl cysteine is a precursor to glutathione.

Alpha lipoic acid, a fat-soluble molecule found in every cell of the body and that cleans up your glutathione and helps it get back to work, is a potent antioxidant, protecting your skin and balancing blood sugar. It is used for toxin-related illnesses and detoxifying mercury. Sources of alpha lipoic acid include dark green leafy vegetables, animal foods, and organ meats.

Yum, Algae!

Blue green algae, like spirulina or chlorella, have an abundance of nutrients that help to cleanse and detox the body by chelating heavy metals. This protects against DNA mutations and increases the levels of NK cells in humans.[12] Chlorella is a unicellular green algae that contains high levels of powerful nutritional components such as proteins, vitamins, minerals, and dietary fiber. Animal studies have also found it useful in removing toxins such as dioxins, cadmium, lead, and radiation exposure.[13] Spirulina is a great nutrient-dense detoxifier. It enhances the microbiome, protecting the body from radiation and heavy metals. It eliminates candida,[14] improves immunity, and helps fight off infections and chronic illnesses such as cancer.[15] It benefits the body by reducing inflammation and curbing hunger. When purchasing chlorella, look for organic, and make sure to buy "cracked cell wall chlorella," otherwise it is difficult to absorb. If you are eating a lot of fish, you may want to take blue green algae, in order to prevent mercury from getting stored in your tissues. But if you are eating a lot of fresh greens, you are likely already detoxing.

Need Extra Help?

For those with high toxic load, it may be beneficial to add supplements to optimize healing. It is important not to detoxify too early, as you need a healthy gut and adrenal system for detoxification not to backfire. As discussed previously, probiotics and digestive enzymes (specifically with lipase) optimize gut healing and improve digestion of fats. Glutathione (600–1,200 mg acetyl-glutathione daily), or N-acetyl cysteine (600–1,800 mg daily), along with vitamin C (2000 mg daily), and a liver support blend with alpha lipoic acid (300–600 mg daily) and milk thistle (150 mg twice daily)—all can be taken on an empty stomach.

If you are a diabetic, be aware that ALA can lower blood sugar levels. If you have cancer, on chemo or radiation, this may theoretically decrease the effectiveness of medications. Doses of 1,200 mg per day or more can cause urine to have a strong smell. A small amount of people have been shown to have allergic reactions like hives or itching. With higher doses of 1,200 mg or more, take with a multivitamin containing biotin, as alpha lipoic acid can interfere with its absorption. R-alpha-lipoic acid is more active and better absorbed.

Step 4: Swap Out Toxic for Clean

Environmental toxins are bad for your body and the planet. Unfortunately our food, water, air, homes, and body care products are often the source of hidden toxins that we are interacting with daily. We talked about clean eating and drinking in the last section, now let's talk about how we can minimize daily environmental toxin exposure to optimize health instead of swimming upstream.

Home

Living in a toxin-free environment starts at home. Your home is your environment, where you can control most of what you are exposed to daily. Start with one thing and switch out toxic for clean. Here are some strategies:

- Decorate your home with house plants. Plants like spider plants, aloe vera, weeping fig, Chinese evergreen, bamboo, gerber daisies, English ivies, and chrysanthemums can all help to detoxify your air.
- Switch out your chemical cleaners with natural nontoxic or "green" household cleaners, including soaps and dishwashing detergents. Vinegar, baking soda, and hydrogen peroxide can take care of most of what you need done.

- Over time, replace synthetic carpets, rugs, window treatments, furniture cloth, or bedding (as they can gradually release synthetic materials into the air you breathe) with natural, untreated fibers like wool, bamboo, organic cotton, and hemp. Avoid flame retardants.
- Paint with a low- or no-VOC for indoor surfaces, and say no to air fresheners.
- Clean heating systems.
- Don't spray pesticides around or in your home.

Kitchen

- Change the cookware. Better choices are pots and pans made of glass, ceramic, noncoated stainless steel, or cast iron. If using ceramic pots, look for lead free, unglazed/unvarnished.
- Ditch the plastic and limit cans. Eliminate all plastics (especially if they contain the numbers 3, 6, and 7) in the kitchen replace with glass or ceramic, replacing with wooden utensils, porcelain spoons, wooden cutting boards, glass teapot, steel or glass water bottle. Store everything in glass or ceramic containers. Cling wrap usually contains PVC, so using unbleached parchment paper is important. Canned items mostly contain BPA, so make sure to look for the label that notes specifically BPA free.
- Minimize the use of the microwave, and never put plastic in the microwave

Bathroom

- Natural soaps, like castile soap, and essential oils like tea tree oil have a mild antibacterial quality.
- Say no to hand sanitizers.
- Change vinyl shower curtains that release PVCs to PVC free materials like organic cotton or hemp curtain liners.

Laundry

- Change laundry detergent to a nontoxic and green cleaner, and avoid fabric softeners. One cup of baking soda in a load acts like a natural fabric softener. Instead of bleach, use a cup of white vinegar.
- Look for 100 percent organic cotton sheets.
- Between loads, keep washer door open to prevent mold formation.
- Dry cleaning exposes you to so many toxins, so look for clean, organic, and eco dry cleaners.

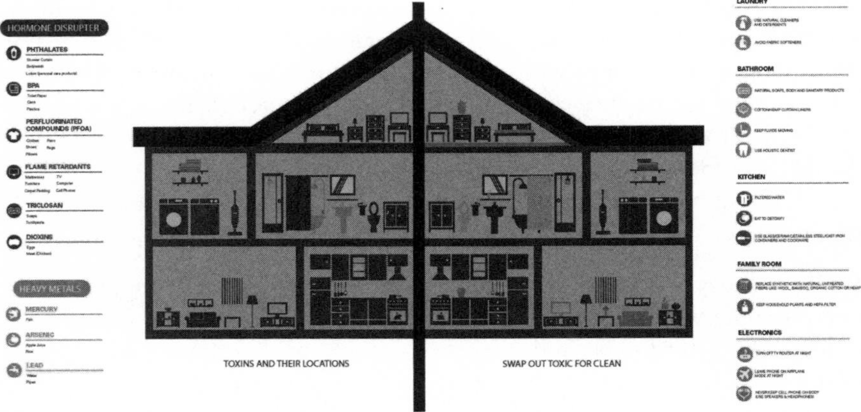

Figure 2.7. The Healing Home

Personal Care Products and Cosmetics

The average woman applies 515 synthetic chemicals in a single day.[16] What you put on your skin is as important as what you eat, as the skin is an excellent delivery system for chemicals.

Choose organic, gluten free nonallergenic skin-care, cosmetics, and feminine hygiene products and cosmetics with no preservatives. Look for a natural brand of deodorant that doesn't contain aluminum, but a light dusting of baking soda can also work.

Water

It is best to consume and expose yourself to purified water. A reverse osmosis unit, preferably with a triple filtration process, is important to reduce the amount of toxins/drugs in your tap water. But before you install a filter, it is easy to purchase filtered water in glass bottles. Consider buying a whole house purification system and a fluoride filtration system. The water filter should remove heavy metals, bacteria/viruses/parasites, nitrates, VOCs, sediment, medications, and copper. Trace minerals are necessary and provide flavor to the water, so these can be added back to the water if needed.

Oral Health

Most procedures done by regular dentists can pose a threat for toxin exposure, so be sure to see a holistic or biological dentist who will look to make sure the biocompatible materials are safe and right for you. Say no to amalgam fillings, replace all metal fillings with white resin (though it is plastic, but better than mercury) or zirconium. Always ask if they use a rubber dam and amalgam separator when removing the mercury filling to keep everyone protected. After the procedure, rinse with activated charcoal. Look into what other precautions they use to protect the staff. Always ask your functional practitioner for a referral and/or go to wwwdaomt.org, the website of the International Academy of Oral Medicine and Toxicology to find a reputable practitioner.

Electronics

We live in day where we are constantly surrounded by electronics, but that doesn't come without its hazards from charged electromagnetic fields, computers, TV, cell phones, and microwaves. Limiting exposure can optimize health and healing. Simply turning off the TV router at night, never carrying a cell phone on your body, switching it to airplane mode anytime you can (especially at night) and using the speaker or headsets at all times are great places to start.

Mold

If after a couple months you still do not feel adequate, despite doing all the above, or perhaps you develop an autoimmunity, mold might be causing inflammation. Mold is most common in damp and humid areas like the bathroom and basement, especially in older homes and in homes with basements, known leaks, crawl spaces, flat roofs, and those built on a hillside. Some molds are easy to detect, like black mold, but others are not so easy to find. Mold can also be found under floorboards, anywhere there's a crack in the wall or window frame, making it even harder to detect. Mold can also be ingested, like on pistachios, cashews, peanuts, aged cheese, vinegars, pickled foods, dried fruit, and mushrooms. Symptoms may be depression and other mood disorders, ADHD, skin rashes, headaches, autoimmunity, sleep issues, fibromyalgia, or fatigue.

Testing is tricky, as the typical mold test only focuses on the air quality and the level of mold spores. Sometimes it is best to find a mold-free place to stay for a while and see if you feel better. If you feel better away from home, and if you feel worse when you return home, you could be reacting to mycotoxins. If this is the case, all the approaches in this book will be helpful. But also carefully clean out your home with tea tree oil, distilled white vinegar, and grapefruit extract including air ducts and purifying the air. Hire a certified mold remediator. Take 300 mg of glutathione up to three times per day and glucomannan 1.5–3 g twice a day to help bind toxins and get you back on the road to recovery. Be cautious with supplements grown on aspergillus, medicinal mushrooms, sacchromycessaccharomyces, and kombucha. Avoid peanuts, raisins, dried fruit, nuts, coffee, and alcohol and focus on a low mold diet.

Detoxify Your Whole Self

Just like the rest of the foundations of good health, even detoxifying isn't a separate entity, but a combination of the whole. Optimizing digestive health, eating anti-inflammatory nutritious food, reducing stress with relaxation, and improving sleep, our social lives, and our soul by practicing forgiveness and meditation are all key in healing.

I'm Too Toxic

If you feel you have a high toxic load, it can be very difficult to do a detox program on your own, so find a professional. A professional can test for genetic mutations or other errors in liver detoxification that can also slow the recovery, like single nucleotide polymorphisms (SNPs) (MTHFR [no I didn't just swear], GSTMI, and COMT SNP gene mutations). If any level is positive, then taking large doses of a premethylated B vitamin (B6, B12, and folinic acid) and glutathione will help optimize function and detox, along with everything else above. B12 also is needed for proper functioning of the brain and nervous system. Chelation, by your practitioner with dimercaptosuccinic acid (DMSA), may need to be done, especially if you have constant yeast infections, spent time in China, have amalgam fillings, eat tuna more than once a week, work with toxins regularly, or have SNPs. Make sure you have fully healed your gut before chelation.

Again, knowledge is power. The knowledge about what is lurking in your environment allows you to take control and get back in the driver's seat of your and your family's health. Don't spend your time worrying about what you can't control. Just by optimizing gut health, eating to heal, and limiting these toxins, you allow your body to be well prepared when toxins do enter. So bring 'em on and keep them out!!! You can do this!

DIGESTIVE HEALTH AND DETOXIFICATION Rx AT A GLANCE

The Gut Rx

- Focus every meal on veggies, clean protein, and healthy fat.
- Follow the elimination diet for about four weeks, or until your symptoms improve or resolve: Remove grains, dairy, sugar, processed foods, and starchy veggies; and if needed remove legumes, soy, nuts, eggs, alcohol, nightshades, caffeine.
- Add bone broth (at least one cup per day).

- Concentrate on probiotics (watch for die-off reaction) and prebiotics.
- Add Epsom salt baths.
- If still no improvement, then add other supplements and consider further testing.

The Nutrition/Supplement Rx

- Balance all meals, focusing on nutrient-dense foods that will heal the gut and keep glucose and insulin stable.
- Fast in between each meal for about three to four hours.
- Don't eat three hours before bed time.
- Intermittent fasting as appropriate.
- Add if needed: probiotics, vitamin D/cod liver oil, magnesium, omega 3 fatty acids, vitamin K2.

The Detox Rx

- Confirm that you're toxic.
- Identify toxins.
- Keep the fluids moving!
- Eat your vegetables and fruit to keep your body alkaline.
- Clean up your environment—swap out toxic for clean.
- Optimize with supplements, if needed
- Detoxify body and mind. Laugh, play, and experience joy.

• 3 •

The Four Big S's

Stress, Sleep, Social Health, and Spirituality

CALMING THE STRESS MONSTER

Congrats! You made it this far, and I probably completely stressed you out. That was the plan (aren't I terrible) because now I can teach you how to manage it—the next step in the foundations of good health. So exciting! Stress causes more than 80 percent of complaints that patients present to their doctors, as it can exacerbate almost any chronic illness. Managing stress is essential in any healing and disease-prevention program, as your thoughts, feelings, and emotions have an effect on physical health, and physical health affects spiritual, emotional, and overall psychological well-being (who would have guessed that everything was connected?). Having a regular practice of mind-body techniques—such as breathing techniques, guided relaxation, and guided imagery—can have a powerful positive effect on health. Such a routine helps to maintain a balanced inner world, developing a more measured response to stressful situations and helps to keep damaging hormones at bay. Optimal stress management to teach our bodies to be a little calmer plays a large role in preventing and/or reversing chronic illnesses.

The Monster under Your Bed

We have all been there. That feeling when your heart races, blood pressure rises, muscles tighten, and you start to breathe faster—the stress response. When your body feels threatened, the hypothalamic-pituitary-adrenal system releases hormones, like cortisol, trying to protect you and prevent injury, also known as the "fight-or-flight" mechanism. Once the threat is over, dopamine is released, giving you a sense of accomplishment. This response can be lifesaving in emergency situations, where you need to act immediately, but it starts to wear your body down with the constant bombardment of stress in our everyday life.

Cortisol continues to be secreted until the stressor resolves, your adrenal glands tire out (a state normally referred to as adrenal fatigue), or you learn to manage stress effectively. Short-term stress can lead to fatigue, weight gain, constant illnesses, hair loss, and skin, mood, digestive, hormonal, and sleep issues. With chronic stress, our body feels like it is constantly under attack, with limited downtime between stressors, and this disrupts the healthy state of equilibrium, leading to suppression of the immune system, inflammation, and chronic illnesses.[1]

Chronic Stress Does a Body No Good

Chronic stress is a serious issue and can affect every organ, not just the mind. Studies have shown that stress can double the chance of becoming obese,[2] can cause diabetes,[3] can lead to a five-fold increased risk of dying from heart-related problems,[4] a 65 percent increased risk of developing dementia,[5] an increased risk of breast cancer,[6] and a 70 percent increased risk of disabilities in later life.[7] The *Journal of the American Medical Association* found that too much stress can be as bad for your heart as smoking and high cholesterol.[8]

Stress and Your Hormones

Severe and acute stress leads to high cortisol levels; raises your blood sugar levels, triggering leptin and insulin resistance;[9] promotes weight gain[10] around the middle; and may ultimately cause full-blown diabetes and further inflammation.[11] Stress can also create imbalances in reproductive hormones, leading to increased polycystic ovarian syndrome, which prevents ovulation and causes infertility.

Stress and Your Gut

The vagus nerve is a thick bundle of nerves that runs all along your spinal column connecting your brain to your digestive system.[12] This is known as the gut-brain-microbiota axis.[13] The gut, known as the second brain, also contains its own receptors that react to the gut bacteria and its metabolites. It also produces neurotransmitters (brain chemicals that communicate information between the brain and the body), specifically about 90 percent of the body's serotonin and 50 percent of the body's dopamine (your "feel good" chemical). Stress can also affect good bacteria negatively, lowering our level of probiotics,[14] even in acute stress—promoting overgrowth of the bad bacteria in the small bowel. These pathogenic bacteria interfere with the production of these vital neurotransmitters. So the more good bacteria you have, the more neurotransmitters and the less pronounced your response to stress is, as you then are producing an optimal level of neurotransmitters and are experiencing less depression, anxiety, and other mood disorders.

Not only does high cortisol affect the bacteria, but it can also lower the release of hydrochloric acid and affect the activity of digestive enzymes, lower the absorption of nutrients,[15] and increase food cravings to allow the bad bacteria to thrive further. Studies have shown that adding back in good bacteria like B. longum[16] and L. rhamnosis,[17] as discussed earlier, along with the use of prebiotics, can relieve stress, lowering cortisol.[18]

Stress and the Immune System

Stress suppresses secretory IgA, an immune molecule,[19] releasing substances like adrenaline and norepinephrine into the gut and making the lining of the digestive system more permeable (i.e., think leaky gut) and inflammatory.[20] Even short bouts of stress can trigger or worsen leaky gut/intestinal permeability[21] and make you susceptible to the reactivation of infections (specifically Epstein Barr virus) that may lead to autoimmunity.

Calm the Stress Monster

A daily practice of relaxation techniques can help decrease anxiety, lower blood pressure and heart rate, keep damaging hormones at bay, change gene expression, improve blood circulation and digestion, and enhance the overall immune system, having a powerful positive effect on you and your health.

Now comes the fun part! Managing stress is easy. So how can you make this happen? First identify what your stressors are and then find a strategy that works for you. It isn't impossible! It's so easy and cost-effective (so exciting!). Let's get you relaxing! Yay!

Look Deep Within, Then Go Deeper

In order to manage stress, it's important to first become aware of it by assessing what your stressors may be. They can be external, like personal life challenges, or internal, like emotional issues, unrealistic expectations, low self-esteem, fears, guilt, and mood issues. Make a list of any past, current, and future stresses that may be external or internal. Are you taking care of yourself (imbalanced diet, lack of sleep, too many medications, and deficiency of nutrients)? How are you currently managing your stress?

Remember to think way back to your childhood, as sometimes a chronic stress response can be hardwired in us from birth or early life. Any childhood stress or trauma that creates subtle shifts of your microbiome early in life can alter your healthy HPA axis, cue your body to produce more cortisol and fewer good bugs, leading to increased stress response later in life and inflammation. By assessing your stress, you can see where your deficiencies are and then target them accordingly.

Relax, Renew, and Revive

Helping your nervous system to reestablish equilibrium is key in lowering inflammation. Relaxation techniques can bring your nervous system back to a balanced, silenced state from the inside out, creating a deep calmness and allowing you to be fully present in life despite facing its challenges and stresses, for now and the future. These relaxation activities can trigger the vagus nerve and help support the function of the peripheral nervous system[22] helping you be more physically, emotionally, and spiritually resilient. Research has shown that toning down the fight-or-flight response can help decrease the inflammatory response in autoimmune conditions like rheumatoid arthritis.[23]

Practice Makes Perfect

The relaxation response is a mentally active process (so sitting in front of the TV or computer doesn't count) that leaves the body relaxed, calm, focused, and content. Most relaxation techniques can be incorporated into your existing daily schedule, like at lunchtime, during commutes, or at bedtime, as you only need about ten to thirty minutes a day. As you learn relaxation techniques, you'll become more aware of muscle tension and other physical sensations of stress. Once you know what the stress response feels like and you have mastered the skill, you can use this when you start to feel stressed, anxious, or overwhelmed and can prevent the stress from getting out of control.

Find a Method That Works for You

There are so many relaxation techniques that can help you bring your nervous system and emotions back into balance by producing the relaxation response. The ability to relax improves with practice and is a skill. If one strategy doesn't work for you, then try another. Everyone is different! Stick to one that works for you!

Stress Relief Strategies

Managing stress is all about taking care of the most important person in the world. Below are other strategies that can be used to lower the stress response.

The Power of Your Breath

You take it everywhere you go, every second for as long as you bless the world with your presence. Focusing on your breath is the easiest, fastest, and most powerful way to immediately destress and is a great weight loss aid. Practicing a simple technique like belly breathing for five minutes two or three times a day will help establish your equilibrium.

Here's what you should do: Lie on a flat surface with either your legs straight or your knees bent; or sit up in a comfortable position. Place one hand on your upper chest and the other on your abdomen—this will enable you to feel whether you're using your diaphragm instead of your chest muscles to breathe; your belly should rise more than your chest.

Close your eyes and breathe in slowly through your nose counting to 4, letting your stomach expand against your hand. Hold your breath for a count of 7. Exhale though your mouth slowly and steadily to the count of 8. Let your stomach fall back inward as you exhale all the air from your lungs. Again, the hand on your upper chest should remain as still as possible. Pause for a count of 1 and then repeat the cycle for ten breaths. Make your breaths as deep and slow as possible.

Visualization or Guided Imagery

Visualization is a relaxation technique where you take a visual journey to a peaceful and calming place in your mind to relieve stress. Sit in a quiet spot, loosen any tight clothes, close your eyes, and imagine your restful place, a place where you are completely content and at peace. Picturing it vividly with all your senses (smell, sound, touch, sight) and enjoying the feeling of deep relaxation, focus on your breath. When ready, gently open your eyes. Creating this "mental escape" enhances coping skills by releasing all tension and anxiety, creating harmony between the body and mind.

Progressive Muscle Relaxation

In this relaxation technique, you focus on slowly tensing and then relaxing each muscle group. This helps you become aware of your body and helps you counteract the first signs of muscle tension that accompanies stress. When your body relaxes, so will the mind. I recommend that my patients combine deep breathing with progressive muscle relaxation for an additional level of stress relief.

There are two steps:

1. Deliberately tensing muscle groups
2. Releasing the tension in muscle groups

Simply loosen your clothing, take off your shoes, and get comfortable. Take a few minutes to relax, breathing in and out in slow, deep breaths. When you're relaxed and ready to start, shift your attention to your right foot. Take a moment to focus on the way it feels. Slowly tense the muscles in your right foot, inhaling, squeezing as tightly as you can. Hold for a count of 10. Relax your right foot. Focus on the tension flowing away and the way your foot feels as it becomes limp and loose. Stay in this relaxed state for a moment, breathing deeply and slowly. When you're ready, shift your attention to your left foot. Follow the same sequence of muscle tension and release. Move slowly up through your body, contracting and relaxing the muscle groups as you go. It may take some practice at first, but try not to tense any muscles other than those intended. The most popular sequence runs right foot, then left foot, right and left calves, right and left thighs, hips and buttocks, stomach, chest, and back, right, and left arm and hand, neck and shoulder, then finally your face, forehead, and lips. If you are left-handed you may want to start with your left side first.

Other Lifestyle Techniques

As I stated earlier, following the foundations of good health in its entirety will help to lower stress, as it will help to balance yourself and your emotions and allow you to effectively deal with what is at hand. So let's recap here:

1. **Heal the gut.** Taking probiotics will help to add good bugs back in to help balance your peripheral nervous system.
2. **Eat an anti-inflammatory diet and stay hydrated.** Adopt an anti-inflammatory diet and focus on balancing your foods with veggies, protein (especially those that are high in B12 like grass-fed beef, fermented foods, and wild-caught salmon), healthy fats, and plenty of water. Try to avoid caffeine and alcohol because these interfere with the sleep cycle, slowing the recovery of your adrenals. Try instead chamomile, nettle leaf, dandelion, and holy basil tea; these will help to ease stress. If you need to drink caffeine, one serving before noon is less problematic. Some may also need additional supplementation to cope (see later in this chapter).
3. **Live in a clean environment.** By lowering the toxic burden inside and outside our bodies, we can lower the stress from within. For added relaxation, add lavender oil to your detox baths. Spending time in nature will also help you detox your breath and increase your sense of peace, allowing you to even digitally detox or to spend time away from computers and other electronic devices.

4. **Cultivate positive relationships and have fun**. Spend time with those who will listen, support, and encourage and don't give you more stress. Simply smiling and laughing will lower cortisol and boost brain chemicals like endorphins, which will help your mood. Massage is also a therapeutic touch that is healing and is a great way to relieve inflammation and stress. Just doing what you love and scheduling fun rest days during the week will allow your liver, body, mind, and soul to detox and distress.
5. **Optimize sleep**. Sleep is important in healing and rejuvenating, improving stress levels.
6. **Connect with your soul—find your higher purpose.** Meditation and gratitude will help you to develop a positive attitude and reframe your stress and tackle it better.
7. **Time manage and organize**. You are the master of your own time. Plan, prioritize, create daily reminders for tasks, and delegate tasks to others. Learn what causes you stress and what is important to you. Learn to say no, and remove guilt from the situation. Declutter your life, and that includes your physical environment and your electronic environment, like your emails and messages. Never "should" on yourself. These simple techniques will empower you to take back control of your health and time.
8. **Exercise.** One of the biggest stress busters is exercise. Let's discuss this in a little more detail.

Exercise Can Heal

Regular exercise is crucial for the foundations of good health, as it lowers markers of systemic inflammation.[24] Not only is exercise an amazing stress reliever, but it also has great benefits in reducing cravings, regulating appetite, improving insulin sensitivity, improving self-confidence and digestive function by increasing microbial diversity, improving detoxification, boosting happy chemicals in the brain, sharpening memory, reducing the risk of fractures and helping build healthy bones, and keeping chronic diseases at bay and overall lowering inflammation.[25]

Choosing the Right Kind of Exercise

Moderate exercise is safe for most, but if you have a chronic illness, speak with your doctor before starting a new exercise program. When designing your personal fitness program, you should first consider your fitness goals.

Tips on Exercising

- Take time to stretch every morning, before and after exercising. Stretching can improve range of motion, boost circulation, and keep muscles loose and flexible. Remember to breathe while stretching.
- Find an exercise you will enjoy, and exercise for at least thirty minutes every day.
- Key is not the amount but the intensity of exercise.
- Have a mix of aerobic, strength training, core support, and fascia work.
- Don't overdo it—listen to your body.

Aerobic Exercise

Aerobic exercise like spinning, interval training, dancing, bicycling, running/jogging, walking, or swimming are all great stress relievers. For all my patients, I have them start off with walking. One step in the right direction is better than no steps in the right direction. Wearing a pedometer will help motivate you to try to aim for getting about ten thousand steps per day. Extra bonus points if you can do it outside, while taking deep cleansing breaths.

Shorter workouts like high-intensity interval training or burst training with short speed bursts are also another option. Studies show that you can boost metabolism and burn more calories all day, even after you complete the exercise (no, that doesn't mean you can eat more). It is characterized by a short period of exertion followed by a rest period then back to exertion (getting your heart rate up to 70–80 percent of its maximum). An example of interval training includes doing a five-minute warm up, with a ten-minute interval to bring your heart up for thirty seconds, then down to target heart rate for ninety seconds, and finishing with a five-minute cool down.

Strength Training

Strength training helps to increase lean muscle mass, makes your bones stronger, boosts metabolism, and burns more fat at rest. Yoga, tai chi, lifting weights/tubing are all great options and should be done two to three times a week. Yoga reduces anxiety and stress and improves flexibility, strength, balance, core support, and stamina as it involves a series of moving and stationary poses, combined with deep breathing, strengthening the relaxation response in your daily life. Both yoga and tai chi help to reduce stress by calming the mind and conditioning the body, by focusing on the breath and paying attention to the present moment. Incorporate fascia work in your workouts, as it can help to relax the bands that connect your tissues and keep you flexible.

Can't Exercise Make Inflammation *Worse*?

Exercise definitely reduces inflammation, but in some instances it can increase it, mostly when an exercise has the potential to become chronic—it induces a state of chronic inflammation.[26] Strenuous exercise itself causes increased intestinal permeability. Exercise as long as you feel good and energized afterward. If you feel exhausted or worse after exercise or your symptoms worsen—you're doing too much.

Other Relaxation Techniques

- Hypnosis
- Biofeedback
- Art therapy
- Neurofeedback
- Tapping/Emotional Freedom Techniques
- Float tank
- Binaural beats
- HeartMath®
- Relaxation apps

Stress-Reducing Supplements and Herbs

In times of chronic stress, your body requires extra nutrients to support the adrenals, as stress in and of itself can deplete vital nutrients like magnesium, the B vitamins (can help to reduce homocysteine, a toxic amino acid), omega 3s, and vitamin C. Certain plant compounds known as adaptogens can help balance and modulate the stress response, helping to lower some of the negative effects of chronic stress. Ashwagandha lowers cortisol and balances hormones and can be taken in supplement form 500 mg once or twice daily. Other adaptogenic herbs are Asian ginseng root extract (200 mg twice daily), Rhodiola root extract (50 mg twice daily), Cordyceps (containing both cordycepic acid and adenosine, 400 mg twice daily), and holy basil. Homeopathy and acupuncture are also great options.[27]

When You Might Need Extra Support

If, despite all your efforts, you still don't feel good, then it's time to seek professional help. This is true especially if you start to notice warning signs like inability to sleep, depression, using drugs or alcohol to cope with stress, negative and self-destructive thoughts or fears that are beyond your control, or thoughts of suicide.

Stress is inevitable, but it doesn't have to take control of your health. Bad relationships, financial hardships, work stress—these can all be appropriately managed to limit stress. Do what works for you. The important thing is to find activities that you enjoy and that give you a boost. Don't let stress take over your life and your health. Any little bit is better than nothing! You can do it. See? Aren't you already a little relaxed?

GETTING A QUALITY SNOOZE

With all the relaxing that happened in the last section, WAKE UP, let's take it one step further. One of the most critical aspects to keep our body regulated is not what we do during the day, but what happens at night (get your mind out of the gutter, even though that is also really important). I'm talking about how we sleep. Even though most of us try to scrape by with as little as we can, getting enough sleep normalizes cortisol levels, improves memory, and helps to control weight and overall inflammation.[1] Our body doesn't consume much energy while we sleep, so it leaves more energy available over eight or nine hours per night for the body to remove toxins, make hormones, activate cellular repair, boost the secretion of growth hormone, mend injury, and fight infections. So we all need sleep!

If You Don't Snooze, You Lose

As a mother of four, I am not very familiar with the word *sleep*, but I keep this on my top priority list, and here's why: When we fail to get enough sleep, our bodies are unable to put out the effort needed to do all the important tasks like removing toxins, leading to hormonal imbalances and inflammation. In the short term, sleep deprivation can cause mild symptoms of tiredness, irritability, a decrease in the quality of your life, attention deficit, depression, anger, and anxiety. One is also susceptible to decreased performance and alertness, impaired cognition and memory, increased appetite because of stimulated ghrelin (a hormone that tells the brain you are hungry), suppression of the hormone leptin (which tells the brain you are full), and holding on to fat. Just by decreasing your sleep for one night by only one and a half hours could reduce your daytime alertness by as much as 32 percent!

Sleep helps to regulate most of hormone production. Fifteen percent of our DNA is controlled by our circadian rhythm, including our body's repair mechanism. Lack of good circadian rhythms is also associated with numerous serious medical illnesses, including mental and emotional disturbances (like being twice as likely to feel depressed or anxious[2] and encounter other mood issues), quadrupling your risk of cancer, doubling your chance of obesity[3] and being linked with diabetes,[4] insulin resistance, increase in an inflammatory marker called hsCRP (which is a strong predictor of heart disease[5]) and an increase in your risk of heart disease and stroke.[6] Not getting good sleep is also related to something known as frontal lobe syndrome, which involves confusion, impulsivity, poor judgment, an inability to perform tasks, and catatonia.

Optimizing Your Snooze

Assess

In order to target sleep issues, one first needs to assess what the possible causes behind the sleep issues can be. Stress and disease can lead to inflammation, causing sleep issues that further worsen the problem. So targeting the root cause is the key to better sleep.

- For short-term insomnia, any stress like an upcoming exam, jet lag, change in work schedule, emotional stress, or a sleep hygiene problem can lead to insomnia.
- Chronic diseases, like sleep apnea, restless legs, chronic pain, and narcolepsy can hinder sleep.
- Medications can also lead to insomnia: antidepressants, cold and flu medications that contain alcohol, pain relievers that contain caffeine (Midol, Excedrin), diuretics, corticosteroids, thyroid hormone, high blood pressure medications (beta blockers, calcium channel blockers), anticonvulsants, bronchodilators, decongestants, and stimulants.

Sleep Hygiene

No, I'm not talking about how clean your sleep is. Sleep hygiene[7] includes practices that when implemented promote better quality of sleep. Let's talk about this in detail. Your sleep is a treat, not a punishment. This is your special time that you deserve after putting in a hard day's work and will allow you to be more efficient during your day (a win-win situation!).

Create a Restful Sanctuary

In order to get amazing, restful, deep sleep, you need to prepare for success by creating an environment that is conducive to the best sleep of your life. Set the night room temperature to about 68 degrees Fahrenheit, complete with hanging blackout curtains on the windows, clearing the clutter, and limiting noise or using a white-noise fan to block background noise. Changing your mattress pad can regulate your body temperature. Socks can help to keep your extremities warm. Adding a household plant to your room can improve the air quality and inhibit electromagnetic fields (EMFs). Keep this room for sleep and sex only, and leave your office out of your bedroom.

Bedtime Routines Are Not Just for Babies

Just like for children, a sleep routine is very important for our adult bodies. Go to bed the same time (or around thirty minutes within the same time) every day and wake up around the same time 365 days a year (yes, even on the weekends); this can deviate by about an hour. If you are short on sleep one day, get back on schedule immediately, instead of sleeping in or taking a long nap. Going to sleep around 9:00 to 11:30 pm helps to promote the best hormonal environment for sleep, fat burning, and regeneration. Start winding down about two hours before bedtime by taking time to relax, using either meditation or other stress relieving strategies. Take a warm bath with Epsom salt and lavender oil. Set aside time to write down your worries. Turn off electronics at least ninety minutes before bedtime, as this will allow your melatonin and cortisol levels to normalize; minimize blue lights from electronics and use amber lights or glasses to filter the blue light. A f.lux program can be used for your computer, which will change the color of the computer's light from blue to orange as the sun sets; the same is true for other electronic screens. Flip switches to turn off your Wi-Fi, put your phone six feet away on airplane mode, and turn off notifications to limit EFMs. Try using earthing sheets, which stimulate a similar reaction as if you were in direct contact with the ground and allows you to receive energy that helps you sleep. Try not to eat for about ninety minutes before sleeping; if you have to eat, it should be high in fat and low in carbohydrates, to limit the insulin spike. Also, if you can't fall asleep after forty-five minutes, get up and try again in one hour—don't just lie there.

Live the Morning Right for a Successful Snooze

What you do during the day can determine how you sleep—starting from the moment you wake up. Lowering overall inflammation will help to improve your sleep. Daytime sleep disrupters are caffeine, sugar, stress, lack of movement, and too much artificial light or evening exposure to fluorescent light. Foods to help you sleep include walnuts, avocados, and green leafy vegetables. Exercise regularly in the morning or afternoon. Periods of time with direct contact with the ground can help create an internal balance, optimizing sleep.

Stay well hydrated and replace caffeine with relaxing teas like chamomile and valerian (add in a teaspoon of gelatin; yum!). If you need caffeine, limit it to the morning hours only. If you must nap, do so for twenty to thirty minutes before 4:00 pm. Increasing the bright light exposure for at least thirty minutes from 6:00 am to 8:30 am provides natural light cues for your circadian rhythms and keeps you alert. Light boxes or visors and other gadgets can be used to stimulate sunlight even when you're stuck behind the desk. After the sun sets, replace bright white lights with amber bulbs or wear amber glasses; this allows your body to shift into sleep mode. For further sleep help, refer to the insomnia section in the psychology chapter.

Coping with Shift Work

Working irregular or night shifts can disrupt your sleep schedule. Adjust your sleep–wake cycle by exposing yourself to bright light while you're awake and wearing dark glasses on your journey home. Keep your schedule as regular as you can, by bunching night shifts together and avoiding frequently rotating shifts. Get extra sleep before your shift, eat well on the job, and destress when you get home; also, taking adaptogens (like eleuthero) if needed can improve shift work insomnia.

Travel and Jet Lag

If you travel a lot, jet lag can upset your sleep pattern, so leave home well rested. When you arrive at your destination, stay awake until the local bedtime. Melatonin can be helpful.

I know I woke you up and then put you back to sleep by talking about sleep. Listen to your body; if you need a nap before you keep reading, do it! Sleep allows your body to take care of you, so let it! I think I'm ready for a nap.

BUILDING SOCIAL SUPPORT

Everyone loves company, but did you know good company is also great for your health? The feeling of being loved releases a flood of potent hormones into the bloodstream, which not only makes us feel better emotionally, it also significantly strengthens our immune system. In other words, to give and receive love inspires healing—physically, emotionally, and spiritually. Humans are social creatures by nature and need each other to survive, starting when we are very young and learning to depend on each other for survival.

Positive Support and Love Empowers

I'll be your friend for life. I'm here for you unconditionally, and I am your shoulder to cry on. Our relationship, hopefully a positive one, or any other positive relationships from friends, family, or pets, improves your immune system and can be healing. Friends prevent loneliness and give you a chance to offer needed companionship. Positive company can increase your sense of belonging and purpose, boost your happiness and reduce your stress, improve your self-confidence and self-worth, and help you cope with any traumas.

Based on the results of brain MRIs and blood and saliva tests, we know that feeling loved and supported releases hormones into our bloodstream; such hormones include serotonin, relaxin, endorphins, and oxytocin,[1] which keep us happy and healthy. These hormones lower cortisol,[2] improve blood circulation, lower blood pressure and heart rate, improve digestion, clear out toxins, increase natural killer cells and a number of white blood cells, red blood cells, IgA[3] and helper T cells, activity that helps the immune system clear out infections and renew energy to repair cells and fight cancer.

This helps lower inflammation overall, improving sleep, relieving feelings of restlessness, and decreasing chronic pain as muscle tension and pain perception lower. Studies have shown that negative relationships and loneliness can lead to an earlier death, increased cortisol levels, and a depletion of our immune system. Studies have shown that having pets releases the same hormones, and pet owners live longer than people who don't have pets.

Mingle for Optimal Health

So if finding a great social environment is another important tool to improving health, where are we supposed to find positive support?

Join Groups

Joining support groups or taking a class at a local gym or community venue like a library will help you locate those people with similar interests. Then invite acquaintances with a similar goal for a meal or green shake. Finding groups in your faith communities or volunteering at the hospital, place of worship, community center, museum, or other charitable organizations are also great ways to connect, meet new people, and form strong connections with those who have similar goals and mutual interests.

Joining a chat group or online community might help you make or maintain connections and relieve loneliness. Remember to exercise caution when sharing personal information or arranging an activity with someone you've only met online.

Reach Out

Random acts of kindness and generosity include smiling, holding the door open for someone, and reaching out to the ones you love. Chat with neighbors who are out as you take your child or pet for a walk, or pick up the phone to call those you love and tell them you were thinking of them. Call someone else the next day, and continue to repeat the process. Also don't be afraid to ask for help.

Surround Yourself with Positive Relationships

You will meet so many people in your lifetime. Some will try to pull you down, and others will lift you up. Stick with ones that fill your life with positivity and love.

When choosing a potential mate: in order to know whether the person is worth sticking around for, I advise all my patients to hold onto any intimacy, not to cloud the water. If the other person really wants to be with you and truly loves you for your heart, they will respect your decision and wait. This will test to make sure they have the self-control and loyalty you desire in a spouse. You are a gem, and deserve someone who will kiss the ground you walk on, someone who really loves you for you, all of you, not just your privates.

Taking Care of Someone with Chronic Conditions

If you are taking care of someone with chronic conditions, it can be taxing on your relationship and your body. So remember to take time to take care of you. You are an amazing person to take care of someone in need. Patience and love are key on the job. Tenderness and empathy will never fail us. To optimize that relationship, it is important to listen actively and be nonjudgmental, answer questions as they come up, work to clear up misunderstandings, validate and respect their feelings, help them to relax, and always allow for setbacks and regressions. But to get the support you need, it is important to join a support group, so you can continue being the gem that you are—inside and out!

Nurturing Your Relationships

In order to nurture your relationships, first be your own best friend and build that positive self-image and self-esteem—because you are worth it! Take your time to look for quality friendships, focusing on the positive aspects of every relationship. Open yourself up by listening and sharing, but respect boundaries and privacy, accepting others for who they are.

Remember, it is never too late to either build a new friendship or reconnect with old friends, as maintaining a healthy friendship or relationship is always equal give and take. Always let them know they are appreciated. Investing time in finding amazing quality friends is important in healing chronic inflammation and disease. So "make new friends, toss the tarnished but keep the old; one is silver and the other gold," because positive relationships are healing.

CULTIVATING SPIRITUALITY

We are going to talk about a topic that is taboo in most medical offices but so critical in healing and preventing chronic disease—the soul. Numerous studies have indicated a positive relationship between spirituality and health. When a person practices daily meditation and positivity, it not only intensifies calmness but also cultivates optimal physical health. When the spiritual energy begins to flow, blood circulation improves,[1] blood pressure goes down,[2] cortisol and stress levels go down, digestion improves,[3] the body detoxes, unhealthy genes are switched off,[4] and the overall immune system is enhanced.[5] Meditation and positivity can transform your body for the better in a very powerful way, especially if you practice them daily.

Religion isn't the same as spirituality. Religion involves a coded set of beliefs, but spirituality is about your relationship with your soul. A spiritual practice is one that encourages you to feel—in your body and your emotions—a deep sensation of calm and peace. It enhances the sense of connectedness and helps you gain perspective and clarify goals.

Connecting Deep Within Heals

Gratitude is an emotion expressing appreciation for what one has—a universal concept in nearly all of the world's spiritual traditions. In the feelings of gratitude the spiritual is experienced. Giving thanks to a supernatural power, benefactors, or others is one of the most effective way to get in touch with your soul. Being thankful helps create a subconscious world of positivity that governs 90 percent of our thoughts and actions. The positive energy boosts optimism, which in turn helps prevent disease and improves our immune system, well-being, and sense of happiness.[6] Gratitude is not just some feel-good action; practicing it daily, not just around Thanksgiving, is proven to have actual physiological consequences. It helps lower inflammatory markers, influences epigenetics, and even helps the heart, adding years to life. "Heart-felt" emotions—like gratitude, love, and caring—produce sine wave or coherent waves radiating to every cell of the body, all determined through technology that measures changes in heart-rhythm variation and measurements of coherence. Research shows that with "depleted" emotions—like frustration, anger, anxiety, and insecurity—the heart-rhythm pattern becomes more erratic and the brain recognizes this as stress. This in turn creates a desynchronized state, raising the risk of developing heart disease and increased blood pressure, weakening the immune system, impairing cognitive function, and blocking our ability to think clearly.

According to a study published by the American Psychological Association in 2015,[7] a grateful heart is also a happier and healthier heart, literally. They found that higher gratitude scores were proportional to a better mood, higher-quality sleep, more self-efficacy, and less inflammation and improved heart health.

Gratitude makes us optimistic. Being optimistic improves our health and has been proven to improve our immune system and lower inflammation. When we are stressed, gratitude helps us bounce back faster and focus on what is going well in our lives. Cancer patients who were optimistic predicted less disruption of normal life, distress, and fatigue; those who were pessimistic were likely to experience thickening arteries. Optimism has been found to correlate positively with life satisfaction and self-esteem.

Meditation changes the brain, literally—the whole brain. Studies have proven that meditation can change the entire brain by altering gray matter volume, preserving the aging brain, and increasing neuronal activity in emotional areas, frontal areas, and areas related to emotion regulation, self-control, and positive emotions.[8] The way meditation changes gray matter volume is by reducing activity in the "me" centers of the brain and enhancing connectivity between brain regions.[9] Many studies have explored the relationship between mindful meditation and the reduction of symptoms of depression, anxiety (even social anxiety), and pain.[10,11] Just a couple weeks of meditation can help people increase productivity by increasing their focus and memory.[12]

Meditation has the power of improving overall health. It has the ability to reduce the risk of heart attack and stroke in people at risk; it also increases longevity, decreases atherosclerosis in carotid arteries, and increases sensitivity to circulating insulin. It helps alleviate delayed left ventricular enlargement, headaches, migraines, and involuntary movement disorders, such as Parkinson's disease and Tourette syndrome. In addition, the American Heart Association also endorses transcendental meditation as a complementary treatment for high blood pressure depending on circumstances.

So exciting!!! So much to be thankful for. Now excuse me as I go meditate.

Healing Spiritual Practices

It is so easy to become preoccupied with chasing our dreams or working hard just to get by that we can easily become oblivious of our quality of life, how we treat others, how we feel, the moment of now. Stress, work and family responsibilities, and routines can trap us in a pattern of negative thinking that feeds on itself and creates more stress and unhappiness. This cycle can lead to other ailments, as well, including constant fatigue and even depression. Finding ways to focus on the positive can help reprogram thoughts and lower inflammation. How do we do that? Let's talk about it.

Gratitude

Being optimistic, loving each moment as it comes, and embracing thankfulness not only affect our minds but also influence our genetic composition and heart.

Our Subconscious in Control

Our subconscious governs 90 percent of our thoughts, actions, and drives to survive and thrive, shaping our every behavior. We are constantly bombarded with negativity, so training our subconscious to be more positive is crucial. Actually, the subconscious mind is nothing but the "neural pathways" that have been established in your brain as a result of your past beliefs and conditioning. Your subconscious does no thinking of its own but rather relies on your perception of the world around you, listening to verbal and nonverbal cues. When you consciously turn negativity to positivity, from the inside out, the neural pathway associated with negativity will take time to come down fully, so it is critical to continue gratitude regularly. Your thoughts and subconscious are powerful, as unconscious negative thoughts can undermine your health, while positive thoughts can boost immune system and heal disease.

Building Gratitude

You can take charge of your inner world and focus on what is positive by implementing the following:

- *Train your subconscious.* As soon as you wake up in the morning, take a moment to think about ten things you are grateful for. Starting your morning on a positive note influences the rest of your day. It guarantees that you always get up on the right side of the bed and trains your subconscious to think positively. I also recommend you place sticky notes that say "I am grateful for this" all around the house on the objects you are thankful for, creating a zone of positivity to subliminally train your subconscious. You can place sticky notes on photos of people you love, your shoes, your mirror in the bathroom, lights, and so forth. Be thankful for simple things, things you take for granted in your internal and external world, things that go well, people and events from the past that have helped you be who you are today. Focus on happy memories.

- *Journal.* Journaling and writing about what in your life you are thankful for works similarly to the above exercise. Decorate your journal with things that remind you of your purpose in life and help you feel positive, like pictures and inspirational quotes. Write in your journal daily, about two to five minutes. After writing your gratitude list, you can list negative thoughts and then transform them by finding what is positive in those situations. Use gratitude to improve all negative situations.
- *Express gratitude.* Showing appreciation to those who have helped you in your daily life helps you and motivates others, creating a peaceful environment. You can easily incorporate gratitude in any situation, and, especially when you combine it with relaxation techniques, like deep breathing and walking outside, the effects can be powerful.

Meditation

Many of my patients are skeptical when I first tell them that something as simple as meditation could be their best cure. After all, the word *meditation* quite often conjures up the image of someone in the lotus position, eyes closed and looking peaceful, something that likely requires a great deal of practice, patience, time, and effort, and so people put it off. There are so many types of meditation, like mindfulness, transcendental meditation, yoga meditation, zen, seated meditation, and guided meditation, just to name a few. Let's talk about mindfulness, a meditation you can take wherever you go.

Mindfulness

Mindfulness is how you're feeling right now, in THIS moment, internally and externally. Staying calm and present in the current moment will help to bring your nervous system back into balance and decrease stress. Being present helps you to not worry about the past and future, and it limits stress; it can be applied to almost any activity you are engaging in (eating, exercising, walking, meditation, and/or working). Mindfulness allows us to see our internal and external environment clearly, showing us how best to respond and be fully aware of many different levels of perceptions at once.

To practice mindful meditation, choose a quiet, relaxing, and comfortable environment. Keep your spine straight, sitting up. Choose a point of focus—an internal feeling, external word or phrase, a calming imaginary scene, or an object in your surroundings. Eyes can be either open or closed. Develop an observant, noncritical attitude, becoming aware of your physical sensations. If you do get distracted, gently turn your attention back to your point of focus. Concentrate on your breath and be grateful.

One can easily combine a relaxation technique like progressive muscle relaxation; focus on each of the sensations in each body part, and imagine yourself hovering above yourself, allowing your breath to go beyond your body, allowing you to notice how your body feels (also known as body scan meditation).

Forgiveness

Acts that have offended or hurt you can always remain a part of your life, smoldering your health insidiously; these can increase inflammation, preventing you from completely healing from chronic disease. Forgiveness involves a decision to let go of resentment and thoughts of revenge, lessening the hurt, helping you focus on other, positive parts of your life; it can lead to feelings of understanding, empathy, and compassion for the one who hurt you. Learning to forgive is essential to spiritual health and allows peace to emerge within you.

In order to forgive, try to understand others' actions, bringing compassion and passion into the situation. Journaling can also help you turn the negative into positives, helping to assign a new meaning and a new positive label to the hurt. As crazy as it may sound, be grateful for every person who may have hurt you, as they have made you who you are; this is just a perfectly crafted chapter in your unique journey. Eventually, resolve the negative charge attached to the event, allowing you to forgive yourself and others as you surrender the pain to a higher power.

Daily Prayer

Set aside times in a day to pray quietly for at least five minutes. Concentrate on connecting to a divine energy or create affirmations and visualizations. Surrender all your worries and hurt to a higher power. Combining either a walking or breathing meditation with any prayer increases our mental focus, deepening our prayer.

Spiritual Groups

A group setting, like a prayer circle or group meditation, can hold you accountable and provide you with the support to help grow you spiritually.

Other spiritual practices that help to lower inflammation are therapeutic touch, healing touch, and qigong. Reading inspirational books or stories, practicing artistic self-expression, and finding your purpose can all help you heal chronic disease.

Finding a spiritual practice that works for you is key to healing chronic disease. But no matter what you choose, connecting to the spiritual energy is important. Every day our minds are full of worries, thoughts, and dreams, but at a deeper level, the mind begins to quiet, and it is this deeper level that is the core of the spiritual practice. Don't force yourself, though. You can help slow down your thoughts by focusing on something else, like your breath, a special image, or prayer. Find a quiet place, unplug from electronic devices, and free yourself from obligations. Observe your racing thoughts, and then by distracting yourself, you will allow the thoughts to eventually dissipate.

Be easy with yourself, as it is not always about getting it right; let your mind take you where it needs to go. There are many types of spiritual practices and other ways that will allow you to connect with your soul, refresh the spirit and lower inflammation. Find what works for you and do it. So breathe—give yourself permission to heal and be happy. You deserve it! Be thankful for all that is going on right in your life. I am thankful for you!

REALITY CHECK—STAYING MOTIVATED

Now that we've examined the foundations of good health, let's face reality. When one doesn't feel well, the motivation to implement what we just learned is hard—very hard. Taking it one step at a time—preparing your mind, body, and soul—can help you succeed! You got this!!!

Preparation for Success

1. **Cultivate a healthy mindset.** Most people will pass by this book, but because you picked it up, it means you are considering the idea of living a better, happier life. You deserve a happier and healthier life. You are beautiful (or handsome) inside and out! Imagine what you will be able to accomplish when you feel your very best! The opportunities are endless! Let's do this!!!
2. **Discover your reason.** Why do you want to do this now? To be pain free, to achieve your dreams? What do you want to accomplish when you are freed and ready to fly?

3. **Know who's really in control.** We talked about our microbiome and how bad bugs can influence our behavior and our cravings. Those sneaky, pesky little devils are sabotaging you! So ignore the cravings and start making the decision regarding your own health! You are in control!
4. **Out with the old and in with the new.** Now, bid farewell to all the inflammatory foods that keep sabotaging you, remove and dispose of them from all your hiding spots (yes, even the Oreos you hide in the cereal box), and now let's focus the attention on nutrient-dense healing foods. Stock up on lots of raw veggies, low-glycemic fruits, fresh meats, hardboiled eggs, and nuts for snacks (to tame the inner beast). Bake with coconut, nut, or seed flours, and keep baked goods in the fridge for a quick breakfast or dessert.
5. **Set goals and targets.** Setting achievable goals and targets, with set specifications and dates, will help to optimize your success.
6. **Identify your obstacles.** What is stopping you from doing this right now? After identifying those obstacles, come up with a plan of action that will help you overcome them, taking it one day at a time, one obstacle at a time.
7. **Set a routine.**

   a. *Grocery shop once a week.* Find a time when you will go grocery shopping weekly and stay on the outside of the grocery store (going down the list of veggies, clean protein, and healthy fats, as discussed in the last chapter). Keep your fridge stocked for success with veggies, nut bars/nuts, fruit, and clean protein sources. Avoid your weak spots, like the bakery, and never shop when you're hungry, otherwise your bad bacteria might start shopping for you! Take control! You are stronger than these darned microscopic bugs!
   b. *Plan your meals ahead of time.* I spend one day a week cooking for the week, cooking all my veggies, protein, fats, and other healthy carbohydrates. I stock my fridge for success. On the weekend, plan your food for the upcoming week so that you can go shopping and have everything you need.
   c. *Take advantage of every spare moment.* If you have fifteen free minutes anywhere, take advantage of it by taking a walk around the block; do some deep breathing while commuting or waiting for an appointment. Mindfulness and graditude can be done with any activity, even with exercising. Yay! It can't get better than that!

8. **Build your own positive support system and be prepared.** Inform those around you that you are trying to eat healthy, and let them know you want them to help support you. Bring your own food to events and stick with "the list" when you go to any event. Never go completely hungry, and say no to food pushers. Find friends who will hold you accountable.
9. **Don't overwhelm yourself.** Take one meal at a time, one day at a time. Going down that list will make it less overwhelming—it's that simple.
10. **Have fun!** This is an exciting time, as now you are finally in the driver's seat—nerve wracking and exhilarating all at the same time! Yay! Everything you are doing is empowering you for now and forever! Do what you love and makes you happy. Reward yourself when you accomplish the weekly goals (and no, eating a whole apple pie isn't a reward), choosing a reward that will keep you on the right tract. Get creative and imaginative—this can be so much fun!
11. **Setbacks are actually steps forward.** If you find yourself getting off the wagon, it's okay, just get back on. Your setback is the platform for a stronger comeback. Every setback is an opportunity to grow and to realize you are actually human! You are worth it!

You are amazing! Making yourself a priority (yes, even mothers) can cultivate a healthier and stronger present and future. Imagine the possibilities when you can fly! I can't imagine how much you will be able to accomplish! You are worth it, to you and those around you! Now let's fly!

THE FOUR BIG S's Rx

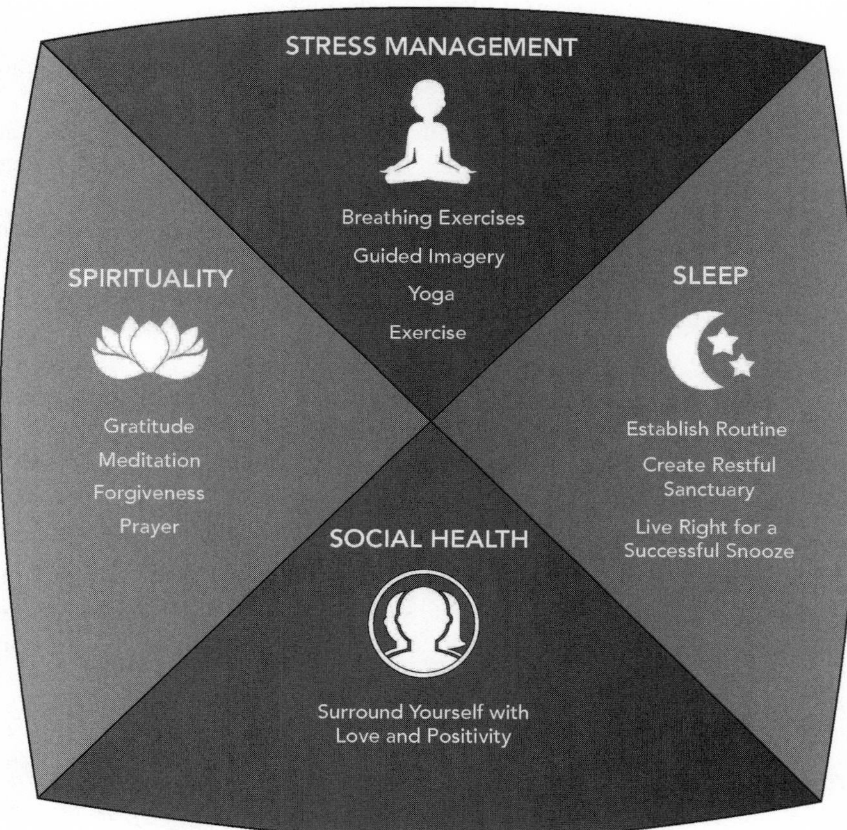

Figure 3.1. The Four Big S's

Part 2

REMEDIES FOR HOLISTIC HEALING

• 4 •

Adjusting *The Holistic Rx* for Your Condition

Yay!!! You've made it through the toughest part!!! Literally, over the years, what I just discussed previously (and likely bored you to death with)—the foundations of good health—is where I start all my patients. Now it's time to get personal and dig a little deeper! But again, make sure you're implementing the following, as that is the key in healing chronic inflammation from the root cause. Find a health care practitioner you click with and is willing to listen and spend the time you need with you, and supplement as you need (especially with vitamin D, fish oil, probiotics, and magnesium). I know you're excited to get personal, but let me summarize the main foundational pieces first! This is my Holistic Rx to you!

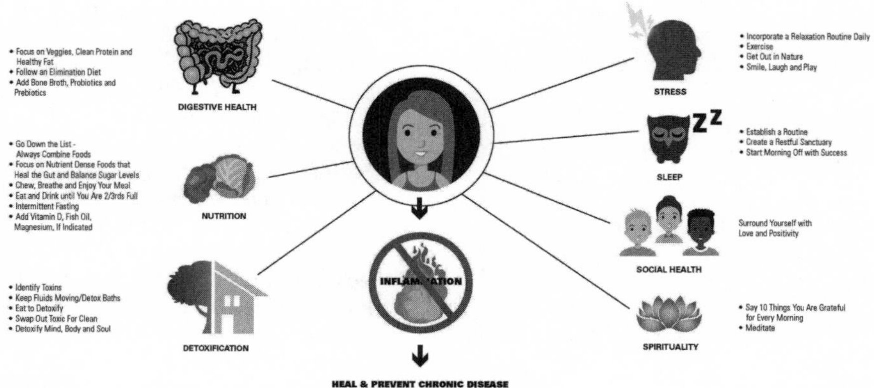

Figure 4.1. The Holistic Rx

LAB TESTS—LET'S GET PERSONAL!

To tailor *The Holistic Rx* to you, work with your primary care provider to get an initial set of lab tests. The following tests are ones your primary care doctor should feel comfortable ordering, and most insurances cover them, if coded appropriately.

There is a difference between optimal and normal. Optimal is what your body functions best at, as normal is anywhere within that large range that doesn't classify as low or high. I have provided the target/optimal ranges that I use and the interventions I typically recommend for my patients. (See Table 4.1.) Your personal physician may work with slightly different targets/optimal ranges and interventions. You are unique and may require refinement of these recommendations based upon your personal health circumstances. To get these tests, just request them from your doctor. These tests can be repeated every one to three months depending on your personal situation.

Table 4.1. Time to Get Personal!

Labs	*Optimal Fasting Levels*	*Interventions*
Complete blood count (CBC)	Normal values for the target range	If anemic, gut healing is stressed.
Comprehensive metabolic panel (CMP)	Normal values for the target range Fasting glucose: less than 90 mg/dL Calcium: less than 10 mg/dL	If fasting glucose is elevated, IR management is stressed. If calcium is higher than 10, carefully dose vitamin D, to prevent parathyroid issues. If liver tests are elevated, look for other causes and improve IR.
Thyroid stimulating hormone (TSH)	Ideally less than 2.5 microiu/mL	If elevated, will need to add free T3, free T4, reverse T3, TPO antibody and thyroglobulin antibody (but if present with anxiety, fatigue, hair loss, or other thyroid type symptoms, I add this in regardless of TSH). Work with your doctor to begin a combination of T3 and T4 medication such as compounded T3/T4 or natural dessicated thyroid.
Free T4, Free T3, Reverse T3 TPO antibody Antithyroglobulin Antibody	Free T4 > 1.1 ng/dL Free T3 >3.2 pg/mL, Reverse T3 <10:1 ratio RT3 to FT3 TPO antibody <9 IU/mL or negative ATA <4 IU/mL or negative	If elevated, address root cause. If reverse T3 is elevated, it can be due to excessive exercise, starvation diets, stress, or heavy metals If the antibodies are elevated, address autoimmunty.

Labs	*Optimal Fasting Levels*	*Interventions*
Magnesium	More than 2 mg/dL	There isn't a great test to check the exact levels in your blood. But we can get a sense that you are deficient and if it is less, need to supplement 1000 mg of Mg for 3 weeks then maintain at 500 mg per day.
25-hydroxy Vitamin D (vitamin D25-OH);	50–80 ng/mL (nanogram/ milliliter)	Adjust vitamin D dose up or down according to level. There are multiple ways to dose vitamin D; work with your doctor to determine how much supplemental vitamin D you will need. Blood level more than 45 ng/mL or for maintenance: 2000–4000 IU daily depending on sun exposure, activity level, age, etc. Levels 35–45 ng/mL, correct with 5000 IU of D3 for 3 months Levels <35 ng/mL correct with 10,000 IU of vitamin D3, duration depending on level. Best taken with food, calcium, and with vitamin K. Too much can be toxic as it is stored in the liver; continue to monitor every few months.
Folate and Vitamin B12	In the top quartile of the reference (range for that lab) B12 >500 pg/mL	Interpret with homocysteine, if lower than 500 add 1000 mcg of B12 × 3 weeks and then maintain 500 mcg every day, but may need more; if you have SNPs, please check with your doctor. B12 should be avoided with Leber's disease.
Homocysteine	4–8 micromole/L	If low, add more protein to diet. If high, switch to the methyl forms of folate (methylfolate) and methyl forms of B12 (methyl B12). Also a vitamin B complex like B-100. Add B12 500 mcg q day, folate 50 mcg q day and B6 50mg q day and recheck in 3 months; some practitioners may add riboflavin and vitamin B9. If still high once folate and B12 are optimized, see a functional medicine practitioner for guidance.

(*continued*)

Table 4.1. *Continued*

Labs	*Optimal Fasting Levels*	*Interventions*
Highly sensitive C-reactive protein (hs-CRP)	Less than 1.0 mg/L (milligram/liter) = low risk (ideal) 1 to 3 mg/L = intermediate risk Greater than 3 mg/L = high risk	If high, follow the foundations of good health. If still high, see your practitioner for further guidance.
Fasting lipids	Triglyceride/HDL cholesterol ratio less than 3	A ratio greater than 3 indicates probable insulin resistance and may indicate need for more fish oil.
HDL cholesterol (good cholesterol)	HDL cholesterol greater than 60 mg/dL (milligram/deciliter)	If HDL is less than 60, decrease carbohydrates, increase vegetables, berries, fish oil, and exercise.
Fasting insulin	Less than 10 mIUL	If higher, concentrate on lowering insulin resistance.
HbA1c	Less than 5.4%	If higher, concentrate on lowering insulin resistance. If it remains elevated despite perfect diet and lifestyle. Have your doctor check a fructosamine (represents a blood sugar level over the previous 2–3 weeks) level.
Extra: Selenium Vitamin A Zinc Iron/Ferritin	Selenium 200–250 mcg/L Vitamin A 0.8-1mg/L Zinc 1,000–1,200 mcg/dL Iron/Ferritin 75–100 ng/mL	If low, add supplement or foods containing the nutrient. Zinc can also be checked via a zinc taste test.

Most patients respond tremendously to the changes listed in Table 4.1, especially within four weeks. Now any change is good change! But if after three months, you still have not seen enough changes, go through the following checklists on Digestive Health and Detoxification and The Four Big S's.

Digestive Health and Detoxification

- I am complying with all the recommendations of the foundations of good health.
- I have followed the Gut Rx or other gut healing diets.
- I am successfully avoiding all trace exposure to gluten and other grains.

- Could legumes/lentils, nightshades, nuts, seeds, and eggs be causing problems? Or could there be other food sensitivities (e.g., histamine or salicylate intolerance)?
- I have double-checked ingredients on supplements, medications, spices, and prepackaged and prepared foods.
- I eat a large variety of vegetables, with other green foods, proteins, and healthy fats at each meal.
- I am drinking broth regularly.
- I am moderating my intake of high-glycemic-load foods.
- I am fasting three hours between meals.
- I am not eating three hours before bed.
- I eat appropriately sized meals with an appropriate amount of time between them.
- I am drinking enough water but avoid excessive liquids with meals.
- I eat probiotic foods or take a probiotic supplement.
- I use sea salt or Himalayan salt.
- My environment is toxin free.
- I have asked my doctor to check genetics and methylation issues.
- I am taking gut healing supplements as needed.
- I am taking the appropriate supplements for optimal general health and organ function support.
- I have identified my possible toxic exposure.
- My fluids are moving.
- I am taking Epsom salt baths as often as I can.
- I am eating to detoxify.
- I have swapped toxic for clean.

The Four Big S's: Stress, Sleep, Social Health, and Spirituality

- I am learning to relax and use my breath.
- I am respecting my boundaries, and say no when I need to and ask for help and accept it.
- I make sure I am having fun every day.
- I practice mindful meditation daily.
- I spend time in nature.
- I am engaging in some sort of mild to moderate intense activity every day.
- I make sure I get eight to twelve hours of quality sleep every night and nap when I need to.
- I practice good sleep hygiene (sleeping in a cool, quiet, dark room and making positive sleep associations).

- I sleep and wake up the same time each day.
- I make time to nurture positive social connections.
- I am practicing gratitude daily.

Work with your doctor to assess food allergies/sensitivities, supplements/medications to support organ function, any persistent infections, liver detoxification/heavy metal poisoning, hormone regulation, and genetic variations.

EVEN MORE PERSONAL?

Once you've incorporated the foundations of good health, it's time to get even more personal (like we already weren't personal enough! I promise I will mind your personal space . . . maybe). The more tools in your very stylish tool belt, the better. Optimizing health with the foundations of good health is key, but one can also accelerate and maintain healing by incorporating other holistic integrative modalities.

Chapters 5 through 21 offer an alphabetically arranged guide to self-directed integrative treatments to chronic illness and conditions, sectioned by subspecialties/organ group. Flip to what your specific condition is. You will notice I first recap the most important pearls of the foundations of good health that pertain to that specific system, and then dive into additional integrative modalities that can be added as an adjunct to the foundations of good health to accelerate and optimize your health. You don't need to apply all of them, but the idea is to know what is out there and ponder, with your practitioner, about what steps you wish to take further. The options are seriously endless! Now if that doesn't give you optimism, I don't know what else will!

Let's start with building your dream team that will help get you off the ground!

Building Your Wellness Team

- *The most important player in your team is YOU!* Be your biggest advocate, educate yourself, and be empowered to get back in the driver's seat of your own health.
- *Work with your physician.* Find a general practitioner who will respect you for taking such an active role in your healing and doesn't get defensive when you ask questions or bring up your own research. Find a practitioner who will have an open mind about nutrition and integrative holistic approaches to healing and prevention and is willing to learn with you.

- *Build your support system.* Find a friend, partner, coworker, basically someone who is supportive and will hold you accountable for the changes you are hoping to make.
- *Find integrative therapies and practitioners.* Once you have found that doctor and your support system, continue to build your wellness team with those who can incorporate these modalities to heal the body from the inside out by returning the body back into balance and homeostasis. Find integrative, functional, and holistic practitioners who will help to encourage your natural self-healing process: biological dentists, nutritionists, psychotherapists, exercise physiologists, health coaches, acupuncturists, energy healers, massage therapists, homeopaths, and naturopaths (a multidisciplinary approach to healing that uses natural resources).
- *Me!* I promise to motivate you to get you to where you need be and higher, cheerleading you every step of the way, leaving no question unanswered, guiding you the best of my ability! Let's do this together! (as long as you can stand my enthusiasm and my sense of humor. . . . oh and I'm a hugger, so be forewarned!)

TAILORING FOR YOU!

Let's briefly discuss the organization integrative modalities that you will see listed under each chronic condition and others that can also be tried to optimize health and wellness.

Digestive Health and Detoxification (D & D): Special Considerations

As I have already discussed this in great detail, here I will only highlight the foods/practices that will optimize that organ system, to pay special attention to those.

The Four Big S's: Special Considerations

Already discussed in great detail within the last section, here I will only highlight the practices that will optimize that organ system and anything to be cautious about.

Chronic Condition

I will give a brief introduction to each chronic condition, including symptoms, signs, and diagnosis.

Additional Integrative Modalities

Supplements, homeopathy, acupressure, and aromatherapy will be discussed for every condition. Discuss the options with your practitioners, to see what fits best for your unique self. Let's discuss the additional integrative modalities in a little bit more detail.

Supplements (vitamins, minerals, nutraceuticals [herbal medicine])

After you have the foundations of good health down, a supplement can be added to fill in the gaps to help maintain health or treat a specific condition. A large majority of chronic health conditions can be helped with fish oil, magnesium, vitamin D, and probiotics, so always consider them first line for your chronic condition (I won't repeat them for every diagnosis). I will discuss the most important first, then under the other category are ones that can also be used to improve the condition. The idea is not to start taking all of them, but to discuss the options with your doctor, and if you find a supplement combination, you will know what supplements will benefit your specific condition.

There are multiple types of nutritional supplements:

Vitamins

These are necessary for producing energy, regulating cell and tissue function, protecting your DNA, and a lot more. There are about thirteen essential vitamins (A, C, D, E, K, B1 [thiamine], B2 [riboflavin], B3 [niacin], B5 [pantothenic acid], B6 [pyridoxine], B7 [biotin], B9 [folate or folic acid], and B12 [cobalamin]) these are divided into fat soluble (A, D, E, K) and water soluble (all the others).

Minerals

These are elements that originate in the earth. The ones that are important to us are calcium, magnesium, phosphorus, sodium, potassium, chloride, and sulfur. The trace minerals (as you only need them in small amounts) are fluoride, manganese, copper, zinc, iodine, molybdenum, selenium, iron, and chromium. In nature, minerals are commonly bound to another substance that can impact its bioavailability and absorption.

Nutraceuticals

Other supplements are "essential" (your body needs them through food or supplement, as it can't produce them), like omega 3 fatty acids and nine amino acids. Other supplements are not essential in the diet but are beneficial, like probiotics, prebiotics, nutrients from plants (phytonutrients), and others that are produced in the body but can be taken as a supplement, like melatonin, collagen, coenzyme Q10 (Co Q10), and glucosamine. All these can be grouped together and referred to as nutraceuticals.

Botanical/Herbal Medicine

This system uses the whole plant to treat or alleviate medical conditions and includes herbs and other remedies like lemon balm, peppermint, and passionflower. Herbs aren't regulated, so educate yourself before buying them. Look for herbal preparations that have been harvested from wild strands or cultivated organically; don't buy the whole herb or those encapsulated powdered herbs, as the dried plants deteriorate upon exposure to the environment, especially when ground into powders. Follow the label instructions, and if you're nursing, pregnant, or have other medical conditions or are on any other herb or drugs, don't take herbs without talking to your doctor, as some may have possible interactions (I will discuss the most relevant as they come up). For example, when you're on blood-thinning medications (e.g., warfarin or aspirin), don't mix these with other herbs that may thin the blood, like feverfew, supplemental garlic, ginger, and ginkgo. Valerian shouldn't be mixed with sleeping medications. Avoid mixing drugs and herbs that have opposite actions. Some herbs may reduce the effectiveness of some drugs by causing them to metabolize too quickly like St. John's wort or immune-boosting drugs, especially if you're on an immunosuppressant. Stop taking any herbs about ten to fourteen days before surgery, as herbs like ginseng and licorice root can affect heart rate and blood pressure, and kava and valerian may increase the effects of anesthesia. Nursing and pregnant women should avoid herbs (besides ginger and echinacea for flu or colds and fenugreek and alfalfa that are safe), as what is safe for adults may not be safe for children. But when in doubt, always talk to your practitioner and/or herbalist.

Homeopathy

Homeopathy was founded in the late eighteenth century and is based on the law of similar, stating that disease can be cured by a medicine that creates similar symptoms to those the patient is experiencing. The remedy can be chosen after taking into account the whole person (mental, emotional, and physical). In each chapter, I have listed the most common symptomatic homeopathics that can be used for that condition. Read down the list and choose the one that best fits your symptoms. The closer the medication matches your symptoms, the higher the dilution (e.g., 30C is stronger than 15C). The remedy can be taken as long as you remain symptomatic or even as prevention. The more severe the problem, the more doses can be taken per day (e.g., for intense pain, a dose can be taken every fifteen minutes; and as the pain improves, the doses can be spread out). Taper down the dosage to once per day as your symptoms improve. Take a 6C, 12C, 15C, or 30C (this will be your symptomatic homeopathic remedy). After your symptoms resolve, you may stop taking the remedy. You will also see homeopathic medications with an "X" dosage; C is more diluted and stronger than X potencies.

Homeopathic medications are all natural and can be used for a wide variety of acute and chronic conditions. For chronic conditions, two types of medication are used: chronic reactional mode medication (see Appendix) and symptomatic medicine (listed under each chronic illness), use both for optimal results. Homeopathics are ultradiluted, so besides an occasional initial worsening of symptoms that can be resolved by adjusting the dosage, homeopathic medications have very limited side effects or drug interactions and are safe to use for children.

There are mixed studies, but more than one hundred clinical trials have shown benefits of homeopathics. If you decide to use homeopathy, there is little risk. Many have reported improvement of symptoms, as I have personally experienced. Obtain your homeopathics from a reputable source, to make sure there is no added heavy metal; liquid homeopathics can also contain caffeine or alcohol so should not be taken when pregnant unless under supervision. They can be purchased in combination remedies and single remedies available at natural food stores. Homeopathics are regulated by the U.S. Food and Drug Administration (FDA), but the FDA doesn't evaluate the effectiveness or safety of each remedy. The North American Society of Homeopaths (NASH) has a directory of practitioners, including their credentials. Look for certification by the American Board of Homeotherapeutics, the Society of Homeopaths, and Council for Homeopathic Certification.

Traditional Chinese Medicine

Traditional Chinese Medicine (TCM) focuses on health as a balance between body, mind, and spirit. TCM has multiple concepts. Practitioners believe that each of our organs, our food, and our tissues have a yin or yang force. When one force overpowers the other, the qi (pronounced *chee*) is imbalanced and our body becomes diseased. Qi embraces all energy, like the world around you, heat, movement, emotion, light, and even your iPad. Unobstructed flow of qi, or "life energy," through the body, along pathways known as meridians and disease is because of obstruction of qi flow.

Two most commonly used types of TCM focus on correcting imbalances of energy in the body by balancing the body's vital energy, which flows through the meridians (these begin in your fingertips and connect your organs), improving blood flow, promoting deep relaxation, lowering stress, bringing the body back into balance, and allowing it to heal.

Acupuncture

Acupuncture involves thin needles inserted into the body, releasing endorphins and stimulating the nervous system. Acupuncture is beneficial for a wide variety of conditions, both physical and emotional. It is increasingly recognized by Western medicine as an effective alternative or adjunct to conventional treatments for pain, musculoskeletal problems like arthritis and back pain, nausea, sinus/ear problems, stroke rehabilitation, headache, menstrual cramps, digestive disorders, blood pressure issues, erectile dysfunction, infertility, and asthma, just to name a few. Common side effects include bleeding and bruising at the site, along with occasional soreness in the muscle. Look for a licensed acupuncturist (L.Ac.) who holds a license in one or more states; a person certified by the NCCAOM (The National Certification Commission for Acupuncture and Oriental Medicine) is called a diplomate of acupuncture (Dipl.Ac.), and there are physicians at the American Academy of Medical Acupuncture (www.medicalacupuncture.org). For more information about professional standards and licensing requirements for acupuncturists, contact the American Association of Acupuncture and Oriental Medicine (www.aaaom.org).

Acupressure

Acupressure uses specific finger placement and pressure over specific points along the body that follow the meridians. I will list these points in detail, as acupressure can be learned as a self-care strategy. To apply pressure to pressure points, locate the pressure points from the illustration. (See Figures 4.2 and 4.3.) Use your finger or knuckle to apply firm and deep pressure directly and steadily on the point; use force that is between pleasant firm pressure to a little painful pressure for at least ten to thirty seconds, repeating the procedure five times. Work points on the right and left, when it applies. Remember to breathe deeply and relax in a comfortable position. Don't continue to press if too painful; pain may diminish when you use the middle finger with index and ring finger on either side. For chronic problems, you can treat once a day. Use caution if you are pregnant or if you have sensitive or damaged areas. You might feel more vulnerable to cold after each session.

Here are some examples of conditions and which pressure points to focus on:

- Digestive problems: ST25, ST28, ST36, CV8, LU3
- Neck pain, gallbladder: 20, 21, 39
- Pain in the elbows and shoulders: LI11
- Back pain: GV3, GV14, GB30
- Stress: LU1
- Anxiety: P6
- Immune system: K3, LV3, SP6, ST36, K27, LI11, CV17
- Detoxification: LV3, SP6, K27, LI4, HP6, CV17, CV6

Following are the standard meridian abbreviations:

- GV Governing Vessel
- SI Small Intestine
- ST Stomach
- LI Large Intestine
- SP Spleen
- H Heart
- CV Conception Vessel
- LU Lung
- B Bladder
- LV Liver
- EX Extra Point
- P Pericardium
- GB Gallbladder
- K Kidney
- HN Heart/Neck
- HP Heart Protector
- TB Triple Burner

Feng Shui

Feng Shui is the ancient Chinese are of placement. Like TCM, both come from ancient Chinese roots and help to restore and increase energy, balance energies, and promote healing. Feng Shui helps to balance yin and yang in the surrounding environment.

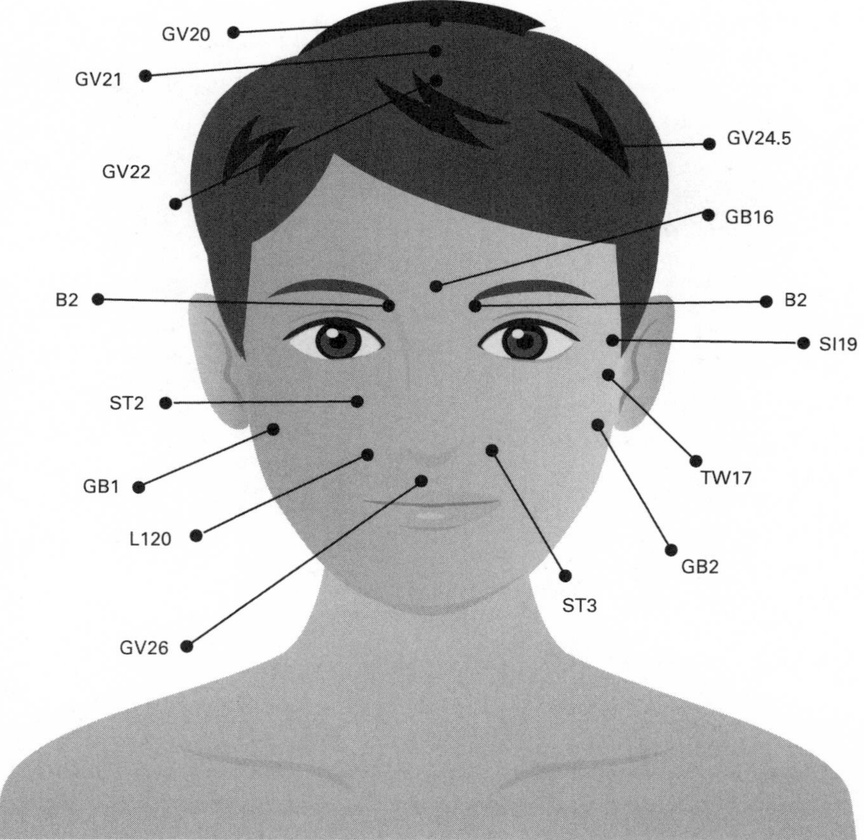

Figure 4.2. Acupressure, Head

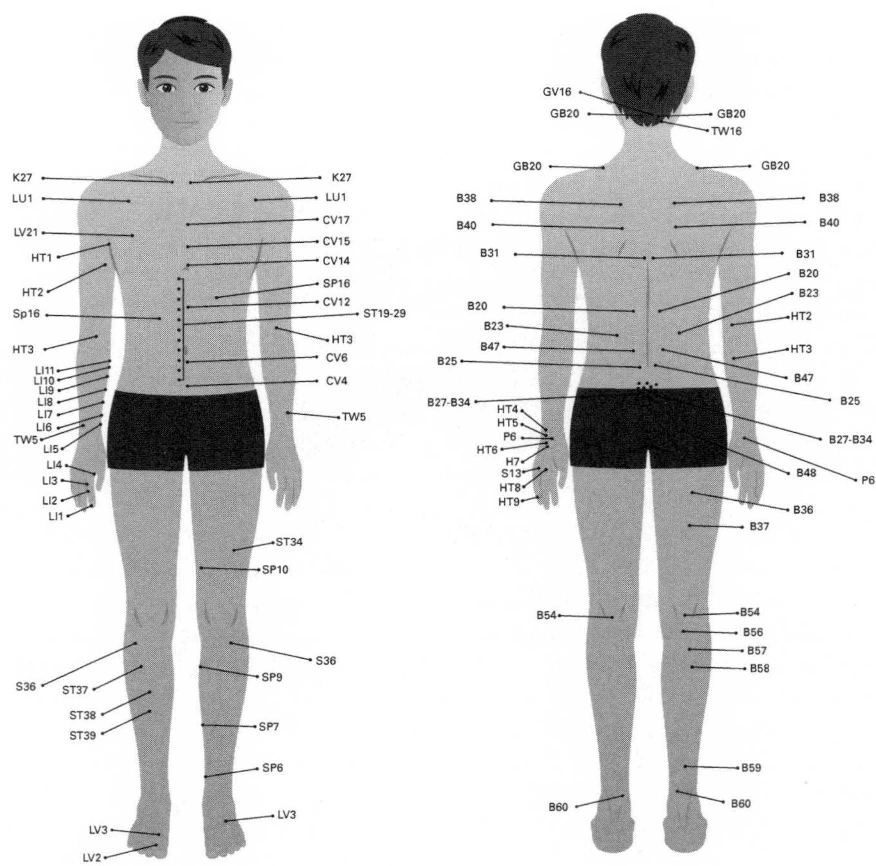

Figure 4.3. Acupressure, Body

Aromatherapy

Aromatherapy is the use of essential oils from leaves, fruit, roots, flowers, or barks. The scents from these oils have a powerful influence on physical and mental health, with great antibacterial and antifungal properties. Aromatherapists dilute essential oils, and when inhaled, these send chemical messages through the nerves to the brain's limbic system, amygdala, and hippocampus, which control mood and emotion, this then subsequently alters emotional and physiological states, which in turn can influence the body's immune, respiratory, and circulatory systems. Essential oils are gaining new attention as an alternative treatment for infections because they have antiseptic properties, relieve pain and inflammation, help detox, enhance well-being and mood, improve concentration, balance energy, relieve stress, balance hormones, and boost immunity. They even help spiritually by enhancing mindful practices.

Aromatherapy can be used for self-treatments, so I have listed the most beneficial for the conditions here. They can be used topically and massaged into skin; inhaled by a diffuser or on a cotton ball; added to personal care products like shampoos, body butter, lip palm, cleaners, and toothpaste; and added to baths, compresses, showers, and saunas. A carrier oil can be used when massaged topically. Examples include unscented, organic, and cold-pressed almond oil, avocado oil, coconut oil, pomegranate seed oil, olive oil, and jojoba oil (for most people, do a 10 percent dilution, five drops of oil per ½ tsp of the carrier). Oils can also be added to a warm bath and hot/cold compresses. Look for oils that are extracted from organic sources. Some of the most popular essential oils are clary sage, lavender, chamomile, rosemary, tea tree, and peppermint.

Essential oils have very few negative effects, but the use of citrus or other oils can cause sun sensitivity, so wait twenty-four hours before going into the sun and forty-eight hours after using bergamot. Oils like clove and oregano should be diluted and shouldn't be used for more than one week. Many essential oils should not be used in pregnancy: clary sage, basil, cinnamon, clove, cypress, fennel, jasmine, juniper, marjoram, myrrh, rose, sage, thyme, German chamomile, and rosemary. Clary sage, cypress, eucalyptus, ginger, rosemary, sage, and thyme shouldn't be used with heart medicines (specifically blood thinners). Some essential oils interact negatively with drugs; these should not be used if you suffer from high blood pressure or epilepsy. Lavender and tea tree oils have effects similar to those of estrogen and should be avoided with tumors that are estrogen dependent. Use essential oils with caution in combination with homeopathics as they may diminish their effects.

When in doubt, talk to a professional. Before using an essential oil on the skin, try a test patch.

Bodywork

Bodywork and manual medicine refer to body manipulation that is used for relaxation and pain relief. Bodywork helps to realign and reposition the body, addressing issues that were causing discomfort and contributing to health problems, to allow natural graceful movement. The various types include the following.

Chiropractic Care

This is comprehensive treatment that uses the hands to manipulate the body, correcting structural misalignment to alleviate discomfort. Such care may also include a variety of therapies like soft tissue mobilization techniques such as massage, trigger point therapy, electromyography, ultrasound, laser-guided therapy, using traction, or applying ice or heat to areas of discomfort. Chiropractors often also provide acupuncture, herbal medicine, and homeopathy in conjunction with their other treatments. Chiropractic medicine, when performed properly, helps to alleviate pain, improve digestion and circulation of blood and nerve flow, and can promote overall health of the body. It is not recommended for people with serious bone problems, such as bone cancer, acute joint disease, bone marrow disease, or bone/joint infections, as rare complications have been reported from traditional high-pressure, low-speed manipulation. Make sure the chiropractor has a degree from an accredited four-year chiropractic college. The American Chiropractic Association and the International Chiropractors Association maintain a database of member doctors as well as information on all chiropractic specialties.

Osteopathic Manipulative Medicine (OMM)

This holistic system, like others, depends on the musculoskeletal system functioning smoothly, treating the whole person (mind, body, and spirit, not just symptoms), encouraging the body to heal itself. It is similar to chiropractic medicine, but osteopathic doctors can do surgeries and prescribe medications like MDs. Osteopathic practitioners believe structure influences function, and if that is affected, other areas of the body can be affected, and once the body is aligned, the organs can function properly. The American Osteopathic Association provides a database of licensed reputable practitioners.

Massage

To enhance a person's health and well-being by eliminating muscle spasms and trigger points and improving relaxation and loosening stiff joints. Massage therapy is a great adjunct to other holistic healing. Focusing concentrated pressure on trigger points allows the muscle to relax, though it may be initially painful. Other types of massage include Shiatsu massage (massage that works with your body's energetic meridians, acupressure, and gentle stretching), Thai (therapist works your body through series of stretches and is great for flexibility), Abhyanga (massage that uses herb-infused oils and applies them specific to your dosha [see "Ayurvedic Medicine" below], correcting its imbalances, and reflexology.

Reflexology

Similar to acupressure, reflexology involves the application of pressure on particular areas of the feet, hands, or ears that relate to a specific muscle groups or organs. It helps the patient to relax, reduce pain, and improve sleep; it relieves depression and anxiety, as nerve endings in the extremities provide a "map" for the rest of the body, improving functioning. I discuss reflexology here because it can easily be done to oneself to optimize healing and relaxation.

To massage your foot, clean your hands and trim your nails. Begin and end each session with relaxing your feet with simple pressing and squeezing or kneading or whatever feels good and pressing and holding the solar plexus of each foot for five to ten seconds for relaxation. Then walk your thumb up from the base of the heel to each toe, pressing the reflex points with the outer edge with the tip of finger or thumb. After you are relaxed, locate the healing zones of the feet that correspond to the specific organs, body parts, or systems that are causing you the most stress, and press the corresponding reflex area or point (e.g., allergies: work lymphatic organs and breathing passages, eyes, nose, throat areas; gynecological problems: work the uterus, fallopian tubes, and ovaries). (See Figures 4.4, 4.5, 4.6, and 4.7.)

End with relaxation and breeze strokes (lightly running your fingers down the entire foot barely touching the skin to help soothe the nerves).

Other more general points are:

- Relaxation and peace: solar plexus/diaphragm
- Detoxification and digestion: liver, colon, kidneys
- To stimulate blood supply to nerves: the entire spinal area
- Improve circulation: hands and feet all over
- For systemic issues: work the entire foot
- For positive thinking and clarity: head/brain
- Balance hormones: pituitary, endocrine glands
- Improve sleep: pineal gland
- Balance metabolism: thyroid
- Release tension: neck/shoulders
- Calm breathing: chest/lungs
- Endocrine problems: thyroid, pancreas, and adrenals
- Improve energy: adrenals, spine, and diaphragm
- Improve mood: pancreas, endocrine glands, head, and solar plexus

Look for a certified massage therapist via the National Certification Board for Therapeutic Massage and Bodywork (NCBTMB) with licenses like LMT, CMT, or NCMT.

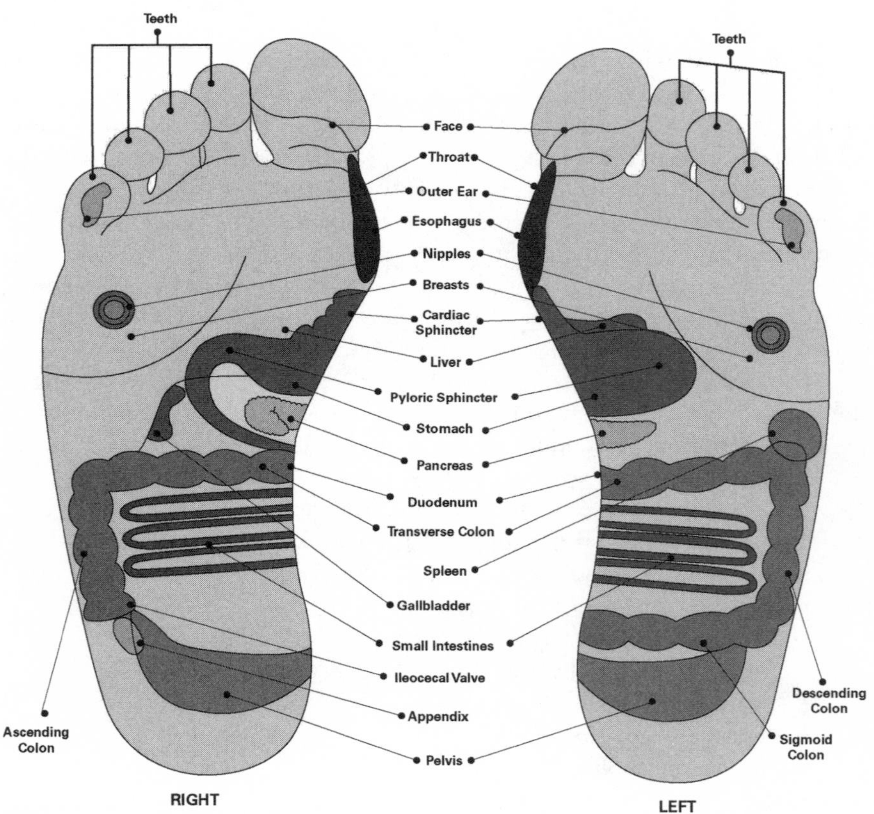

Figure 4.4. Reflexology, Bottom of Foot

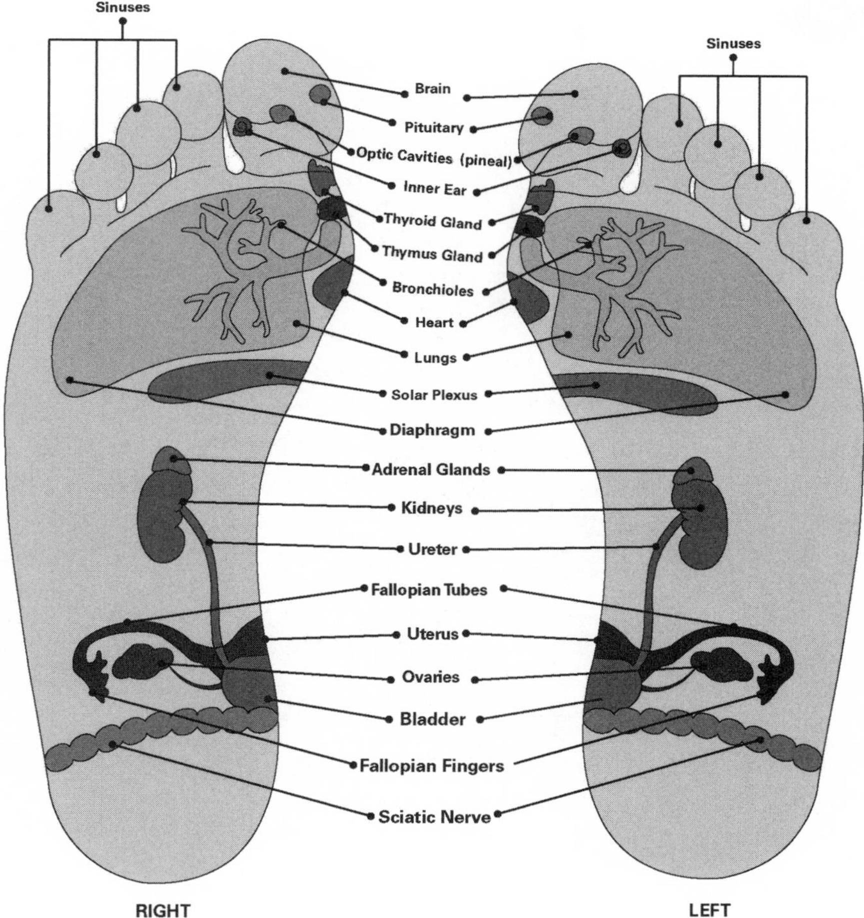

Figure 4.5. Reflexology, Bottom of Foot

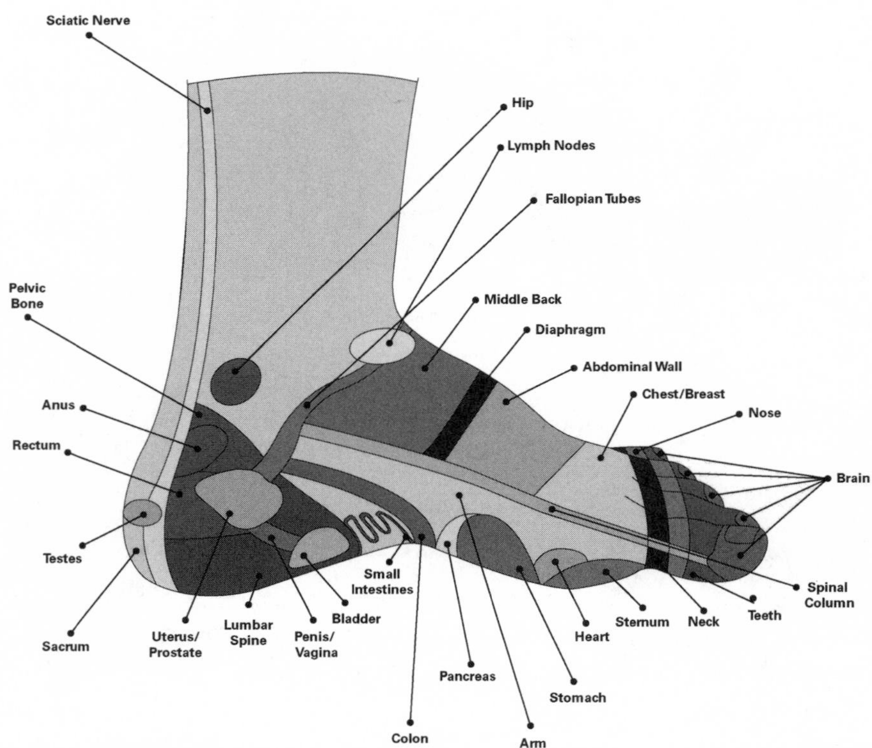

Figure 4.6. Reflexology, Inside of Foot

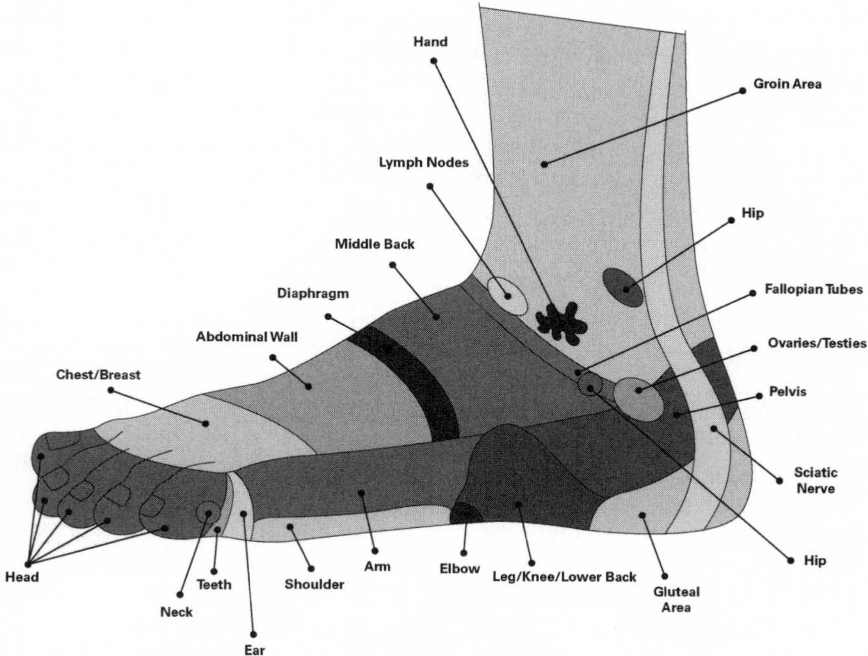

Figure 4.7. Reflexology, Outside of Foot

Craniosacral Therapy

This is a noninvasive form of bodywork that releases compression in the bones of the head, spinal column, and sacrum to alleviate stress and pain. CST uses a very gentle touch looking for abnormal rhythm that may remove any impediments to the flow, improving conditions like depression, anxiety, temporomandibular joint disorder, migraines, and whiplash injury.

Other body work techniques: laser therapy, magnetic therapy, cupping, and physiotherapy.

Hydrotherapy

Hydrotherapy is based on the fact that water has many properties that give it the ability to heal, treat certain conditions, and maintain health. Treatment is provided by a trained hydrotherapist and can be found in a hospital physiotherapy department. It consists of underwater massage, mineral baths, ice, saunas, whirlpools and hot tubs, water jets, and colonic irrigation (can soothe bowel inflammation), which are excellent for relaxation and detoxification. Cold or hot compresses can be beneficial for pain; even alternating them can help with circulation (even for hemorrhoids) and optimize detoxification. Hydrotherapy can be used as an adjunct to help treat conditions like depression, insomnia, pain, fatigue, and other chronic issues. Nasal and sinus irrigation can help to relieve pain and congestion in the nasal passages and sinuses.

With relapsing flares, like in autoimmunity or severe hypertension, avoid hot tubs, saunas, and extreme temperatures. Keep the water temperature between 81 and 83 degrees Fahrenheit.

Ayurvedic Medicine

Ayurvedic medicine emphasizes the prevention of disease, using personal treatments to maintain the balance between body, mind, and spirit. A *dosha* is a unique pattern of living force and energy that controls how our body works; when out of balance, the body fails to adapt and displays abnormal patterns of activities (excess and deficiencies) it manifests in disease. Three doshas are vata (space and air), pitta (fire and water), and kapha (water and earth). Everyone inherits a unique mix of these three doshas, and one is usually more dominant and its balance is needed for overall health and wellness. Ayurvedic medicine helps the body detoxify; yoga, meditation, massage, and other herbal remedies are usually implemented as well. After determining your doshas, the vaidya, or Ayurvedic doctor, will then help you rebalance them by addressing lifestyle habits and digestion. This modality works best with massage, aromatherapy, yoga, dietary recommendations, detoxification/enemas, psychological intervention, and herbal medicine.

Ayurvedic medicine is best as a complement to other healing systems and can be helpful for chronic conditions like digestive issues, allergies, asthma, insomnia, heart disease, autoimmune disease, skin conditions, viral infections, wound healing, and reproductive and overall health. Look for providers with credentials and education from the International Society of Ayurveda and Health. Make sure the practitioner has experience and uses pure remedies free of lead, arsenic, and mercury.

Energy Medicine

Energy medicine helps to improve impeded energy flow that has been blocked (leading to illness) by blending healing touch and heightened consciousness. Examples include Reiki, a Japanese technique that involves touching the patient's torso or head in a specific order to reduce pain, anxiety, depression, fibromyalgia, and cancer, also improving blood pressure and heart rate, treating the whole person, mind, body and soul; therapeutic touch and healing touch that use a sweeping motion head to toe, hovering just above the body, reading clues about the patient's energy fields, modulating the energy to smooth out energy blockages or knots, helping to relieve pain and anxiety; healing touch that involves light touch around the body, acting as a conduit to self-healing; and polarity therapy, which is based on electromagnetic energy current flow through the channels of the body—the more effectively they flow, the better they help the body. Energy medicine also includes stretches, nutritional advice, and emotional counseling.

Biofeedback

Biofeedback uses a series of machines, electrodes, and sensors (feedback devices) that provide information about your body, helping you to use your mind to heal and regulate body functions. Biofeedback is often used as a stress-relieving technique and has been beneficial for headaches, blood pressure, insomnia, digestive issues, anxiety, ADHD, and asthma. Pelvic floor disorders, like prolapsed uterus, and incontinence can also be helped with biofeedback. The Association for Applied Psychology and Biofeedback (aapb.org) can help you find qualified biofeedback practitioners in your area.

THE INTERVIEWING PROCESS—YOU DESERVE THE BEST!

Find a practitioner through a referral from a friend, family member, or your conventional doctor. It is key to always check education and credentials, then set up a pre-appointment phone call or appointments with the practitioner of interest, to get a good idea of the practitioner and the practice. During this interaction, be prepared with a list of questions and concerns, and because most health care plans don't cover alternative integrative modalities, always inquire about any upfront costs. Be cautioned if any practitioner makes excessive claims and insists on signing you up immediately for a specified number of treatments. It is important to be open with your primary care provider about what other modalities you are pursuing and any list of herbs and medications you are currently taking. This will keep an open and honest relationship with all your providers.

Always remember: You may need medications to put out the fire before you control the blaze. As an adjunct to the foundations of good health, apply these additional integrative modalities in conjunction with your doctor, empowering you to optimize healing from the inside out.

YOU GOT THIS!

Right now conventional medicine is telling you that you are going to have to live with these symptoms for the rest of your life. I am telling you that because you have been suffering with these conditions for so long, after applying the foundation of good health, any little improvement in the right direction is a HUGE improvement. Teeny tiny improvements are better than no improvement, and one step in the right direction is better than no steps. Even a step backward can make you stronger! You can do this!! Now let's take this to the next level!!! So exciting!

• *5* •

Autoimmune Disease

Autoimmune diseases occur when your immune system starts to attack your own body. Why would it do that? Does it not love you anymore? Well, it does, but it's just a little confused. Autoimmune disease is essentially the immune system's misguided attack on your own body.

Your body has a complex network of special cells and organs (collectively called the immune system) that defends your body from foreign invaders: germs and all the other "bad guys." To do its main job, it must be able to tell the difference between self and nonself: what's you and what's foreign. Excess inflammation confuses the body and makes the immune system less able to tell what is enemy and what is not. When this happens, the body makes autoantibodies that attack the normal cells. To make matters worse, cells called the regulatory T cells fail to keep the immune system in line. The particular body parts that are affected determine the specific autoimmune disease. There are more than eighty known types, and if you have one, you are three times more likely to develop another.

D & D: SPECIAL CONSIDERATIONS

Digestive health and detoxification is critical for overcoming any autoimmune problems. Along with what we discussed earlier, other possible food sensitivities to watch out for are nightshades (tomatoes, eggplant, potatoes, and peppers), legumes/lentils, eggs, caffeine, nuts, and seeds; so it is best to avoid these. Fix deficiencies like calcium, iron, vitamin D, zinc, B6, B12, and folate. Eat as many vegetables as you can at every meal. Eat foods high in sulfur, including cabbage, onions, garlic, leeks, cauliflower, and asparagus, as it can help to reduce symptoms and optimize healthy fat intake like coconut oil and olive oil. Raw, unprocessed honey can also boost immunity.

For thyroid disease, increase foods with fatty acids, iodine (seaweed, saltwater fish, or a multivitamin), tyrosine (red meat and chicken, seaweed and seafood), selenium (red meats, liver, chicken, turkey, fish and shellfish), zinc (red meats, chicken, seafood and seaweed), iron, omega 3s, vitamin D3, B vitamins (leafy greens, broccoli, beets, red meat, and liver), vitamin A (orange fruits and veggies, liver, kale). Foods like kale and broccoli have been called goitrogens, but there are far more benefits to cause worry. Avoid IV detoxification in all cases of autoimmunity.

THE FOUR BIG S's: SPECIAL CONSIDERATIONS

With autoimmune disease, as with any chronic condition, stress management is key to healing, including exercise—but jogging and heavy weightlifting may be too harsh on your joints. Listen to your body and don't overdo it. If you push yourself too hard, you will do more harm than good. Flexibility, strengthening, aerobic exercise, and body awareness practices like tai chi, yoga, and Pilates can help improve posture, coordination, balance, and relaxation, in turn improving joint and muscular mobility. Seeing an exercise physiologist will help to find what will work best for you.

A WORD ABOUT INFECTIONS

If after three months of following the foundations of good health, including the GutRx, you continue to experience symptoms, especially fatigue and brain symptoms, consider the possibility that an infection is contributing to your problems.

Certain microbes are associated with certain autoimmune conditions. A functional medicine practitioner can test you for the type of microbe that could be associated with your condition. If you do have an infection or coinfection with one or more organisms, depending on the type of infection and your personal health condition, the practitioner may treat you with nutraceuticals, pharmaceuticals, or a combination of both.

Leaky gut, stress, inflammatory food, and other factors that disrupt the balance of your immune system as discussed earlier can reactivate a dormant infection and trigger your immune system. A functional medicine or holistic practitioner can test you for the type of microbe that could be associated with your condition. Locate a practitioner with ample experience, as it may take years to clear the infection, especially if there is more than one infecting agent. I often find that there are other infections in the gut such as parasites, Candida, bacterial overgrowth, and bacterial imbalances that need to be addressed and corrected. To defeat infections, it is important to combine gut healing with the right diet and supplements. Locate a practitioner with ample experience, as it may take years to clear the infection, especially if there is more than one infecting agent. Depending on the type of infection and your personal health condition, the practitioner may treat you with nutraceuticals, pharmaceuticals, or a combination of both. If treating one infection doesn't seem to improve the autoimmune condition, keep working with your doctor to see if there is a coinfection. The following are the most common infections that can trigger autoimmunity. Table 5.1 discusses what infections are most common depending on your unique situation.

Viral Infections

Chronic viral infections can hide out in our bodies in a dormant state, and can then become active and trigger an inflammatory response. Herpes (e.g., 1, 2, 6) is one virus that can do this, and once you're infected, it stays in your body for life. The Epstein-Barr virus (EBV) is another possible culprit in chronic viral infection. For EBV activity, ask your doctor to check EBV EA-D IgG (early antigen), EBV VCA IgG/IgM (viral capsid antigen), and EBV EBNA-1 IgG (nuclear antigen). The EA-D IgG will tell you if you have an active or reactivated chronic viral infection, EBV-VCA IgG positive means you've had or have an infection, while the IgM is due to a reactivated infection. A positive EBV EBNA IgG means that the result is most likely due to a past infection. The EBNA and VCA will be positive if you ever had an infection and if EBV is actively replicating inside your B cells (a type of white blood cell that produces antibodies). More than one can always be present—for example, hepatitis C.

These can be treated with Lauricidin (1 tsp three times daily), an acid derived from coconut oil and humic acid (two pills per day), both which lower your viral load. L-lysine (500 mg) can be taken for prevention, and 1–4 g per day with food during an outbreak.

Other herbal treatments to consider are Lomatium (can lead to a one time rash), Cordyceps (750 mg two capsules, three times daily for ninety days) or Olive leaf extract (one capsule, two times per day for sixty days). You can add NAC (1800 mg per day), a thymic protein A, adaptogens, vitamin D, vitamin C (500–3000 mg per day) or lysine for additional support.

Bacterial Infections

Certain bacterial infections can go along with autoimmune conditions. See Table 5.1 for types of bacteria that may be implicated; examples include Yersinia enterocolitica (not a good conventional test but a specialized stool test), H. pylori (can be identified using a breath test, stool antigen test, or blood tests), SIBO (breath test), Chlamydia pneumoniae, and Bartonella or Mycobacterium avium subspecies paratuberculosis (MAP).

If you're diagnosed with a bacterial infection, you'll need a combination treatment that includes antibiotics, probiotics, caprylic acid, an enzyme supplement containing cellulase, hemicellulase, xylanase, beta glucanase (to prevent yeast overgrowth), and other gut-healing supplements. Treatment for H. pylori naturally is a combination of zinc, berberine, bismuth citrate, mastic gum, and even oil pulling and cranberry juice (see Gastroenterology [chapter 11] for more detail). Yersinia can be treated with a combination of sweet wormwood, grapefruit seed extract, berberine, black walnut, and uva ursi. Garlic cloves, licorice, quercetin, Coenzyme Q10, turmeric, and oil of oregano also help with infections.

If needed, take probiotics during the course of antibiotics (don't take blindly), but at different times in the day. Antibiotics can be used if absolutely necessary along with probiotics. SIBO can be treated with xifaxan and if methaine predominant add neomycin or tindamax. Chlamydia pneumoniae can be treated with the antibiotic minocycline, 100 mg twice a day for three weeks. Use doxycycline for Yersinia.

If your symptoms don't improve, consider that you might have Lyme disease, an infection caused by Borrelia burgdorferi. It can cause symptoms similar to those of autoimmune conditions, and it can affect multiple organs. Ask that your practitioner use an advanced testing method such as iSpot Lyme or ELISA, western blot and lyme PCR tests. If positive, you might need to discuss antibiotic treatment with your licensed practitioner. Healing foods and supplements for lyme include thyme, lemon balm, zinc, licorice root, L-lysine, lomatium root, reishi mushroom, silver hydrosol, astaxanthin, and ascent iodine.

Fungal Infections

Systemic infection with yeast (Candida) is common in people with autoimmune conditions. It is always important to test for Candida with a blood test and stool analysis for IgG and IgM. If these tests are positive, the recommended treatment is Diflucan (100 mg twice a day for three weeks) or nystatin (500,000 units, two capsules, three times per day for thirty to ninety days), and herbal therapies are discussed in Gastroenterology (chapter 11).

Parasitic Infections

Parasites include toxoplasmosis (can be found in blood tests) and blastocystitis hominis (can be tested with a stool test). Toxoplasmosis can be treated by a specialized physician who can prescribe a medication. Treat blastocystitis either with an antibiotic or herb, like Alinia (1000 mg twice a day for three days, repeated two weeks, then again two weeks later or nystatin (500,000 units, two capsules, three times per day for thirty to ninety days) with Alinia or after treatment to help with possible fungal overgrowth. Herbal treatments include CandiBactin (two capsules, three times per day for sixty days), wormwood-containing antiparasitic (600 mg, two times per day for seven days, repeat in two weeks; don't use with history of liver problems), oil of oregano (150 mg, two capsules, three times per day for sixty days) combined with S. boulardii five to fifteen billion CFUs, two to four times per day for sixty days.

Table 5.1 Autoimmunity and Infections

Autoimmune Disease	*Type of Microbe*
Autoimmunity in general	E. coli, Proteus
Ankylosing spondylitis	Klebsiella
Graves' disease, Hashimoto's thyroiditis	Herpes, EBV, MAP, H. Pylori, Yersinia,
Guillain-Barre syndrome	Campylobacter, cytomegalovirus, EBV
Multiple sclerosis	Chlamydia pneumonia, EBV, measels
Rheumatoid arthritis	Citrobacter, Klebsiella, Proteus, Porphyromonas, EBV, E.coli, Hepatitis C, mycobacterium
Rheumatic fever	Streptococcus pyogenes
Systemic lupus erythematosus (SLE, or Lupus)	EBV
Autism	EBV, Cytomegalovirus, Herpes 1 and 2, 6, Measles
Uveitis	Cytomegalovirus, Herpes 1 and 2
Keratitis	Herpes 1
Autoimmune hepatitis	Herpes 1
Polymyositis	EBV
Psoriasis	Cytomegalovirus
ITP	EBV, Cytomegalovirus
IgA nephritis	EBV, Cytomegalovirus
Glumerulonephritis	EBV
Pemphigus	EBV
Sjogren's syndrome	EBV, Herpes 6
Type 1 diabetes mellitus	EBV, Cytomegalovirus, coxsackievirus
Myasthenia gravis	Hepatitis C, Herpes 1 and 2

If you do have a chronic infection, treating it is critical in healing autoimmune disease. Focusing on improving immunity with the recommendations in Part 1 is key in eliminating infections and lowering the infection's load. Always discuss with your physician to tailor what will work best for you.

Other Recommendations

Low-Dose Naltrexone

As an opioid antagonist, naltrexone can enhance immune function by increasing endogenous adrenaline production, reducing inflammation, and increasing the amount of regulatory T cytokines and IL-1 and TGF-B, so it can be helpful in conditions like cancers and other chronic illnesses. It can be helpful for those that have multiple autoimmune conditions or symptoms and have very high antibodies.

For autoimmunity, only low doses are used, like 1.5 to 4.5 mg per day to push the immune system in the right direction toward healing. Patients should start low, about 1.5 mg per night. This shouldn't be your first line of defense, but use it only after implementing the above and if you still have symptoms.

CELIAC DISEASE

Celiac disease occurs when the body forms an autoimmune reaction to gluten. Typical symptoms include recurrent bloating, cramping, abdominal pain, brain fog, changes in weight, sleep issues (including insomnia), fatigue and headaches, delayed puberty, pale, foul smelling stool, peripheral neuropathy, joint pain and mood changes, thinning hair and pale sores inside the mouth, tingling of hands and feet, vomiting, unexplained weight loss, unexplained infertility or recurrent miscarriage, and skin rash (dermatitis herpetiformis). Testing includes for IgA anti-gliadin antibodies, IgG anti-gliadin antibodies, IgA anti-endomysial antibodies, tissue transglutaminase antibodies, and total IgA antibodies, as well as genetic testing like HLA DQ2 and HLA DQ8.

Additional Integrative Modalities

Supplements

- Supplements that heal leaky gut are key.
- Digestive enzymes: in order to enhance digestion, add a pancreatic enzyme with amylase (see gut healing section in great detail).
- Probiotics.
- B vitamins like B2, B3, B6, B9, and B12.
- Calcium.
- Magnesium.
- Zinc.

- Other gut healing supplements like L glutamine, N-acetyl-D-glucosamine, and gamma oryzanol.
- *Children*: start off with digestive enzymes and probiotics.

Homeopathy

Early constitutional treatment from an experienced homeopath will help improve symptoms. A remedy is chosen based on one's personal symptoms, especially the most distressing. Issues related to celiac disease that can be helped with homeopathy include constipation; increased frequency of bulky, offensive smelling stools; allergies; gastroenteritis; and emotional issues.

Acupressure

- P6, SP6, CV12

Aromatherapy

Essential oils beneficial for gut bacterial imbalance are caraway, lavender, and bitter orange. These oils will harmonize well with beneficial bacteria in the body. Peppermint oil and cumin may benefit the digestive symptoms. Oils that protect the stomach and improve the digestive process include ginger and turmeric. Peppermint and ginger work well together for alleviating nausea.

GRAVES' DISEASE

Graves' disease is an autoimmune disorder characterized by an overproduction of thyroid hormone. Symptoms range from changes in mood, heart racing, muscle pains, insomnia, digestive issues, tremors of hands and fingers, increase in perspiration or warm, moist skin, enlargement of thyroid gland, irregular periods, changes in skin texture (thickening of the skin on the lower legs or red bumps; pretibial myxedema), eye problems like bulging (exophthalmos), pain, redness, and vision loss. Tests include TSH, free T4, free T3, thyroid stimulating immunoglobulins (TSI), and TSH receptor antibody.

Additional Integrative Modalities

Supplements

- B-complex (50 mg twice daily).
- L carnitine (start with 2,000 mg per day and work up to 4,000 mg per day as needed) can help reduce thyroid symptoms like heart palpitations, tremors, insomnia, and anxiety.

- CoQ10 (100–400 mg per day with a meal with fat) can help the muscle weakness and pain.
- Plant sterols balance the immune system.
- Selenium (200 mcg per day); may slow the progression of eye symptoms.
- Magnesium (400 mg per day) will help to prevent arrhythmias.
- Calcium citrate 1,000 mg (ages nineteen to fifty); 1,200 mg (women fifty-one and men over seventy-one), with optimizing vitamin D.
- Buggleweed (start with 2 mL three times daily and can increase after three days to 4 mL and three days later to 6 mL) can prevent thyroid damage and calms the thyroid, preventing the antibodies from binding to your thyroid.
- Motherwort liquid extract (start with 2 mL daily and after five days, increase to 4 mL) helps to improve thyroid symptoms like palpitations, sleep issues, appetite issues, and anxiety. Be sure to talk to your doctor, and don't take with sedating medications.
- Lemon balm (start with 300 mg and after seven days increase to 600 mg) inhibits the antibodies from binding to the thyroid gland.
- Glucomannan (start with 1.5 gm twice daily and then work up to 3.0 gm twice daily) decreases levels of circulating thyroid hormones in your body.

Homeopathy

- Iodium 30C is for the patient who feels very hot, is always in a hurry and obsessive and is dark-haired and dark-eyed.
- Natrum mur 30C is for palpitations and constipation. It is used for people who look anemic, are weak, and crave salt.
- Lycopus 30C is for the racing and pounding heart, which is felt due to nervous irritation and exophthalmos.
- Lodum helps to control palpitations that are worse even with minimal exertion.
- Sulphur can help with heat intolerance in those with hyperthyroidism.
- Pulsatilla is for those who can't tolerate heat and have no thirst.
- Lachesis helps those who can't wear tight clothes with hot flashes.
- Lodum is used for those who are losing weight despite having an increased appetite. They feel extremely hot and seek coolness.
- Lycopodium helps with weight loss, more in the upper body, and those who crave warm drinks and sweets.
- Phosphorus is for extreme weakness and stool that is excessive and offensive.
- Others that can be used are Kali iodatum, Ferrum metallicum, Luricum acidum, and Spongia tosta.

Acupressure

- GV17, ST9, P6, HT7, LI4, ST30

Aromatherapy

Essential oils can reduce stress and improve thyroid function. Frankincense (two drops daily on roof of mouth) and myrrh (on the thyroid area twice daily) can help, along with anti-inflammatory oils like lavender, rose, and tea tree oil. When combined with coconut oil, these can soothe the irritated skin.

HASHIMOTO'S

Hashimoto's is an autoimmune disease of the thyroid. Symptoms include fatigue, depression and mood disorders, weight gain, feeling cold easily, digestive issues, muscular pain, stiffness and swelling in the joints, hair loss, frequent urination and excessive thirst, and changes in menstrual period. Assessment includes TSH, free T4, free T3, antithyroglobulin antibody, antithyroid peroxidase antibodies (this can start to appear decades before it affects the TSH level), reverse T3, and ferritin. Others that can be checked are vitamin A, selenium, and zinc. Landmarks of healing include feeling better or eliminating all symptoms, reducing antibody count first under 100 then under 35 and regenerating thyroid tissue.

Additional Integrative Modalities

Supplements

- Probiotics.
- Multivitamin with vitamin A (5,000–10,000 IU per day).
- Vitamin E (400 IU).
- B vitamins like riboflavin (50 mg per day), niacin (200 mg per day), B6 (50 mg per day), folate (800 mcg per day), B12 (1,000 mcg per day of methylcobalamin), and biotin (5,000 mcg), B1 (600 mg per day) specifically for fatigue.
- Iodine (150–300 mcg per day).
- Zinc (25–50 mg per day).
- Magnesium (500 mg per day).
- Vitamin C (1,000 mg per day).
- Iron glycinate (25 mg per day [keep level between 50 and 100, if you are still menstruating]).

- Omega 3 fish oil (1,000 mg twice daily with food).
- Selenium (200–400 mcg) has been shown to regulate the hormones.
- Others: Antabine is a supplement that has been shown to reduce TPO antibodies by preventing the inflammatory immune system from responding. Can also add curcumin, Thytrophin PMG, or Drenatrophin PMG.
- *Children:* Hypothyroidism: iodine (50–900 mcg daily), selenium (20–200 mcg daily), tyrosine (500 mg daily), vitamin A (200,000 IU in one dose), seaweed (kelp) (2 tbsp daily).

Homeopathy

- Arsenicum 30C to be taken every twelve hours for up to five days while constitution remedy is found.
- Calcaria carbonica helps those with constipation (first part hard and soft stool) and perfuse menses.
- Sepia can be used with patients who are weak, have a pale yellow face, feel cold, and feel sensations of bearing down; it helps to control excessive hair loss. These patients crave acid foods and pickles.
- Lycopodium can be used for those who suffer from gastric problems with excessive flatulence, crave hot foods, and are weak and irritable.
- Graphites can help those who tire easily, are obese, become sad easily when listening to music, and are constipated and timid.
- Nux vomica is a remedy for those who have hypothyroidism and are easily offended, have constipation, are bloated after eating, have excessive desire for stimulants, and crave fatty foods and spicy foods. These people also feel cold.

Acupressure

- ST36, P6, KD3, GV7, KD7, SP6, LI10, LI11

Aromatherapy

Frankincense can help to lower thyroid antibodies when used in conjunction with other modalities. Peppermint oil can help to reduce brain fog, depression, headaches, and digestive issues. Lavender and myrtle may help to restore hair and calm anxiety. Others that can help with symptoms of hypothyroidism are lemongrass, myrrh, clove, basil, marjoram, rosemary, grapefruit, and clary sage.

MULTIPLE SCLEROSIS

Multiple sclerosis (MS) is a potentially disabling disease of the brain and spinal cord. It occurs when the immune system attacks the protective sheath (myelin) that covers the nerve fibers, damaging the nerves permanently. This causes communication problems within the nervous system. Signs and symptoms depend on the amount and location of nerve damage and may include fatigue, dizziness, slurred speech, prolonged double vision, involuntary movement of the eyes (nystagmus), tremor, problems with bowel and bladder function, lack of coordination, numbness or weakness in one or more limb or trunk (typically on one side of the body), and electrical shock sensations with certain movements (Lhermitte's sign). Diagnosis includes imaging and a spinal tap.

Additional Integrative Modalities

Supplements

- Vitamin E (400 mg of mixed tocotrienols or mixed tocopherols daily).
- Vitamin B complex use the higher potency (B-100) per day, including B6, B7 (biotin), and B12.
- Cyanocobalamin (1,000 mcg sublingually each day).
- L-methylfolate (levomefolic acid) (1,000 mcg daily).
- Coenzyme Q (200 mg daily) (doses up to 2,400 mg per day have been well tolerated; some note heartburn, digestive upset, and headaches with doses more than 600 mg per day; may reduce effectiveness of blood thinning medications).
- Digestive enzymes with protease, bromelain, amylase, and lipase.
- Algae (two to eight) capsules or up to one teaspoon of powder daily.
- Others include: Alpha lipoic acid (300–600 mg per day) for nerve pain; aged garlic to lower oxidative stress and improve blood flow.

Homeopathy

- Agaricus is most useful when the MS is accompanied by symptoms of uncoordinated eye movement, muscle spasms, twitching, and poor coordination. They may feel like sharp shooting pains, and your movements may be very weak and shaky.
- Alumina is for symptoms of weakness, progressive paralysis, heaviness of your lower extremities, confusion, and digestive issues like constipation. They may also have dry skin or mucous membranes. Symptoms

improve in open air and damp weather. They are worse in the morning, when you first wake up, and in a warm room.

- Argentum nitricum is for progressive paralysis, poor coordination, and loss of balance. Trembling is common in those who would benefit. They may always be in a rush, with multiple phobias.
- Arsenicum album benefits people who are more anxious, pessimistic, and restless. There may be progressive paralysis and burning sensations.
- Causticum is indicated when there is slow, progressive paralysis of the limbs, numbness of hands and feet, problems with breathing, swallowing, and speech, and incontinence issues. There may be numbness of the hands and the feet. Restlessness is present at night.
- Cocculus is for patients who have paralysis accompanied by dizziness when trying to focus on moving objects. You may have painful contracture of the limbs and trunk, and feel too weak to talk loudly.
- Conium is for paralysis of the eye muscles and ascending paralysis that begins with weakness and heaviness in the thighs and lower limbs. Symptoms are worse in the morning.
- Gelsemium sempervirens is helpful with trembling and weak muscles. The eyelids are heavy, and you may experience double vision and numbness of the face and tongue. Symptoms improve after urination. They may feel dizzy and drowsy.
- Ignatia amara will help when multiple sclerosis is accompanied by twitching and spasms, especially if the condition presents itself after grief. They may feel emotionally upset, and all their senses may become noticeably more acute.
- Kali phos is helpful when there is weakness in the back and limbs that becomes worse with exercise. This then leaves you in pain and very fatigued, and possibly unable to move the extremity.
- Lachesis is best when jealousy or anger worsen symptoms. Symptoms are more left-sided. Symptoms worsen during the premenstrual phase or start with menopause.
- Natrum muriaticum helps when optic neuritis (eye pain and temporary vision loss) is present, along with numbness throughout the body. Symptoms are worse in the sun; they may come on after grief. Their mood may be low. There are symptoms of awkwardness, such as dropping things.
- Nux vomica helps when they crave alcohol and stimulants. They may also be irritable, highly driven, and intolerant to contradiction. Paralysis is accompanied by muscle spasms, cramps, twitching, and spasmodic digestive signs.

- Magnesia phos is helpful when there are painful spasms of twitching or jerking, and symptoms are improved by pressure, friction, and warmth.
- Phosphorus is best used when there are problems with vision and incontinence. Numbness in the hands and the feet are also present. These patients may also crave ice-cold drinks. Their reflexes are exaggerated, they tend to faint easily, and episodes are linked to any emotional upset.
- Plumbum is for progressive paralysis, heaviness and wasting of the muscles, especially in the legs.
- Tarentula is useful when there are very jerky movements of the hands, feet, and tongue.

Acupressure

- GV20 (this point helps with headaches, poor memory, mental disorders, ringing in the ears, fatigue, and poor sleep)
- GV26, P6, LU9, GB34, LU1 (if you feel anxious or depressed)
- GV26 (reduces muscle spasms and relieves dizziness)
- ST36 (improves digestion)
- SP6, H7, B2, B23, B13, GB20, and LV3

Aromatherapy

For people with MS, relaxing oils are important, along with those that support the neurological system. Find the ones that work the best for you and then rotate them as needed. Frankincense and helichrysum support the neurological system. Frankincense can be taken internally, two drops three times per day for three weeks, then take one week off, and then the cycle can be repeated. Helichrysum can be applied to the neck or temples two times per day. Basil oil and cypress oil can reduce MS symptoms by improving circulation and muscle tone. Other good choices are lavender, jasmine, neroli, geranium, ylang-ylang, and rose.

Systemic Lupus Erythematosus (SLE or Lupus)

Lupus is a chronic condition in which your body's immune system attacks your own tissues. It may affect many different body systems, including your skin, brain, heart, lungs, and blood cells.

Symptoms vary from person to person, and no two cases of lupus are exactly the same. Signs and symptoms may come on suddenly or develop slowly and may be mild or severe, temporary or permanent.

The signs and symptoms of lupus that you experience will depend on which body systems are affected by the disease. The most common signs and symptoms include fatigue, joint pain, dry eyes, sensitivity to the sun, skin lesions that appear worse in the sun, chest pain, butterfly-shaped rash on the face that covers the bridge of the nose and cheeks, fingers and toes that turn white or blue when exposed to stress or cold weather (Raynaud's phenomenon), headaches, confusion, and memory loss. Diagnosis can be made via history, physical exam, and laboratory testing.

Additional Integrative Modalities

Supplements

- Plant sterols and sterolins (20 mg three times daily on an empty stomach).
- Methylsulfonylmethane (MSM) (2,000–8,000 mg daily) has natural anti-inflammatory benefits. Reduce the dosage if diarrhea occurs.
- Digestive enzymes (1 or 2 capsules of a full-spectrum enzyme product with each meal).
- Green superfood supplement chlorella and spirulina are key in alkalizing and detoxifying the body.
- Boswellia (1,200–1,500 mg of a standardized extract containing 60–65 percent boswellic acids two to three times daily) anti-inflammatory effects.
- DHEA: this supplement helps support your adrenal hormones. Have your doctor measure DHEA-S in the blood, and take supplements of DHEA to get your levels over 100 mcg/dl. The usual dose I recommend is 25 mg, but you should have your DHEA-S level checked to make sure this is the right dose for you.
- Indole-3-carbinol (DIM), broccoli extracts, and sulforaphane: all of these help detoxify estrogens.

Homeopathy

- Arsenicum album helps for anxious and restless individuals, and have a sensation of burning in their joints that feels better when warmth is applied.
- Belladonna is best when pain and swelling come on suddenly. The joints are hot and red, with a burning sensation that feels worse with motion.

- Sepia is for women with lupus who find that their symptoms flare up near their menstrual cycle and experience constipation, depression, irritability, and a tendency to be cold. They may crave sweet, salty, and sour foods.
- Pulsatilla works best when the symptoms improve with cold and if the pain wanders from joint to joint.
- Rhus toxicodendron is for those who have pain that increases with rest and is worse in the cold and the damp. A major symptom is stiffness of joints that improves with some movement and warmth.
- Sulphur is suitable if you have strong cravings for spicy foods and ice-cold drinks. They get overheated easily and have burning pains that are relieved with cold applications.

Acupressure

- S13 (stiff neck, headaches, ringing in the ears, weakness of the arms and spasms/back, ache of the back muscles)
- GV26, SP10, SP4, SP6, SP21, LI4, LI11, LV3, LV5

Aromatherapy

Use essential oils that promote relaxation, help with digestion, and support the neurological system. Some good choices to start with are lemon verbena, lavender, rose, jasmine, and geranium. Black pepper and ginger encourage blood flow and will help revive tired joints and muscles. For digestive issues, you may take three drops of ginger oil internally two to three times daily. Frankincense essential oil is effective at reducing inflammation and immune reactions. Helichrysum oil supports the nervous system. For skin inflammation, lavender and geranium oils work well. Lemon balm or juniper in a hot bath can help to detoxify the body, lowering inflammation.

RHEUMATOID ARTHRITIS

Rheumatoid arthritis (RA) occurs when inflammation attacks the lining of your joints in addition to a wide variety of other body systems, including the eyes, lungs, heart, blood vessels, and skin. Signs and symptoms of rheumatoid arthritis may include fatigue, fever, weight loss, joint stiffness (usually worse in the morning and after inactivity), and tender, warm, swollen joints (early on it can affect your smaller joints and then may progress to larger joints like wrists, elbows, shoulders, knees, and hips). Diagnosis is made via history, a physical, and lab work.

Additional Integrative Modalities

Supplements

- Gamma linoleic acid (GLA) (450–500 mg per day).
- Curcumin and boswellia reduce pain and inflammation in the joints. You can use curcumin alone or in a combination product.
- Turmeric (1,000 mg once a day).
- Fish oil (1–3 g of EPA/DHA per day).
- Others: bromelain, MSM, glucosamine, vitamin C (500–1000 mg per day), selenium (200–400 mcg per day), vitamin E (200–400 IU per day), ginger (100–200 mg three times per day) and choosing one of the following- grapeseed extract (100–300 mg per day), pinebark extract (100–300 mg per day), or antioxidants.
- *Juvenile RA*: 5 MTHF (200–400 mcg daily), vitamin C (500–1,000 mg daily), calcium (1,000 mg daily), vitamin D (1,000–4,000 IU daily), CoQ10 (10–250 mg daily), vitamin E (200–400 IU daily), fish oil (2–4 g of EPA daily), zinc (10–20 mg daily), selenium (20–200 mcg daily), castor oil applied topically to the joints daily.

Homeopathy

- Bryonia is for severe pain that is made worse by movement, the slightest touch, or heat, and is relieved by cold applications.
- Pulsatilla is for pains that pass from one part of the body to another and are made worse by warm environments. It's suitable if you have a hard time digesting fatty food and tend to feel sad.
- Causticum is for pains that are accompanied by muscle spasms and tend to improve in wet weather or with warmth.
- Rhus tox is for stiffness that tends to wear off with movement, thereby causing restlessness. The aching and stiffness are worse in cold and damp weather, after rest, or in the morning.
- Colchicum is for stiffness and pain that is worse in the winter and during the nighttime hours.
- Dulcamara is for stiffness and pain that is worse when you are overheated, and in cold or damp weather.
- Mercurius is for aches and pains that are worsened by heat and cold, worse at night, and accompanied by offensive sweat.
- Ruta is useful when you have pain that especially affects the tendonous insertions of muscles and large joints.
- Rhododendron is for aches and pains that are worse in cold weather and during electrical storms. Pain is located in the muscles and ligaments.

- Calcarea hypophos is for sharp pains in the wrists and hands.
- Aconite is for the sudden onset of sharp pain, worse in cold and dry weather, with general feelings of restlessness and anxiety.

Acupressure

- The Yang Lin Qian point (for inflammation and joint pain)
- LI4, LV2, LV5, GB 41, GB34

Aromatherapy

Ginger essential oil has anti-inflammatory and analgesic effects; other helpful oils include juniper, vetiver, ylang-ylang, turmeric, frankincense, myrrh, and orange essential oils.

• *6* •

Cardiology

Love cures all. Without our heart, there is no love. Let's extinguish the flames in our heart, to allow unconditional love to penetrate deep into the cracks of the world, as love knows no boundaries.

D & D: SPECIAL CONSIDERATIONS

Almost all cardiac risk factors are related to lifestyle, environment, and inflammation, so treating insulin resistance and lowering inflammation are the cornerstones of preventing and healing heart disease. Adding herbs and spices like turmeric, garlic, ginger, cinnamon, curry powder, rosemary, thyme, basil, chili peppers, and coriander, and focusing on fiber and healthy fats are important for anyone suffering from cardiac illnesses. Drinking tea like green tea, black tea, and oolong tea is great for the heart as it contains flavonoids and has an anti-clotting effect. Increase fiber up to 50 g per day, eating foods like nuts, seeds, berries, and veggies. High-potassium foods like avocados, melons, spinach, broccoli, squash, and apple cider vinegar (which helps keep the body alkaline) have been shown to improve blood pressure; omega 3 foods like grass-fed beef, wild-caught salmon, chia, and flax are great for the heart. Other foods to focus on are pomegranate juice (8 oz)/seeds, watercress, goji berries, apples, capers, olives, onions, green pepper, and scallions. Limit/eliminate alcohol and caffeine and eat about an ounce of dark chocolate daily (Yay!). Detoxifying your environment from lead, cadmium, and mercury is important.

THE FOUR BIG S's: SPECIAL CONSIDERATIONS

Stress has the ability to raise blood pressures as it constricts blood vessels and worsens heart disease, so adopting a daily relaxation technique is important, as previously discussed. Moderate exercise helps you lower your insulin resistance, inflammation, and blood pressure. Consulting a doctor before starting an exercise program is important, as some may have special needs that need to first be addressed. Chiropractic care can improve cardiovascular problems.

CORONARY HEART DISEASE

Coronary heart disease is a chronic disease where plaque (a waxy substance) builds up, over many years, inside your coronary arteries, which supply oxygen-rich blood to your heart. Signs and symptoms are pain in the chest or radiating into the upper extremity, neck, jaw, or back; this may even feel like indigestion and include shortness of breath, sleep issues, and fatigue. Pain can be triggered by stress and gets worse with activity. If you are having any pain, go to the nearest emergency room immediately. Once the acute issue is over, preventing another attack can be accomplished with lifestyle changes.

Labs that can be done to further assess overall heart health and risk are micronutrient testing, carotid doppler, stress testing, and coronary artery calcium scoring and carotid intima media thickness test for anyone with a risk of early heart disease, especially once they reach the age of fifty, especially if they smoke, have high cholesterol, or have a family history of vascular disease. Those who want to know where they stand with high cholesterol or already have heart disease can obtain an Endo PAT testing.

Advanced lipid testing breaks down lipoprotein particles by size and subclasses, and gives you more insight into if your elevated levels are problematic, small and dense, or safe and fluffy and also looks at oxidative stress, endothelial dysfunction, and markers of inflammation. The small damaged particles will sneak through the blood vessel cracks and lead to plaque buildup; the smaller the LDL, the more prone to oxidation, similar to HDL, which can be damaged from sugar and toxins.

Comprehensive nutrition panels, like ION panel testing, are very helpful for coronary vascular disease prevention and treatment. This evaluates amino acids, vitamins, minerals, antioxidants, fats, urinary organic acid (evaluates how effective your body can turn food into energy), and heavy metals, as deficiencies may lead to chronic illnesses and endothelial dysfunction. Once these deficiencies have been addressed, one can significantly reduce cardiovascular disease risk, as long as you're also addressing lifestyle modifications, as discussed previously.

Obtaining a lipoprotein alpha test will help to detect early cardiovascular disease, especially in the presence of an abnormal calcium score and thick carotid artery scan. Always look at the entire picture and don't concentrate on just one value itself.

Additional Integrative Modalities

Supplements

- Fish oil (one tablespoon daily).
- B vitamins with B1, B3 (niacin 500 mg two to three times daily), B6 (50 mg per day), B9, and B12.
- Taurine (3 g twice daily).
- Coenzyme Q10 (100–300 mg daily) this nutrient is an antioxidant that protects the heart and blood vessels from the damaging effects of free radical damage and helps to stabilize blood sugar.
- Garlic (Allium sativum) (1,200 mg per day) antioxidant and natural blood thinning properties it reduces cholesterol and homocysteine.
- Curcumin (500–1,000 mg per day).
- Magnesium (500 mg daily) for improved circulation and reduced blood pressure.
- Carotenoids.
- Vitamin C (250–500 mg twice daily) Do not take vitamin C when you're going to have lab tests; more than 300 mg of supplemental vitamin C within twenty-four hours of testing can interfere with numerous lab tests.
- Vitamins D, E, and K.
- Carnitine tartrate to produce ADP and power the heart (500–1,000 mg twice daily up to 3 g twice daily).
- Other supplements: quercetin (250–1,000 mg per day), choline (no drug interactions, do not exceed the upper limit of 3,500 mg per day, and make sure you are taking with other B vitamins, particularly pantothenic acid), grapeseed extract (300 mg per day), L-citruline (500 mg per day), sytrinol (150 mg per day), ALA (300 mg twice daily), PQQ (20 mg per day), pterostilbene (50 mg per day), ribose (5 g two to three times daily; enhances mitochondrial energy production), NAC (600 mg per day), reversatrol (250 mg per day), alpha lipoic acid, l-theanine, green tea extract, ashwaganda, berberine (500–1,000 mg per day), selenium, red yeast rice (1,200–2,400 mg daily; lowers LDL cholesterol

and reduces heart-related deaths), and hawthorn (500–900 mg daily) improves circulation to the heart and reduces blood pressure. Glucomannan capsules can help to bind toxins. Branched-chain amino acids (leucine, valine, isoleucine 4:1:1 ratio; 5,000 mg per day), phosphatidyl serine 300–600 mg twice daily.
- Plaque stabilization and reversal/reduction: Vitamin K2 (Menaquinone-7) (100–500 mcg per day) and MK4 (1,000 mcg per day), omega 3 (5 g per day), aged garlic extract (600–1,200 mg twice per day), curcumin (1,000–5,000 mg per day), quercetin (500 mg twice daily), vitamin C (1,000 mg twice daily).

Homeopathy

If you have cardiovascular disease, see a licensed homeopath for a constitutional remedy. If any of the following remedies seem appropriate for you, try them, but only on a temporary or emergency basis. After that, see a homeopath for further help. Homeopathy may help you recover from a heart attack. Once you've received emergency help and are under a doctor's care, consult with a naturopathic or homeopathic practitioner. If you have symptoms of a heart attack, call 911 and follow the responder's instructions. While you're waiting for the ambulance to arrive, you can take a 30C potency every two or three minutes.

- Aconitum napellus is for numbness and pain in the left arm. The person feels very fearful and anxious.
- Arnica is helpful when you have the sensation that your heart is being squeezed or you feel a bruising pain.
- Cactus can also ease the pain of angina. Take it if you feel as if a band is tightening around your chest.

Acupressure

- H3, H4, H7 (stimulates circulation)
- GV 24.5 (produces sense of calm)
- CV17 (reduces sadness or anxiety)
- P3 (eases pain)
- P6 (improves anxiety caused by heart palpitations)
- SP4
- B15
- Chest pain: HP4, HP7, HP6, K27, CV14, CV17

Aromatherapy

Essential oils can help heal inflammation and symptoms related to heart disease, as they contain anti-inflammatory components and help to reduce oxidative stress. Some include ylang ylang, lemon oil, frankincense, lemongrass, ginger, and helichrysum. To improve poor circulation, a stimulating rosemary massage can be used, by combining almond oil, thyme essential oil, black pepper oil, ginger oil, rosemary oil, and clove oil.

HYPERLIPIDEMIA

One in three Americans is dealing with elevated cholesterol. Cholesterol plays an important role in our body, but we are constantly demonizing and looking toward statins as our savior. Statins block the enzymes (HMG-CoA reductase) that reduce the cholesterol production in the liver that thereby lowers the cholesterol in our blood. Studies show that among people who take statins for five years, only one in eighty-three lives are saved; one out of one hundred develop diabetes; one out of ten suffer from muscular damage; and 18 percent develop undesirable side effects like liver dysfunction, memory loss, increased cancer risk, anemia, and sexual dysfunction. Statins also block CoQ10 (an enzyme that acts as an antioxidant, plays a key role in cellular energy production, is needed for your heart to work effectively, and maintains blood glucose levels). Though some can benefit from a statin, always talk to your doctor about risks versus benefits, as alternatives are present, depending on your condition and unique situation.

Additional Integrative Modalities

Supplements

- Fish oil (1–2 g of EPA/EHA per day) helps to reduce cholesterol and triglycerides.
- CoQ10 (200–300 mg daily) especially if you're on lipid-lowering meds.
- Red yeast rice (start with 600 mg twice a day to 1,200 mg twice daily at bedtime); take 25–100 mg of CoQ10 when using this product to prevent possible deficiency. Look for a citrinin free product.
- B vitamin like niacin (1,500–3,000 mg per day, if diabetic); high doses of niacin can lead to increased blood sugar levels.
- B5 (pantothenic acid).

- Chromium.
- Choline.
- Phytosterols, plant sterols, and stanols: (2,000 mg per day).
- Others: Garlic (500 mg per day) lowers cholesterol and increases HDL; berberine (500 two to three times per day), guggul (daily total of 1,500 mg standardized to 5%; guggulsterone (equivalent to 75 mg of guggulsterones) increases HDL and reduces cholesterol; two to four capsules of glucomannan fifteen minutes before meals with a glass of water; artichoke extract (500 mg three times daily); acetyl l carnitine (1,000 mg daily) for high triglycerides.
- *Children:* fish oil (EPA/DHA 1–2 g daily), pycnogenol 50–100 mg daily, vitamin B3 (5–20 mg daily), green tea (decaf 4–6 cups daily), psyllium (6 g daily), plant sterols (2–2.5 g daily).

Homeopathy

- Allium sativum is a remedy for those who eat excessive meat, with symptoms of belching, burning, and increased appetite.
- Aurum metallicum can help those with a rapid pulse, depression, or anger over any contraindication with pain behind the sternum, especially at night.
- Baryta muriaticum is indicated for those who are elderly with symptoms of vertigo and heaviness.
- Nux vomica can be used for those who crave alcohol and fatty foods.
- Calcarea carbonica is a remedy for those who are overweight, sensitive to cold, and have continuous perspiration on scalp and tightness in chest with palpitations.
- Lycopodium helps when patient desires sweets and has symptoms of flatulence and other digestive symptoms.

Acupressure

- Liver point, LI11, LI4 and LV3

Aromatherapy

Essential oils can lower cholesterol levels, as they decrease emotional stress, improve circulation, and have cardio supportive and antioxidant properties. Essential oils like lavender, cypress, and rosemary oil can help overall health.

HYPERTENSION

Hypertension, or high blood pressure, refers to the amount of resistance to blood flow in your arteries and the amount of blood your heart is able to pump. Most individuals don't have symptoms, but some can have headaches, nosebleeds, or even shortness of breath with severe hypertension. Diagnosis is made with a history and measuring your blood pressure during an office visit.

Additional Integrative Modalities

Supplements

If you are already taking BP medication, talk to your doctor, as it may lower it further and can be very dangerous.

- Omega 3 fatty acids (1,000–2,000 mg daily of EPA and DHA); has been shown to reduce blood pressure when taken long term.
- Magnesium (500 mg daily); helps to relax smooth muscles.
- Coenzyme Q10 (100–300 mg daily); studies show that this nutrient reduces blood pressure and is a great antioxidant for supporting heart health. If taking warfarin, you should be monitored as it lowers warfarin levels. Side effects are gastrointestinal symptoms.
- Garlic (600 mg aged extract).
- Others—Vitamin C (600 mg daily) induces sodium dieresis; L arginine (4–8 g per day), or L-citrulline (2–4 g per day); Hawthorn (Crataegus oxycanthae) (250 mg of a standardized extract three times daily), dilates the artery walls and decreases blood pressure; Hibiscus (1.25 g in tea form, mixed in 240 ml of water, three times daily).
- If on meds like diuretics, take calcium (750 mg), potassium (100 mg), vitamin B1 (300 mg), P5P50 (50 mg), zinc (25 mg), magnesium glycinate (240 mg per day), or if on a beta blocker, then start CoQ10 (start 200–300 mg per day) and melatonin (6 mg at bedtime).
- *Children:* fish oil (EPA/DHA 1–2 g daily), magnesium (200–400 mg daily), arginine (1–2 g daily).

Homeopathy

Atherosclerosis

- Arsenicum album can be used in those who are pale, thin, and cold sensitive. They can present with alternating weakness and vascular lesion.

- Arsenicum iodatum can help to prevent sclerosis of the artery, both as a preventative and curative effect (five pellets daily to once a week).
- Baryta carbonica is a remedy for elderly individuals who have high blood pressure, memory disorders, headaches, fatigue, palpitations, and possibly an aneurysm.
- Sulphur is for hyperphagic individuals with a psoric reaction mode with congestive or hypersensitive manipulations.
- Thuja occidentalis patients are usually obese in the truncal areas.
- Natrum sulphuricum 15C is indicated when the trunk, shoulders, and hips get heavy and when there's a tendency to joint pain, bronchitis, and frequent diarrhea.
- Natrum muriaticum is for those with high blood pressure that begins after an emotional upset, who crave salt, have incredible thirst, and dislike the sun. Such persons desire to be alone and often experience headaches, heart palpitations, and insomnia.
- Phosphorus can help those with bouts of labile hypertension, who crave salt, feel nervous and high strung, and present with frequent fainting spells.
- Vanadium is a remedy for those with frequent fainting spells, dizziness, feelings of compression, confusion, general mental deterioration; the heart feels like it is being compressed in the chest, and liver problems are present.
- Glonoinum can be used for those with pounding sensation in the artery accompanied with attacks of tachycardia, congestion, and a tight headache, with flushed face and throbbing pains in the carotids that get worse with heat and sun exposure or from alcohol.
- Arnica helps to limit hemorrhage and edema and prevents thrombosis, as it acts specifically on the capillaries.
- Arsenicum metallicum (9C daily) can be taken if you are anxious, depressive, have hypertensive vascular erethism with palpitations, extra systoles, hot flashes; improvement occurs with hot air.
- Aconitum hypertension occurs in acute attacks with congested face, tense pulse, severe headaches, and palpitations; patient is anxious and agitated.
- Argentum nitricum is a remedy for symptoms that occur with stress and patient craves salt and sweet foods.
- Belladonna is a remedy for a flushed face and pounding headaches; patients feel immediate heat, but hands and feet are cold; they are sensitive to light.
- Lachesis is prescribed for general symptoms of suspiciousness, jealousy, and talkativeness. The person feels warm, congested, and is intolerant

to anything touching the neck. Patient has a tendency toward bruising and is susceptible to hypertension during menopause; symptoms improve with blood flowing, like menstrual periods or a nosebleed.

- Nux vomica is for high blood pressure that occurs from the effects of stress. The person feels irritable and impatient and has a strong desire for stimulants such as coffee, as well as alcohol. The person overeats, drinks a lot, has digestive issues, is usually chilly, and is prone to constipation; symptoms improve after a short nap.
- Ignatia is for those with sudden increases in blood pressure and who are hypersensitive to worries and frustrations.
- Arsenicum album (15C) is for lipid disorders.
- Calcarea fluorica is indicated with early onset of atherosclerosis and for those who have hyperlaxity of ligaments.
- Lycopodium is useful for those with heart disease, cholesterol issues, liver disorders, uric acid, or kidney disorders.
- Plumbum metallicum is indicated for those with renal insufficiency, thin arteries, and the elderly.
- Silicea helps those who are thin, have a tendency toward osteoporosis, and have chronic supporations.
- Calcarea carbonica (15C) helps when obesity runs in the family; the person has a tendency toward diabetes, polyposis, and kidney or vesicular stones.

Acupressure

- ST36, H7, LI11 P6, LV2 (acute stage)
- LV3 (during remission)
- GB 20, K3, B38, CV17 (if feel chest tension when stressed)
- GV 20, LI4, K1, GB34

Aromatherapy

Essential oils help to decrease emotional and oxidative stress, dilating arteries. Lavender, ylang-ylang, frankincense, geranium, mandarin, marjoram, eucalyptus citriodora, yarrow, and clary sage calm your body, bringing down your blood pressure. Massaging with juniper oil will help break down the fatty deposits in your body and arteries. Others that can be tried for hardening of the arteries (atherosclerosis) are lemon, ginger, black pepper, basil, linalool, rosemary, cineole, and juniper.

• 7 •

Dental Health

We underestimate the power of a single smile. A smile has the potential to change another's life forever, healing from the inside out. So wear your smile proudly!

D & D: SPECIAL CONSIDERATIONS

Healing the gut, keeping blood sugar regulated, and creating an alkaline environment is key in healing tooth decay and getting you on the path to remineralization. Four things can contribute to tooth decay: lack of minerals in the diet, like magnesium, calcium, and phosphorus; lack of fat-soluble vitamins like D, A, E, and K; too much sugar consumption; and too much phytic-acid-rich foods. Limiting foods with phytic acid—like grains, nuts, seeds, and legumes—especially when starting off the process of remineralization, and incorporating soups with gut-healing bone broth should be practiced daily. Also eat high amounts of fat-soluble vitamins and healthy fats from fermented cod liver oil, grass-fed organic raw dairy (if tolerated, eat butter), seafood, and coconut oil. Focus on bone broths and organ and gland meats like bone marrow and liver help to boost the endocrine system and balance hormones. Monitor your sweet intake, including maple syrup, fruit, and honey. Activator X is important in tooth mineralization and is found in primarily grass-fed butter and raw milk, needed for bright white healthy teeth. Aim for 1–1.5 tablespoons per day of grass-fed butter if tolerated. Other foods to incorporate for healthy teeth are zucchini, string beans, kale, chard, seaweed, vegetable juice, and fermented foods. Cranberry juice has anti-adhesion properties and can decrease bad bacteria in your mouth. Adding a remineralizing or special probiotic toothpaste and practicing oil pulling can help to support tooth and gum health. To help prevent gum disease, aim at the gum line while brushing. Charcoal can help to whiten teeth. To optimize oral health further, use colloidal silver (swish and swallow with one teaspoon three times per day for sixty seconds) and spray xylitol on your gums three times per day.

THE FOUR BIG S's: SPECIAL CONSIDERATIONS

Lowering stress and getting enough sleep have a large impact on oral health. Doing these things can stabilize hormones and optimize calcium and other nutrient levels in the body. Practicing gratitude daily will keep you smiling.

TOOTH DECAY

Additional Integrative Modalities

Supplements

- Fermented cod liver oil (total of ½–1½ tsp per day).
- Magnesium.
- Gelatin.
- Vitamin C.
- Vitamin D.
- B vitamins like B6, B9, B12.
- Vitamin K.
- CoQ10.
- Omega 3.
- Oral probiotics.
- Zinc.
- Calcium.
- For added fat-soluble nutrients add skate liver oil (⅛–¼ tsp two to three times per day).
- Butter and fermented cod liver oil mixtures.
- *Children:* 25 lbs—¼ tsp per day; 35 lbs—⅓ tsp per day; 45 lbs—½ tsp per day; 55 lbs—⅔ tsp per day.

Homeopathy

- Mercurius is a remedy for tooth decay that is black and loose with bleeding gums and excessive salivation.

- Silicea is indicated for those with multiple teeth that are decayed, and is especially used for thin children with a large head.
- Calcarea helps those who are overweight, prone to head sweats, and decays in many teeth.
- Kreosotum is indicated for those with black tooth decay with a foul smelling breath, and the patient is usually constipated.
- Sulphur is best for those with tooth decay and are sensitive to touch; teeth are black and hurt after food or drink.

Toothache:

- Plantago is used for a tooth pain that improves with eating and worsens with cold air or pressure. Mouth is full of saliva. Tooth pain feels nervy.
- Coffea is for pain that is improved with cold and worse with heat.
- Chamomilla is indicated for unbearable pain, accompanied with a sore head, pain worsened with food, drink, coffee at night and by cold air.
- Mercuris is for tooth pain that shoots up to the ears, loose teeth, tender gums that bleed easily with bad breath. This patient is very thirsty.
- Staphisagria is a remedy for tearing toothache, with red cheeks and a disintegrating black tooth. Pain is worse with pressure, food, and cold air.
- Pulsatilla is indicated for tooth pain that is improved in open air and cold water, worsened with hot food or drink. This person isn't thirsty.
- Arnica is for pain after a filling or an extraction.
- Belladonna is indicated for a developing boil of the gums that leads to throbbing pain and a dry mouth.
- Apis is a remedy for those with burning, stinging toothache. The gums feel swollen and tight.
- Bryonia is indicated for teeth that feel too long with pain that is improved on lying down on the painful side and when pressure is applied. Pain is worse with hot food and drink and movement.
- Calcarea is for toothache that is worse with food or cold drinks and pregnancy.
- Magnesia phosphorica is for electric-shock-type pain that is soothed by warmth.

Acupressure

- LI4, ST6, ST7, ST36, TW13, ST44, K3, SJ2, SJ5, GV14, SI18
- Lower jaw: ST6, ST5, TB17
- Molars: TB23, GB2
- Distal parts: L11, LI4, ST40, B60

Aromatherapy

Essential oils can reduce gum inflammation; for example, myrrh and clove have a numbing effect to help relieve pain and soreness. Oregano can reduce bad breath as it is an antibacterial. German chamomile and lemon can also be used for a toothache. Others that are good for mouth and gum care are cistus, cardamom, fennel, tea tree, peppermint, and nutmeg. You can use peppermint oil, along with tea tree oil, added to your toothbrush for natural whitening.

• 8 •

Dermatology

Beauty is actually microbiome deep! By extinguishing the flames in the body, we can take you to a whole new awe-inspiring level. You are truly beautiful (or handsome), inside and out!

D & D: SPECIAL CONSIDERATIONS

Your skin is your body's largest living and breathing organ. Just like your digestive system, your skin also takes in nutrients from your blood, processes and detoxifies it, and contains its own microbiome. Wait! Did you think that was only in the gut? Nope, your skin is also covered with trillions of organisms like bacteria, fungi, parasites, and yeast that live in and on your body, even after you take a shower! Acne, rosacea, and other rashes are due to bacterial overgrowth or imbalance, at least in part. Regulating your blood sugar level and healing your gut are important vital steps in managing and treating rashes, breakouts, and other chronic skin conditions. Elevated blood sugar can also increase acute inflammation, leading to an inflammatory response—a pimple.

A diet rich in antioxidants helps to neutralize all the damaging effects of free radicals—protecting your skin and slowing down aging. So choosing red, yellow, and green fruits and veggies can get you the antioxidants you need.

Adding healthy oils and fatty acids can help to protect your skin, leaving it soft and supple. Excellent sources of omega 3s are salmons, sardines, flaxseeds, Brazil nuts, walnuts, and almonds and alpha linolenic acid from olive oils, and seeds. Add foods like broccoli, egg yolks, onions, and red pepper, as they are important for collagen production for proteins, magnesium, copper, and zinc and high in cysteine for optimal hair and nails. Also add in silicon-rich foods like green beans and spinach. Other foods great for skin are plums, green tea, spinach, peas, and apricots. Optimize hair health with foods like healthy fats, eggs, shrimp, kale, pumpkins, squash, and strawberries. Watch your salt intake, as it can lead to puffy eyelids, swollen legs and ankles, and the iodine can lead to acne flare-ups. Sometimes a diet with low histamine can make a difference (low in avocados, eggplant, spinach, tomatoes, bacon, and dried fruits). And hydrate, hydrate, and hydrate some more for healthy and vibrant skin that glows!

What you put on your skin is as important as what you put in your body. Use all natural/organic skincare products and even take off makeup with olive, sesame, coconut, grapeseed, avocado, and sunflower oil.

THE FOUR BIG S's: SPECIAL CONSIDERATIONS

Flare-ups of skin inflammation often occur after a stressful event, so relaxation and even changing your attitude about stressful situations will decrease flares and optimize healing. Optimal sleep helps give your body time for skin repair and rejuvenation.

ACNE

Your pores are open to allow your hair to grow and to allow secretion of your sebum (oil) from the sebaceous (oil glands) glands. When these pores get blocked, the excess oil builds up and triggers the rapid growth of a bacteria called propionibacterium acnes, but when it grows too quickly a pimple forms. Your pores can get blocked by dead skin cells, overactive oil glands, the bacteria p. acnes (the more you have, the more you break out), and inflammation. These clogged pores can lead to whiteheads, blackheads, and cysts. Diagnosis made via history and exam.

Additional Integrative Modalities

Supplements

- Zinc (50 mg twice daily with meals for three months, then can be reduced to 50 mg daily); can take copper (3–5 mg) along with the zinc; zinc sulfate isn't easily absorbed.
- Nicotinomide (750 mg, Zn 25 mg, Cu 1.5 mg, folic acid 500 mcg per day, vitamin B6 daily for four to eight weeks) can reduce pimples.
- Tea tree oil (5% solution diluted in water, dabbed on blemishes twice daily) can act similarly to benzoyl peroxide.
- Vitex (chasteberry) (160 mg of a standardized Vitex extract) reduce acne formation.

- Others: Vitamin A (2,000–4,000 IU daily) reduces oil and keratin production (going over the upper limit can be a problem as it can be dangerous for pregnant women; prenatal vitamins should not contain more than 3,000 IU of performed vitamin A), Burdock root (Arctium lappa) (300–500 mg of the capsule form/thirty drops of tincture/1 cup of tea three times daily).
- Topical steam treatment: pour boiling water over strawberry leaves, eucalyptus, thyme, and wintergreen; place towel over head and lean over the bowl for ten to fifteen minutes.
- Natural clay mask: tablespoons of Bentonite clay or Fuller's earth with a rose water to form a paste 10 minutes.
- *Children:* Acne: vitamin A (1,000–5,000 IU daily), B3 (4% niacinamide wash applied topically daily), zinc (10 mg daily).

Homeopathy

- Antimonium crudum helps acne associated with digestive disorders.
- Calcarea sulphurica can help chronic or cystic acne that presents with a yellowish discharge.
- Hepar sulphuris calcareum helps acne that is filled with pus and is painful when touched, improved with warmth.
- Ledum palustre helps with pustular acne on the nose and cheeks that feels better with cold.
- Pulsatilla is for those with acne associated with hormonal changes.
- Silicea is for chronic white pustules.
- Selenium is best for acne accompanied with hyperseborrhe and hair loss.
- Sulphur is for those with inflamed, sore, red acne, worsened with heat. Patient also experiences impatience, irritability, and mood swings. Washing or heat can aggravate the symptoms.
- Nux vomica is indicated in acne that is aggravated by excessive consumption of medications, stimulants, or rich food.
- Kali bromatum is for teenagers who are easily depressed and anxious and have acne. Anxiety is shown by nonstop movement.
- Eugenia jambosa is for acne with a little white suppuration spot in the center.

Acupressure

- LI4, LU5, CV9
- Others: GB14, SP10, B23, B47, ST2, B10

Aromatherapy

Lavender oil, germanium, and bergamot (an astringent and antidepressant) can help to improve inflammation. When the skin improves, apply a lotion made with diluted water, lavender, and orange blossom to reduce scarring. Others that can be helpful are clove, geranium, lavender, and tea tree oils. Clary sage, juniper, lemongrass, mandarin, and lemon can help with blackheads.

ECZEMA

Eczema is a chronic skin condition, where an itchy, red rash appears all over the body. Symptoms include dry, red, inflamed, sensitive skin, intense itching, recurring rash, scaly areas, and rough, leathery patches that can be accompanied with oozing or crusting. Diagnosis made via history and physical.

Additional Integrative Modalities

Supplements

- Essential fatty acids (1–2 g EPA/DHA daily or 2 tbsp of flaxseed oil daily).
- Evening primrose oil (3 g daily) or borage oil contains GLA that can be used orally or topically.
- Vitamin E (400 IU) helps the body use the fatty acids and promotes wound healing.
- Others: Burdock root (Arctium lappa) (300 mg capsule or 1 ml of tincture form) helps to cleanse the skin; vitamin C with bioflavonoids (1–3 g daily) improves the immune system; natural creams with chamomile; licorice root gel 2% (to reduce inflammation and itching); zinc (50 mg three times daily for six weeks); copper (2 mg daily); black cumin seed oil (20–40 mg daily per pound of body weight) (can take orally or mixed with lotion onto skin); Neem oil; quercetin (500–1,000 mg three to four times daily) as an anti-inflammatory; and turmeric, which is also anti-inflammatory. Improve wound healing with B5, C, zinc, and fatty acids.
- *Children:* fish oil (EPA/DHA 1,000–4,000 mg daily), probiotics, vitamin D (1,000–4,000 IU per day), zinc (10–20 mg daily).

Homeopathy

Depending on the stage of the eczema, a different homeopathic is used. First, an erythematous eruption precedes the appearance of vesicles, which will rupture before oozing and scaling. Then, a phase can occur in which fissures predominate.

- Remedies for the erythematous phase: apis, urticaria urens, belladonna.
- Remedies for the vesicular phase: rhus toxicodendron, rhus vernix or rhus venenata, mezerum, cantharis, anagallis arvensis, croton tiglium.
- Remedies for the exudative phase: graphites, mezerium, etroleum, antimonium crudum, Viola tricolor.
- Remedies for the desquamative phase: arsenicum album, arsenicum iodatum, natrum sulphuricum, berberis vulgaris, hydrocotyle asiatica.
- Remedies for the phase of fissure formation: nitricum acidum, graphites, Antimonium crudum, petroleum, sepia.
- Remedies for itching: staphysagria (when itching is located on eyelids and genitals), cistus canadensis (red, oozing, and scabby lesions on cheeks and dorsum of hands), manganum aceticum (itching of the articular creases; scales or fissures), radium bromatum (burning and itching on thick skin), dolichos pruriens (itching with constipation), chamomilla (itching causes behavioral disorders).
- Arsenicum album is best used for tender skin eruptions that are also very dry and itchy and swollen; condition is worse in the winter; itching is intense between midnight and 2:00 am. Patient feels restless.
- Alumina is for skin that is dry and itchy and the person is constipated.
- Calendula can be used for affected inflamed areas and can be applied to skin to soothe.
- Calcarea carbonica helps people whose eczema is worse in the winter, have clammy hands and feet, and crave sweets and eggs. Great remedy for cradle cap.
- Graphites is for those with eczema mainly affecting the palms and areas behind the ears. The skin is dry, thick, and has a honey-like discharge from the skin. A warm bed intensifies itching.
- Hepar sulph is for skin that is easily infected and sensitive, worse in the cold.
- Medorrhinium helps those who have been suffering from eczema since very young. They tend to be warm, sweat easily, and crave ice and oranges.
- Mezereum is for blistering eczema that oozes and forms a crust. The open air and the cold makes the skin feel better.
- Petroleum is for dry, cracked skin with itching worse at night and with warmth of bed. Areas affected are the palms and hands.
- Psorinum is for eczema that looks dirty, is irritated, and is prone to infections. These patients scratch until the eczema bleeds. They experience general chilliness.
- Rhus toxicodendron is for itchy eczema that blisters and improves with warmth and movement. The person craves cold milk. The blisters itch more at night or in damp weather.

- Sulphur is helpful when the skin is red, rough, itchy, and dry. The person has diarrhea that gets worse early in the morning. Symptoms are aggravated by heat and washing.

Acupressure

- LI11 (helps with itching)
- B40, SP10, B23, B47, ST36, B10, LI4, LU9, B13
- Weeping eczema: SP9, B52, CV9
- Severe itching: LU7, SP10, LV5, B13

Aromatherapy

Essential oils can help to soothe inflammation and itching. These include juniper, peppermint, bergamot, carrot, jojoba, lavender, frankincense, thyme, benzoin, sweet marjoram, geranium, and chamomile.

Other Recommendations

Other therapies, like biofeedback and climatotherapy (uses water and sunlight as therapy), can be helpful.

HAIR LOSS

Hair loss, or alopecia, can occur in all ages and genders and can be due to multiple causes, including medication side effects, hormonal issues, and nutritional deficiencies (e.g., ferritin). Diagnosis can be made with a detailed history, examination, and testing, including biopsy.

Additional Integrative Modalities

Supplements

- Saw palmetto (320 mg daily) improves hair growth.
- Pygeum (100 mg twice daily) slows hair loss and improves prostate health.
- Pumpkin seed oil (8 g or 1 tbsp daily).
- Aloe vera juice (½ cup twice daily).
- B vitamins like biotin (2,000–3,000 mcg daily) and pantothenic acid (100 mg per day).
- Others include: silicon (Orthosilicic acid); MSM (1,000–3,000 mg daily), which promotes hair development; bamboo extract (900 mg twice daily).

- *Children:* stimulate hair growth—vitamin C (500–1,000 mg daily), vitamin D (1,000–4,000 IU daily), l–carnitine (500–1,000 mg daily), zinc (20 mg daily).

Homeopathy

- Alopecia areata: eberthinum, paratyphoidinum.
- Postpartum: eberthinum.
- Totalis: Thallium metallicum.
- Seborrheic: Selenium metallicum.
- Arsenicum album is helpful when hair loss is the result of stress. The person is very fearful and restless.
- Aurum muriaticum helps those with hair loss associated with headaches and boils on head and symptoms are worse at night. These patients have a high likelihood of being depressed.
- Fluoric acidum helps those who suffer from brittle hair that falls out in little tufts.
- Selenium helps those with painful and sensitive skin and loss of body hair as well.
- Arnica is for hair loss associated with severe injury.
- Kali carbonica helps with hair loss that is associated with dryness of hair and scalp.
- Baryta carbs will help hair loss in an elderly, mentally slow person with poor circulation.
- Ignatia amara is for hair loss that comes on with acute grief or an emotional trauma.
- Lycopodium clavatum is for hair loss after childbirth and premature balding and graying of the hair.
- Natrum muriaticum is for hair loss with dandruff and white crusts on scalp with depression and cravings for salt.
- Phosphoric acidum is for hair loss after extreme emotion and grief. Patient is fatigued and indifferent.
- Sepia is for hair loss associated with hormonal changes like after childbirth or at menopause.
- Silica (Silicea) is helpful when there has been a chronic illness, accompanied by hair loss. The hair is brittle, and the person tends to be thin, chilly, and easily fatigued.
- Phosphorus helps with hair that falls out in handfuls.

Acupressure

- Paihui point (improves blood circulation), hollow point, ST36

Aromatherapy

Rosemary, lavender, clary sage, and cypress can stimulate hair growth; jasmine, rose, and geranium have relaxing properties. Can be added to homemade shampoos.

PSORIASIS

Psoriasis is an autoimmune condition of the skin, characterized by thick plaques on the skin. Diagnosis is via history, examination, and possible biopsy.

Additional Integrative Modalities

Supplements

- Digestive enzymes (one to two capsules at each meal) help to digest effectively.
- Hydrochloric acid (one to three capsules with each meal, decreasing dose if a burning sensation occurs), helps with protein digestion.
- Optimize vitamin D and B12.
- Others: Milk thistle (70–210 mg three times per day), sarsaparilla (250–500 mg three times per day) reduces bacterial toxins effects; a good multivitamin with 25,000 IU of vitamin A (as it is a critical nutrient for healthy skin), 400 IU of vitamin E, 800 meg folic acid, 200 meg selenium, 200 meg chromium, 25 to 50 mg zinc, and other antioxidants; burdock root, cleavers, barberry, calendula, and oil of anise. Topical aloe vera (0.5%) cream has been effective for psoriasis. Creams that help are ones that contain avocado oil, B12, and Oregon grape (10%) cream. Others you can also try are creams with vitamin E, A, zinc, sarsaparilla, and goldenseal.
- Psoriatic arthritis: Evening primrose, Borage, fish oil, curcumin, bromelian, and quercetin.
- *Children:* fish oil (1–2 g EPA/DHA per day), vitamin A (1,000–4,000 IU daily), vitamin D (0.005% applied topically three times a day), aloe vera gel (three times daily), Oregon grape root (10% cream applied three times daily).

Homeopathy

- Arsenicum iodatum helps for dry, scaly, and itchy skin that leaves behind large scales when exfoliated, leaving a raw, exuding surface behind. The person feels weak and exhausted and sweats profusely.

- Kali sulphuricum is indicated in the treatment of scaly dermatosis.
- Arsenicum album helps those patients with psoriasis who are restless and anxious. The plaques are dry, itchy, and scaly, and it feels like the skin is burning. Symptoms improve with warm applications.
- Belladonna can treat rectal psoriasis.
- Calcarea carbonica is for a person with dry, scaly plaques that often open up. Person is fatigued, overwhelmed, anxious, overweight, and chilly. They also crave eggs, dairy, and sweets.
- Graphites may help those with psoriasis that affects the skin behind the ears, back of the hands, scalp/head, and on the genitals. These lesions ooze a honey-colored pus, and symptoms are worse at night.
- Kali arsenicosum helps those that are affected with extremely scaly lesions, which are aggravated by warmth.
- Petroleum is for a person whose condition is aggravated by cold and is worse in the wintertime. These people are generally dry and itchy, and symptoms worsen with the warmth of the bed.
- Mercurius solubilis will help those who tend to have swollen lymph nodes and greasy-looking skin, which can become easily infected. These people are introverted, with strong emotions, sensitive to changes to temperature.
- Mezereum is for psoriasis that is fine, white, and scaly that covers large areas of the body. These lesions crust and itch, feeling better with cold.
- Rhus toxicodendron helps psoriasis that is raw, itchy, red, dry, and chapped and that improves with heat or baths. The person craves milk and is restless.
- Sepia is one of the most common homeopathic remedies for psoriasis. There is a thickening of the skin, with circular eruptions and dryness. This remedy is recommended for women with a hormonal imbalance. They feel chilly and irritable. The psoriasis is often on the elbow.
- Staphysagria helps when the psoriasis affects the scalp and erupts after suppressed grief or emotions.
- Sulphur helps those with dry, scaly, red, and itchy/burning patches, often moist and oozing, that worsen after baths and from warmth. Used for psoriatic arthritis and if the person often feels too hot.

Acupressure

- GB20, LI4, LV3, ST36, and B10

Aromatherapy

Essential oils can help to bring relief to inflamed areas of skin and help support the healing process. Examples include lavender oil (especially for stress and inflammation), frankincense, tea tree, myrrh, geranium, and carrot seed oil (scalp psoriasis). Coconut oil can be used as the base oil. Always check a small test patch to make sure you aren't reacting to that specific oil. Juniper baths maybe helpful.

ROSACEA

Rosacea is a chronic inflammatory condition of the skin on a person's cheeks, chin, eyelids, nose, or forehead that becomes inflamed and red. There are often small red bumps or pustules on the affected areas, small spider-like blood vessels on the face, a red nose, and a tendency to blush or flush easily. Over time, it can give the nose a swollen, waxy look. Common triggers are emotional stress, hot or cold weather, sunshine, consumption of spicy food, MSG, vinegar, cinnamon oil, alcohol, occasionally some skin care products, even links to Candida have been noted. High doses of B6 and B12 can trigger rosacea. Diagnosis can be made via history and exam.

Additional Integrative Modalities

Supplements

- Betaine hydrochloride (one to three capsules with each meal; if there are symptoms of burning, reduce dose) improves digestion.
- Licorice can help to reduce inflammation and soothe irritation.
- Feverfew helps to reduce redness and dryness. Choose feverfew parthenolide-free extract.
- Nicotinomide combo (750 mg, Zn 25 mg, Cu 11.5 mg, folic acid 500 mcg) helps to improve symptoms after four to eight weeks.
- Zinc (60–70 mg per day for no more than three months, then 15–20 mg per day).
- Others: Azelaic acid topical cream (3–10% cream), Gentian root (300 mg or ten to twenty drops five to fifteen minutes before meals to improve digestion), Burdock root (300 mg or 3 ml three times per day) improves detoxification and hormone balance; natural progesterone has anti-inflammatory benefits and improves skin conditions, B vitamin (50 mg twice daily), especially B12 (400–800 mcg sublingually daily), pancreatin (350–500 mg before meals), and brewer's yeast or nutritional yeast (1½ tsp daily). Turmeric, ginger, aloe vera gel, and raw honey applied to the skin have also been shown to improve symptoms.

Homeopathy

- Arsenicum album helps those who are anxious, get cold easily, and have lesions that are hot, dry, and flaky. They prefer warm drinks.
- Pulsatilla is for rosacea that feels better in the fresh air and worse with warm rooms. The symptoms are associated with hormonal changes like puberty or menopause. These individuals are weepy and sensitive, craving sweets.
- Sepia is for rosacea associated with hormone changes, but the woman is fatigued and irritable and craves salty, sour, and sweet foods and has a tendency toward depression.
- Sulphur helps those with chronic redness and inflammation, aggravated by the heat, sun, and warmer climates. The person prefers coolness.
- Carbo animalis is for facial lesions of rosacea.
- Arnica montana is a remedy for those with papulo-pustules.
- Sanguinaria canadensis helps when rosacea is accompanied with burning sensations and itching, hot flushes with redness of the cheeks, aggravated by heat.
- Eugenia jambosa is indicated for rosacea that is common in alcoholics. They often have cramps in the feet.
- Calcarea fluorica helps those who have severe telangiectasias.
- Lachesis mutus is prescribed for rhinophyma, especially if symptoms are aggravated with hormonal changes.
- Thuja occidentalis helps those with rosacea with varicose veins on the cheeks.

Acupressure

- The Yin Tang point, LI20, SI18, ST4, LI4, ST36, SP10, ST3, B10 (helps with anxiety and stress)

Aromatherapy

Tea tree oil, eucalyptus, geranium, chamomile, rose, rosemary, thyme, and lavender essential oil can help to relieve skin inflammation. Try applying it to your skin with a cool compress.

• 9 •

Ear, Nose, and Throat

Can't stop the faucet from running? Lowering inflammation will turn off the faucet and keep the house from flooding. Unless you like floating in your own thick mucus, who am I to judge?

D & D: SPECIAL CONSIDERATIONS

Lowering overall inflammation will allow your body to heal and improve ear, nose, and throat symptoms. Garlic and onions can help to boost the immune function, as they are high in vitamin C, help to speed up recovery, and improve blood circulation. Other foods that are anti-inflammatory are flax, chia, and cold-pressed oils. Apple cider vinegar (1 tsp mixed with water with some lemon juice) can help you lower inflammation at the first sign of an allergy attack.

Nutritional deficiencies can lead to symptoms like dizziness, so optimize green leafy veggies to increase sources of B vitamins. Caffeine and alcohol can lead to worsening immune function and dizziness. If you have a tree pollen allergy, you might try to limit fruits like apples, peaches, pears, kiwi, plums, and nectarine, and veggies like carrots, fennel, green peppers, and celery, along with nuts (almonds, walnuts, and hazelnuts) and spices like basil, paprika, and coriander. If you suffer from a grass and weed pollen allergy, avoid melons, bananas, cucumbers, echinacea, chamomile, parsley, paprika, dill, oregano, tarragon, and pepper.

Detoxing your environment can help you avoid allergens. Keep in mind, especially if you suffer from pollen and have a forced hot air furnace, getting a room humidifier with warm mist during dry conditions will be beneficial. Air duct cleaning should occur every two to three years, and the furnace filter should be changed monthly during winter. Use negative ions or an air cleaner especially with moldy air and air-conditioning. Clean your carpets regularly with a HEPA or water capture vacuum cleaner with environmentally friendly cleaning agents. Avoid the outdoors if the pollen levels and pollution are high. Also, cold temperatures can minimize pollen. Leave the pollen at the door and follow a no shoes policy, and place dirty clothes in the hamper with a cover. Check the pollen count by checking the local TV weather report or newspaper or go to pollen.com to find out what's going on in your area. Pollen levels are higher on the sunny, dry, and windy days and lower on windless, cool, and moist days; mornings are usually worse for allergy sufferers as the grasses tend to pollinate early in the day. Sunglasses keep the pollen out of your eyes. Keep windows and doors closed, and wash your bed linens in hot water at least once a week. Trimming the fur of your animals can help to reduce allergens. Avoid fans that draw in air from outside, and use an air-conditioner in your home. If you suffer from year-round allergies, use blinds instead of curtains, cover your pillows with dust mite covers, and use area rugs on hardwood floors so they can be washed with hot water. Follow the recommendations in chapter 2 to clean your water, air, living environment, kitchen, and body. Flushing out the pollens can aid in easing sinus pressure, congestion, and inflammation. Using a neti pot in the morning and before bed with 8 oz of warm water (never use tap water) mixed with ¼ tsp of salt or premixed saline can ease symptoms.

THE FOUR BIG S's: SPECIAL CONSIDERATIONS

Stress can lead to a worsening of inflammation, so managing stress is key to healing.

Release negative emotions! Energy medicine healing modalities like Reiki, qigong, craniosacral therapy, and therapeutic touch can help.

ALLERGIC RHINITIS

In allergic rhinitis, or hay fever, your body overreacts to a substance that you inhale by making antibodies, releasing IgEs and other inflammatory chemicals like histamines into your airways leading to inflammation. This varies from person to person; it could range from anaphylaxis to minor irritation. There are two types: seasonal and perennial (occurs year round). Some present with symptoms of hay fever that is accompanied with sneezing, runny nose, itching of the nose, roof of the mouth and eyes, swollen eyelids, post nasal drip, facial pain or pressure, fatigue, dark circles under the eyes, headaches, and loss of hearing, taste, and even smell. Diagnosis can be made via history and physical. Blood tests, like a RAST testing, or scratch test can be implemented to determine what the specific allergens maybe. Blood eosinophils can be elevated in those with allergic rhinitis symptoms. It is wise to determine if the symptoms are indeed due to allergies or something else. Causes are environmental, like pollen, mold, smoke, and even dust mites.

Additional Integrative Modalities

Supplements

- Raw honey (2 tbsp per day).
- Stinging nettle (300–500 mg twice daily) has antihistamine activities (can either be taken as a herbal or eaten as a green).
- Butterbur (500 mg per day) has been shown to reduce mucus.
- Quercetin (1,000 mg daily).
- Bromelain (250 mg daily) can decrease sinus and nasal swelling.
- Vitamin C (2,000 mg per day) is an antihistamine and antioxidant.
- Soil-based probiotics.
- Others: Spirulina (1,000–2,000 mg per day) can stop the release of histamines; Tinospora cordifolia (300 mg three times per day) (don't take if you have an autoimmunity or are pregnant or nursing); Epicor yeast (dried saccharomyces cerevisiae fermented product; 500 mg per day); astragalus (160 mg two times per day) (don't take if you have an autoimmune condition, take lithium or other immune suppressing meds); methylsulfonylmethane (MSM) (3,000–5,000 mg daily) reduces allergic and inflammatory responses; eyebright (Euphrasia officinalis; one capsule three times daily) or apply as a solution to irritated eyes by putting five drops of the tincture form in a half ounce of saline and apply it to the eyes twice daily.
- *Children:* Allergic rhinitis: bromelian (80–320 mg daily), probiotics (2–10 billion CFU daily), mixed carotenoids (1,000–5,000 IU daily), quercetin (200–400 mg divided into two to three doses daily), mixed tocopherols (100–400 IU daily), vitamin C (500–1,000 mg daily), stinging nettle leaf (100–500 mg daily).
- Allergy: Bromelain (200–500 mg daily), flavenoids (200–400 mg divided into two to three daily doses), quercetin (250–500 mg divided into two to three doses daily), vitamin C (500–1,000 mg daily), eu-

phrasia (50–200 mg daily), skullcap (250–500 mg daily), stinging nettle leaf (250–500 mg daily), turmeric (100 mg daily).

Homeopathy

- Allium cepa is a remedy for frequent sneezing, tearing eyes, and a lot of irritating, burning nasal discharge. The patient feels incredibly thirsty, and symptoms worsen with warm food or drink. Lights hurt the eyes.
- Nux vomica helps those with dry, ticklish, scraping sensations with watery nasal discharge, stuffiness, and sneezing upon waking up. They are impatient and irritable. Eyes are sensitive to light, ears itch, and their breathing is obstructed. They crave tobacco, sweets, and other stimulants.
- Euphrasia is indicated in those with thick, burning, and irritating tears, with stinging and nasal discharge that worsens when the patient lies down and is indoors.
- Arsenicum album helps those who feel restless, fatigued, and anxious, with stuffiness and violent sneezing. The copious nasal discharge burns.
- Sabidilla is indicated for those with violent sneezing, watery eyes, runny nose, sore throat that is soothed by warm drinks, and headache that feels like your head is shrinking. Patient feels cold.
- Arsenicum iodatum can be used for those with thick, honey-colored discharge from nose followed by three to four days of sneezing and a burning sensation inside the nose. Other symptoms are burning throat, dry skin, anxious personality and irritating cough. Symptoms worsen with warmth.
- Arundo is indicated with those who have allergies, with no discharge but itchy nose, ears, and roof of mouth, along with sneezing. Can be used early in the hay fever season.
- Psorinum is for the person who feels cold, has bland or burning nasal discharge, wants to lie down, and has breathlessness that is relieved by raising arms away from body.
- Gelsemium is indicated for those who are apathetic, feel dizzy and shaky, and have nonstop watering and sneezing accompanied by puffy and heavy eyes.
- Pulsatilla is for those who are tearful and have yellow discharge from eyes and nose; the nose gets congested at night and is better with the open air. Allergies are worse in a warm room.
- Silicia is indicated for those who generally feel cold, have a stuffed nose, especially upon waking, and their sinuses feel tender. Their

allergies manifest as upper respiratory tract infections, and they are usually tired.

- Dulcamara is a remedy for those who feel cold after exertion and have constant sneezing, stuffy nose, swollen watery eyes, which all worsen in the outdoors and damp weather.
- Sanguinaria can be used for those with nasal polyps, dry congested nasal membranes, and chronic rhinitis; if this rhinitis is with asthma, Arsenicum iodatum, iodum, arsenicum, kali iodatum, and sabadilla can be used.
- If the rhinitis is worse with body exertion or warmth, use silicea or pulsatill.
- For early hay fever symptoms, use arundo and/or wyethia.
- For stuffy nose with constant blowing (symptoms are not relieved) use lachesis, psorinum, naja, sticta, or kali bichromium.
- Homeopathic mixtures like Sabidil can be used to alleviate symptoms.

Acupressure

- LI20, ST20, B2, LI4, SP5, B13, GB20
- Others include: B10 (fatigue, headaches and swollen eyes), ST36, and TW5.
- Nambudripad Allergy Elimination Technique (NAET) can help to rebalance your body's immune system.

Aromatherapy

Essential oils have the ability to help you overcome hypersensitivity and chemically support the body by boosting the immune system, fighting against common infections/harmful toxins, and helping the body detoxify. Peppermint oil can help to unclog sinuses and acts as an expectorant; basil oil supports the adrenals, lowers inflammation, and helps the body detoxify. Eucalyptus oil can improve circulation, thereby improving symptoms, and it acts as an expectorant, helping the body detoxify. Lemon oil helps to relieve symptoms by supporting lymphatic system drainage. Tea tree oil has anti-inflammatory properties, is an antiseptic, and destroys pathogens. A eucalyptus inhalation can help to open up the airways; mix with ravensara (decongestant), lavender (decreases stress), and peppermint oil. Using chamomile in a balm can help to trap pollen, is anti-inflammatory, and soothes irritated skin. Frankincense essential oil can boost the immune system and optimize health.

Others include: bergamot, chamomile (German), cinnamon, clove (bud), helichrysum, juniper (needle), lemon, niaouli, peppermint, ravensara, rosemary cineole, rosewood.

SINUSITIS

Sinusitis occurs when the inflammation is located in the sinuses. This can lead to pain, pressure, nasal congestion, nasal discharge or post nasal drip, toothache, sore throat and cough, headaches, loss of smell, and fatigue. Sinusitis can be due to infections, obstructions, changes in air pressure, injury, and/or allergies. Diagnosis is made with a thorough history, physical, and imaging if needed, like X ray, CT scan, or MRI.

Additional Integrative Modalities

Supplements

- Use a multivitamin twice daily with selenium (100–200 mcg per day), zinc (20–40 mg per day), magnesium (400–600 mg per day), calcium (1,000 mg per day and 1,500 mg per day during menopause), chromium (200 mcg per day), bee propolis (500 mg three times per day) and vitamin E.
- Grapefruit seed extract (spray four times daily) has antiviral properties and anti-inflammatory and anti-aging properties. It may slow hepatic metabolism of some drugs like statins.
- Oil of oregano (500 mg four times a day) has antibacterial and antiviral properties.
- Vitamin C (1,000 mg three times per day) can help to boost the immune system.
- Garlic (500 mg twice daily) improves immune function but can enhance the effect of anticoagulants.
- Echinacea (1,000 mg two to three times per day) can help to fight infections especially if taken at the first sign of symptoms.
- Others: nettle for allergies (freeze-dried 300 mg three times per day); quercetin and bromelin (500 mg daily between meals); licorice (ten to twenty drops three times per day), pantothenic acid (500 mg three times per day) and hydrochloric acid (1–2 capsules after protein-based meals), which optimize gut health. N-acetylcysteine (500 mg three times daily) helps thin the mucus to drain sinuses; colloidal silver (spray four times daily for acute sinusitis and twice daily for

chronic) and Pelargonium sidoides are helpful. A Chinese herb called yin chiao can be used three times daily, as well as astaxathin (4 mg per day to twice a day) and vitamin B (50 mg twice daily).

- To treat fungal sinusitis and candida overgrowth: garlic or Allimax/Allimed (100% pure allicin) (beginning with 720–900 mg three times a day and gradually tapering to 180–450 mg once daily over three months) plus Candex/Candisol (two capsules twice per day on an empty stomach). Use a combination of several antifungal supplements such as sodium caprylate, oregano leaf, Pau D'Arco, berberine, grapefruit seed, ginger root, chamomile, biotin, and zinc.
- *Children:* bromelain (80–320 mg daily), multivitamin one per day, fish oil (1 g of EPA/DHA per day), NAC (100–600 mg by mouth daily), nasal lavage (can add goldenseal, five drops, and NAC, five drops, to the salt solution for an added benefit).

Homeopathy

- Belladonna is a remedy for those with a face that is hot and red, temperature is higher than normal, and frontal sinuses are affected, with throbbing pain especially on the right side of the sinus. This pain is worse when lying down or bending head forward and with slightest pressure. Can be taken at the first sign of infection.
- Pulsatilla can help those who are weepy, pain is above the eyes, thick yellow or green discharge is present with nausea and vomiting that is worse indoors and improved with open cool air, cool compresses, and pressure. The right maxillary and frontal sinuses can be involved. They have jumpy neurological pain on the right side of the face.
- Bryonia alba helps those with sinus pain that occurs with any movement of the head downward.
- Hepar sulphuris is indicated for those with yellow mucus for later stages of sinus inflammation. Face is tender; sneezing occurs; and pain is concentrated between the eyes and worsened with cold, dry winds. Person feels cold and irritable.
- Kali bichromium is a remedy for those with feelings of fullness, and congestion on either side of the nose. The mucus is stringy, thick green or yellow, and can lead to pain at the roof of the nose.
- Mercurius solubilis helps those with thick, foul-smelling green discharge that may present with a little blood. Symptoms worsen with open air, eating, drinking, and extreme cold or hot. They may be feverish and have pain that extends to the teeth.
- Silica (Silicea) is indicated in those with tearing, throbbing pain that is felt deep, with an itchy tip of the nose; pain is worse in the right

eye and worsens with light, cold air, movement, noise, and mental concentration.

- Spigelia is a remedy for those with sharp pains on the left side of the face relieved by cold compresses or cool water and worsened by light, movement, noise, and warmth.
- Others: Aurum muriaticum, Medorrhinum, Natrum muriaticum, Thuja occidentalis, and Kali sulphuricum (30C, each three times daily can be used).

Acupressure

These points can lessen sinus pain and pressure by opening up cavities to allow drainage:

- ST3, LI20, B2, LI4 (relieve pain in your sinuses)
- B2 (relieves sinus congestion and headaches)
- SI18, yintang, yu yao point
- GB20 (helps relieve nasal congestion)
- EX HN8
- Frontal: GB14, B2, and EX HN3
- Maxillary: ST2, SI18
- Ethmoidal and sphenoid: GV16, GV20

Aromatherapy

Essential oils can help to open up the sinuses and clear mucus, eliminating infections. Eucalyptus oil has clearing properties that help to relieve blocked sinuses and can be used in a steam inhalation by inhaling, or in a bath or by massaging it in. Combine with peppermint, rosemary, and thyme. Tea tree oil can aid in fighting off infection to aid in sinus relief. Lavender can help you sleep and stimulates your immune system.

Others are: Canadian balsam, helichrysum, hyssop, lavender, marjoram (sweet and Spanish), myrtle (green or orange), niaouli, pine, rosemary (cineole and camphor), cedarwood, revensara, and cajeput.

TINNITUS

Tinnitus, or ringing in the ears, is a sensation of hearing whistling, ringing, buzzing, sizzling, or other sounds, and it may be intermittent or continuous. Sounds may change, can stop and go, or get louder and faster. Tinnitus can be caused by infections, blockages in the ear, or inner ear damage and can be improved once the underlying cause is treated. This can be accompanied with interference with your ability to concentrate, brain fog, and confusion. Diagnosis made by history and physical.

Additional Integrative Modalities

Supplements

- B complex (50 mg per day) support healthy nerves.
- Melatonin (1–3 mg per day).
- Pycnogenol (100–150 mg per day).
- Bioflavonoids (200–800 mg per day).
- Coenzyme Q10 (100 mg three times daily); this may be helpful for those low in CoQ10.
- Magnesium (250 mg twice daily) to support normal hearing.
- B12 (1,000 mcg daily) to support healthy nerves (get your B12 levels tested).
- Others: Ginkgo biloba (120 mg twice daily of a 24% extract) improves circulation through the inner ear; zinc (90 mg daily with 2–3 mg of copper under the supervision of a doctor) may be helpful for those with a zinc deficiency.

Homeopathy

- Salicylic acid can be used for roaring in ears and deafness.
- Carbon sulph is indicated for blocked feeling of ears and tingling accompanied with roaring.
- Kali iodatum helps those with symptoms of longstanding ringing, with no additional symptoms.
- Calcarea cabonica is a remedy for those with crackling or pulsing sensations in the ears. These patients are easily cold, fatigued, overwhelmed, and anxious.
- Lycopodium can be used for those with roaring or humming in the ears, like an echo. These patients have a tendency toward infections with discharge and digestive issues.
- Chinum sulphuricum can help those with roaring, buzzing, hissing, or ringing that impairs the person's hearing and can be accompanied with vertigo.
- Graphitis is a remedy for tinnitus that is accompanied with deafness. The patient also has skin eruptions, poor concentration, and constipation.

- Others that can be used are Carbo vegetabilis, sulphur, Chenopodium anthelminticum, Lachnanthes tinctoria, cimicifuga, Coffea cruda, Kali carbonicum, Natrum salicylicum, and Salicylicum acidum.

Acupressure

- TW7, TW17, TW21, TW 22, SI19, GB2

Aromatherapy

Juniper berry, lavender, cypress, and helichrysum essential oils can be helpful in treating tinnitus.

VERTIGO

Vertigo is a symptom or sensation of dizzy spells that may feel like the environment around you is spinning or you are spinning. Causes may be benign paroxysmal positional vertigo, Meniere's disease, labyrinthitis, or vestibular neuritis (inflammation in the inner ear around the nerve). Other causes can be injury, medications that lead to ear damage, stroke or tumors, migraines, or multiple sclerosis. Other symptoms are feelings of swaying, pulling in one direction, and just feeling unbalanced. There may be associated feelings of nausea, headache, sweating, fullness and ringing of the ear or hearing loss. Diagnosis made by history and physical.

Additional Integrative Modalities

Supplements

- Ginkgo biloba (60 mg two or three times daily) increases blood flow to the brain.
- Cayenne (300 mg twice daily) increases blood flow.
- Coenzyme Q10 (100 mg daily).
- Turmeric (500 mg twice daily) improves blood flow and lowers inflammation.
- Ginger root (500 mg twice daily or 1 cup twice daily in a tea form).
- Vinpocetine (15 mg daily) will improve inner ear circulation symptoms.
- Others: Ashwagandha (1,000 mg twice a day) and Panax ginseng (100 mg two to three times daily with 4–7% ginsenosides) improves adrenal function.

- *For Meniere's disease:* Magnesium (1,000 mg per day) can help to improve the tinnitus and also protect the ears from damage, B vitamins (500 mg B1, 250 mg B6, 500 mcg B12) and vitamin C (1,000 mg three times a day) with 250 mg of bioflavonoids can help to improve symptoms, as well as ginkgo biloba (80–120 mg per day) and teas like fenugreek and chamomile. Other herbs that can be tried are dandelion (decreases the amount of fluid present in the inner ear; thirty drops twice per day or 1 tsp of root or infuse 2 tsp of leaves in a cup of water and drink twice a day), burdock (boil 1 tbsp of seeds or root in a cup of water and take thirty drops of tincture twice a day; helps to improve circulation and release excess fluid from the body, licorice has an anti-inflammatory effect, but it's not to be taken if you have elevated blood pressure or kidney failure (boil 1 tsp of root in a cup of water and drink twice a day, or use sixty drops of tincture)

Homeopathy

- Borax is a remedy that can be used when patients feel worse by downward movement of the head.
- Theridion is indicated when loud noises stimulate symptoms and for Meniere's-type symptoms.
- Calcarea helps those with symptoms that worsen by looking up.
- Conium is indicated when a patient complains of whirling sensations while lying down and on head rotation. A patient complains of whirling sensations.
- Gelsemium is a remedy for dizziness accompanied with trembling and the dizziness may be caused by a viral infection, accompanied with being drowsy; it can be used for dizziness for post-stage-fright. Symptoms can be accompanied by anxiety, mental dullness, trembling, and visual disorders.
- Kali carb helps those who feel worse when they turn, read, or walk and feel better in the open air.
- Nux vomica is indicated for those with symptoms that are worse by flickering bright lights, being in a crowded space. The symptoms may be accompanied with vomiting, nausea, and feelings of being hung over. Symptoms are worse in the morning and improve as the day goes on, and with lying down.
- Tabacum is a remedy for those whose symptoms for vertigo improve with cool air and by closing the eyes and worsen with motion, accompanied by symptoms of fainting, cold and clammy feelings,

nausea, feeling like a tight band around the head, and excessive saliva in the mouth before vomiting.

- Cocculus is for those with symptoms that worsen by lifting the head, looking out the window, traveling in a car, and sleeping and are worse in the morning. Sitting may relieve symptoms. Other symptoms that may be present are nausea, vomiting, anxiety, palpitations, feelings of being ill and sad, and loss of hearing.
- Bryonia helps those with dizziness in a sitting position, movement of head, or bending over. Patient craves cold drinks.
- Pulsatilla can be used when you feel worse with lying down and comes on in a congested and warm room, with improvement from the open air and/or walking.
- Aconitum napellus can be used for those with sudden dizziness with a rapid pulse, shock, and feelings as if you are going to die, with utter panic.
- Argentum nitricum can be helpful for those with symptoms that are accompanied by headaches and trembling. Vertigo can be brought on by phobias, agitation, or when the patient is in a hurry.
- Lachesis mutans is when symptoms are triggered by the feelings of being congested (claustrophobia) and symptoms improve by discharge.
- Phosphoricum acidum is a remedy for those with vertigo accompanied with headaches and malaise or follows an emotional shock.
- China is indicated for those with ringing in the ears with anemia and fatigue.
- Salicylicum acidum can be helpful in those with vertigo that can be associated with ringing in the ears and deafness.
- Chininum sulphuricum is indicated for those with hearing loss, ringing of the ears, and vertigo.
- Chenopodium anthelminthicum can be a remedy for sudden Meniere's disease with accompanying hearing loss, hepatic pain, and migraines.
- Others that can be used are: Carboneum sulphuratum, Bufo, Magnesia carbonica, Oleander staphysagria, Aurum muriaticum, Cyclamen europaeum, Glonoinum, Phosphorus and/or Sulphur.

Acupressure

- TW17, SI19, and TW16
- Others: P6, GV20, GV19, GV21, GB20, GB21, Tai Yang, LV2, ST36, K1, GV26, B23, B47, ST9, LV3

Aromatherapy

For mild vertigo, aromatherapy can improve sensations of dizziness or vertigo. Peppermint oil, black pepper, rosemary, eucalyptus, and cypress oil help to improve blood circulation and oxygen to the brain. Cypress oil can help to open up breathing passages. Others that can help are basil oil, lavender oil, rose oil, rosemary oil, lavender, and tangerine oil. Ginger oil can relieve nausea.

• 10 •

Endocrinology

Happy hormones = Happy you! Go away inflammation, I need my happy hormones back!

D & D: SPECIAL CONSIDERATIONS

Lowering inflammation and maintaining a balance of glucose and insulin is key in optimizing endocrine function and help with weight loss. Add the superfoods of coconut, olives, avocados, fatty fish and other proteins, nuts and seeds, and Himalayan or Celtic sea salt. Eating fat or protein with every meal and limiting carbs helps stabilize blood sugar and improve endocrine function. Increase fiber and vinegar in your diet as these can stabilize blood sugar. Foods high in chromium can naturally balance blood glucose; these include broccoli, grass-fed beef, and green beans. Other healing foods are cinnamon, ginger, rosemary, green tea, cranberries, blueberries, lemon balm, fenugreek, holy basil, neem, bay leaves, turmeric, gymnema sylvestre, and bitter melon. Grapefruit, Romaine lettuce, celery, curry powder, asparagus, aloe vera, and flounder all help with weight loss. Caffeine can be problematic to those with compromised adrenals, as it may prevent you from sleeping.

After an initial weight loss, some may experience a plateau. Insulin resistance keeps our insulin levels up leading to weight gain or the inability to lose weight (even if you are eating the right foods). Periods of low insulin can help break that cycle which can be achieved by intermittent fasting. Remember, it takes time to get your body to get used to fasting, so give yourself at least a month. Talk to your primary care provider to make sure you are healthy enough to fast. Plateaus can also be due to increasing muscle mass but decreasing fat mass, so measure your fat mass and lean mass, tracking them separately, along with measuring waist and hip circumferences, because your weight may not change, but your measurements will if you are lowering inflammation. Check basal metabolic rate (rate at which you burn calories when you are at rest), get genetic testing, review intolerances and toxins, increase water and sleep, and increase the amount of sweating you do—everybody is different. Focus on the foundations of good health, and once you move to a state of lowered inflammation, your body will also follow through, I promise.

THE FOUR BIG S's: SPECIAL CONSIDERATIONS

Lowering stress and improving sleep can help to restore your hormonal balance.

ADRENAL FATIGUE

The adrenal gland is responsible for producing and regulating your stress hormone, cortisol, and producing sex hormones and neurotransmitters that communicate with all your organs. Adrenal fatigue is a term applied to a collection of nonspecific symptoms leading to adrenal dysfunction, resulting in nutrient and hormonal dysfunction, due to chronic stress. Though not a medical diagnosis, it lies on the spectrum between being normal and having Addison's disease (when 90 percent of your adrenal gland's function is lost).

Symptoms include fatigue, trouble waking up, feeling dizzy when standing, easily irritated and short tempered, frequent infections and colds that take time to clear up, low body temperature, palpitations, mood disorders, muscle weakness, increased allergies, insomnia, decreased libido, hair loss, headaches, always cold, cravings for sugar, low blood pressure, thyroid problems, high energy at bedtime, inflammation, weight gain, muscle tension, light-headed when standing, chronic pain, PMS symptoms, and a reliance on coffee. Diagnosis can occur with a blood pressure test to check for orthostatic hypotension; a pupil contraction test can show whether you have difficulty with contracting your pupils; and it's important to check for temperatures that don't remain stable. Hormone tests can be done that check adrenal hormones, DHEA, adrenal saliva, cortisol, and thyroid function.

Additional Integrative Modalities

Supplements

- Ashwagandha (500 mg once daily).
- Vitamin C (500–3,000 mg daily).

- B vitamins like B5 (300–1,000 mg per day), B6 (30–100 mg per day), and B1 (600 mg per day can help with fatigue); ideal for adrenal support.
- Zinc and Selenium.
- Others: adaptogenic and GABAergic herbs like rodiola rosea (100–400 mg daily); eleuthero (2–3 g of dried root in a capsule daily); reishi mushroom (3–6 g of dried mushroom in a capsule daily); maca (75–100 mg per day, not to be used while pregnant); Phosphatidylserine (100 mg three times per day); passionflower (100–200 mg per day); valerian (100–200 mg per day); lemon balm (100–200 mg per day), which helps to support the adrenals; phosphatidylserine (100–200 mg per day); l-theanine (100–200 mg per day); holy basil (2–3 mg per day), which helps recover adrenal function, Siberian, Panax, or Asian ginseng, used during times of high stress to support adrenal function (100–200 mg of ginseng, standardized to contain 4–5 percent ginsenosides); licorice (50–100 mg per day), great for inflammation, especially arthritis or muscle tenderness; tyrosine (500–1,000 mg daily); adrenal glandular (200–500 mg daily); chromium (200–400 μg per day); DHEA, which is important especially for people with autoimmune diseases such as lupus or Sjogren's, but it should be taken under professional guidance. A few more are schizandra (twenty to thirty drops of extract per day or two to four capsules per day) and shatavarri (2–4 mg per day) that can also support the adrenals.

Homeopathy

- Natrum muriaticum is helpful for those with constipation, dry lips and mouth, cravings for salt, and symptoms worse by the hot sun. Patient usually has a muddy complexion.
- Argenticum nitricum is a remedy for those with tremors, apprehension, and cravings for salt and sweet things.
- Silicea can help with no stamina, and feet that sweat profusely and smell unpleasant. Symptoms are worse in the cold weather.

Remedies for stress:

- Phosphoric acidium can help with stress related to grief or bad news.
- Picric acidium is a remedy for stress due to overwork.
- Ignatia can be used for stress that follows an emotional upset.
- Nux vomica is a remedy for stress that is brought on by bad habits like smoking, eating, or drinking too much or when the person is irritable and very overwhelmed.

Acupressure

- P6 (help calm and balance)
- LI4, GB21, LU1, B10, CV17

Aromatherapy

Therapeutic essential oils can help to promote relaxation and manage chronic stress. Mix almond oil with clary sage, frankincense, and geranium oils and massage into skin. Other stress-relieving oils are litsea, orange, and bergamot essential oils. Ylang-ylang, rose, vetiver, and Roman chamomile can help you sleep.

INSULIN RESISTANCE/PREDIABETES/ METABOLIC SYNDROME/DIABETES

Diabetes is a chronic condition that is marked by abnormally high levels of glucose in the blood because the body either stops producing insulin or can't use the insulin that the body does produce. There are multiple types of diabetes. Type 1 is also known as juvenile or insulin-dependent diabetes, an autoimmune disease that occurs when the immune system destroys the cells that make the insulin; Type 2 occurs when the pancreas cannot make enough insulin to keep blood glucose levels normal and is made worse by poor food choices. Prediabetes occurs when the blood glucose levels are higher than normal but not enough to be diagnosed as diabetes; it is also known as impaired fasting glucose, impaired glucose tolerance, or insulin resistance.

Metabolic syndrome is also called dysmetabolic syndrome X or insulin-resistance syndrome and is a cluster of conditions including abdominal obesity, high fasting blood sugar, high blood pressure, low HDL cholesterol, or high triglycerides. About 85 percent of people with diabetes have metabolic syndrome, so we will talk about all of it together.

Signs and symptoms of diabetes type 1 include abdominal pain, nausea, vomiting, increased urination, increased thirst, fatigue, absence of menstruation. Type 2 presents as excessive urination and thirst, yeast infections, fatigue, impotence, blurred vision, numbness or burning of extremities, and poor wound healing. Diagnosis is made by history, physical, and a blood test.

Additional Integrative Modalities

Supplements

- Chromium (600 mcg daily) helps with insulin sensitivity and balances blood sugar levels.

- Cinnamon (2 tsp per day): add to food, smoothie, or tea to help improve blood sugar.
- Alpha lipoic acid (300–1,200 mg daily) improves insulin sensitivity, reduces symptoms of neuropathy, and prevents diabetic neuropathy.
- Capsaicin used topically can help for neuropathy. Can be applied 4 times per day.
- Fiber powder from veggies and seeds can control glucose levels; for supplements like PGX, take two to four capsules before each meal with 8 oz of water.
- Berberine improves sugar and retinopathy (200–300mg two to four times). Avoid in pregnancy.
- Bitter melon.
- Prickly pear (blood sugar lowering properties).
- B vitamins like B1, B6, B7, B12.
- Vitamin C, D, K.
- Iodine.
- Zinc.
- Melatonin.
- ALA.
- Choline helps to reduce risk of fatty liver.
- Calcium.
- *Metabolic syndrome/Insulin resistance:* ginseng; berberine (also restores intestinal barrier function from pro inflammatory cytokines, reduces vascular inflammation; watch with drugs); bitter melon; holy basil; spirulina and maca root increase the glutathione levels to improve immune system.
- Other: Gymnema sylvestre (400 mg of a 25% gymneic acid extract daily). Gymnema lowers blood-sugar levels. Vanadyl sulfate (100–300 mg daily) improves glucose tolerance in people with insulin resistance; higher dosages should be used under the supervision of a doctor. Biotin (9–16 mg daily) is involved with proper glucose metabolism.
- *Weight loss:* guggul (650 mg twice daily), glucomannan (665 mg before bed), CLA (750 mg twice daily), Forskohlil (385 mg twice daily), sphaeranthus indicus, garcinia mangostana, green coffee bean extract (400 mg twice daily).
- Other supplements: berberine can improve lipid control, diabetes prevention, and improve weight issues and memory; magnesium will manage insulin resistance; pycnogenol (100 mg once or twice daily); reversatrol (100–250 mg daily) for better blood sugar control; high potency multivitamin; an antioxidant supplement to reduce inflammation and prevent damage will contain vitamin E, selenium, and

glutathione or NAC and carotenoids; digestive enzymes; nicotinomide (25 mg per kg body weight) reduces progression of disease in newly diagnosed children; folic acid (800 mcg every day) protects vascular damage; thiamine (50–200 mg daily) can reduce numbness and tingling; apple pectin (500 mg twice daily); banaba extract (450 mg per day); cordyceps (400 mg per day); bitter melon (500 mg per day); fenugreek (500 mg per day); green coffee bean extract (500 mg per day); garcinea (1,000 mg twice daily); cinnamon (500 mg twice daily); cayenne, saffron (100 mg per day); astaxanthin (4 mg per day); coenzyme Q10 (60–200 mg per day); green tea extract (250–500 mg per day); curcumin (500 mg per day).

- *Children:* DM type 1: magnesium (100–400 mg daily), vitamin E (100–400 mg IU daily), alpha lipoic acid (100 mg daily), vitamin B3 (2–30 mg daily), chromium (50–200 mcg daily), vitamin C (250–1,000 mg daily), fish oil (500–2,000 mg EPA/DHA per day), vitamin D (600–4,000 IU per day), milk thistle (80% silymarin [200 mg daily]).
- DM type 2: Alpha lipoic acid (100 mg daily), chromium (50–200 mcg daily), magnesium (100–200 mg daily), vitamin D (400–4,000 IU daily), zinc (5–20 mg daily), cassia cinnamon (1–2 g three times daily), gymnasia (100 mg twice daily), milk thistle (80% silymarin [200 mg daily]), Panax (ginseng root extract 15% ginsenosides [200 mg daily]).
- Obesity: fish oil (1–2 g daily), pycnogenol (50–150 mg daily), psyllium (6 g daily), vitamin B3 (10–20 mg daily), green tea (1–3 cups daily), plant sterols (1.5–2.3 g daily).

Homeopathy

- Phosphoric is indicated for diabetes that is associated with symptoms brought on by nervous exhaustion from grief or working too hard.
- Uranium nitricum can help with symptoms of weakness, bedwetting, and digestive upsets.
- Argenticum nitricum is a remedy for diabetes with the symptom of swollen ankles.
- Codeinum helps relieve diabetes that presents with restlessness, depression, and skin irritation.
- Natrum sulphuricum is for diabetes that is accompanied with gout.
- Silicea is for diabetes with cold, smelly, sweaty feet and loss of stamina.
- Phosphorus: Vascular complications of diabetes.
- Insulin dependent: Natrum muriaticum, Sulphur.
- Non-insulin dependent: Sulphur.

Acupressure

- Obesity: ST25, ST36, ST40, SP6, B20, B21, CV12
- ST36, LI4, B40, H7, P6, SP6, K3, GV24.5, GB21 (improve circulation)

Aromatherapy

Essential oils like coriander and cinnamon can help your liver and pancreas to balance blood sugar levels. Obesity/metabolic syndrome can be helped with grapefruit essential oil that can break down body fat. Cinnamon oil can regulate blood glucose level; ginger oil reduces sugar cravings and reduces inflammation. Others include cypress, fennel, geranium, juniper, lavender, lemon, rosemary. Relaxing oils can be tried: bergamot, jasmine, lavender, rose, sandalwood, or ylang-ylang. Use them in a massage, a bath, as lotions, or any of the other methods.

• 11 •

Gastroenterology

Yay! Now for the diseases of the digestive system and most importantly . . . you and your poop! Yup, I said it! It's amazing how one word can cause an entire room of children to burst into laughter. But seriously what your poop looks like is an important clue to determine what is going on in your body—small pellets are sad and sick poops, while snake poops are happy and healthy poops. So let's talk about how to improve your POOP and digestive system! We love you, poop!!! Laugh all you want, but it's time to make friends with your poop. Let's keep those snakes pilin'!

D & D: SPECIAL CONSIDERATIONS

Healing the gut is key, and eating gut superfoods is essential. Maintaining a high-fiber diet is important for overall gut health. Adding fermented veggies and seeds like flax, chia, and hemp can add bulk to stools. Also good are apple cider vinegar; kombucha; bone broth; healthy fats like coconut oil (powerful antifungal); wild-caught salmon; almonds; squash; honey; cabbage juice (rich in glutamine); green leafy and cruciferous veggies (contain methionine, which can fight against H. pylori); bitter greens like turnip greens, dandelion greens, and mustard greens, which help your body produce acid, bile, and enzymes to break down food; and cranberry juice, which can help prevent H. pylori from adhering to the gut. It is important to eat small meals, only filling your stomach two-thirds of the way, to optimize digestion and digestive health. Herbs and herbal teas can help to aid in digestion and decrease bloating; these include fennel, anise ginger, peppermint, caraway seeds, cardamom, cloves, lemon balm, spearmint, thyme, celery seed, and basil, which can help ease any acute symptoms.

Foods to help eliminate parasites are raw garlic, pumpkin seeds, pomegranates, beets, and carrots. Papaya seeds and papaya extracts (papain) have been helpful in eliminating worms and keeping the intestine in a natural acidic state.

Some patients can benefit from a FODMAPs diet, which minimizes poorly absorbed short chain carbohydrates, including most dairy, corn syrup, wheat products, and vegetables and fruit with a high glucose-to-fructose ratio, such as watermelon and dried fruit.

THE FOUR BIG S's: SPECIAL CONSIDERATIONS

Remove the stress from your bowels by creating a bathroom routine and listening to your body and not ignoring urges. Squatting straightens the anorectal angle and allows for easy passage, and using a stool can have the same effect.

BLOATING

Bloating is the feeling of gas filling up in your stomach or bowels. Digestive disorders, fluid buildup, dehydration, food sensitivities, constipation, hormonal changes, small intestinal bacterial overgrowth, infection, cancer, or even bowel obstruction can lead bloating.

Additional Integrative Modalities

Supplements

Gut healing supplements are optimal for relieving bloating; these include probiotics, digestive enzymes, and even activated charcoal tablets (as they can help to absorb toxins and gases) and chlorophyll, which can be taken with each meal.

Homeopathy

- Carbo vegetabilis helps with bloating and belching.
- Lycopodium is useful for passing gas when constipation is also present, especially when eating onions or garlic.
- Dioscorea is helpful for gas in the presence of diarrhea and abdominal pain that is better by bending backward.
- Ignatia is a remedy for bloating of the abdomen after grief.

- Natrum carbonicum is a remedy that can help those who have trouble digesting foods, associated with heartburn, ulcers, dairy-induced gas and diarrhea. They crave for sweets and potatoes.
- Thuja is indicated for abdominal bloating, chronic diarrhea, rumbling of the bowels, accompanied with lots of gas.
- Others that can be used are Ambra grisea, Arnica montana, Aurum muriaticum, folliculinum, Phosphoricum acidum, and sulphur.

Acupressure

- ST36, SP6, LV3
- Others: ST25, CV6, ST37, ST41, LI4

Aromatherapy

Angelica, cardamom, Roman chamomile, fennel, ginger, lemon, peppermint, and rosemary cineole can help with bloating.

CANDIDA

Candida albicans is one of the most common types of yeast infection found in the vagina, digestive system, mucous membranes, and skin. Candida can overgrow if the immune system isn't working properly; broad spectrum antibiotics, birth control pills, oral corticosteroids, high sugar diet, chronic anxiety, other negative emotions, cancer treatments, and diabetes can cause Candida infections. Symptoms of candidal overgrowth are fatigue, brain fog, sinus issues, bloating, gas, abdominal and joint pain, and other digestive issues, bad breath, sleep and mood disorders, craving for sweets, blood sugar and hormonal imbalances, muscle aches, allergies/sinus issues, loss of sex drive, foggy thinking, recurring infections (especially urinary tract and vaginal), oral thrush, skin and nail fungal infections, food intolerances, and sensitivity to smells, sounds, or light.

Additional Integrative Modalities

Supplements

- Focus on healing the gut and supporting the liver, with probiotics and milk thistle.
- Natural antifungals: oil of oregano (300–500 mg three times per day with meals, minimum of sixty days), berberine, caprylic acid (1,000 mg three times per day), hemicelluloses.

- Spleen support: licorice, gentian (250 mg at beginning of each meal), coptis, gardenia, skullcap, ginseng.
- Others: selenium (decreases oxidative stress), garlic (500–1,000 mg of aged garlic twice daily or two cloves daily), grapefruit seed extract (200 mg two to three times daily), vitamin C (1,000 mg twice per day) and pau d'arco tea, S.boulardii (5–15 billion two to four times per day for sixty days), activated charcoal (two to four capsules per day at bedtime for sixty days; may deplete magnesium, so will need to replace).
- Make sure to start any anti-candidal agent at low dose, increasing very gradually to reduce symptoms of candidal die-off reaction.
- *Children:* Candida: probiotics, baking soda (¼ tsp gargled or swallowed in water or formula four times daily), garlic paste applied twice daily, lemon juice (1 tbsp diluted in 8 oz of water and applied topically, gargled, or swallowed twice daily), lemongrass infusion (applied topically or gargled two times daily), GI-probiotic, black walnut hull tincture (1:1 ratio, one drop for each ten pounds of weight, in a glass three times daily), caprylic acid (250–500 mg daily), garlic (one to three cloves daily), olive leaf (250–1,000 mg daily).
- Fungal overgrowth: oregano, carlic, caprylic acid, grapeseed extract, probiotics, olive leaf extract.

Homeopathy

- Candida albicans (look for 30C).
- Sepia can be used for those with yeast infections with yellowish discharge, bearing down sensation and chronic constipation, itching of the skin, fatigue, but improved symptoms after exercise and sunlight exposure. They are irritable/moody, often chilly but can feel worse in a warm room with limited to no circulation.
- Pulsatilla is a remedy for those who tend to cry easily and are irritable and indifferent. Itching or red skin is specifically on the chest and the abdomen. Yeast infections have discharge that is thick and yellowish green with swelling of the vulva; symptoms improve with open air and worsen with lying down, heat, warm rooms.
- Calcarea carbonica is needed for those with constipation, are overweight, crave sweet and salty, and their yeast infections are thick and creamy yellow with burning and itching; they get increased colds. Other features for this remedy are when the patient has coldness of the top of the head, bottom, and the legs with sweating (especially on back of head) with minimal exertion or from coughing, sleeping, and anxiety.

- Sulphur is a remedy for burning or redness in some area of the body, face, ears, rectum, nose, and vagina. These patients are warm, do worse from heat, and have burning of the soles at night, with diarrhea at 5:00 am.
- Graphites can be used for thick, cracked skin on the corners of the mouth or heels.
- Kreosotum is indicated for irritating discharge that leads to swelling or itching, bad odor, and lots of redness, rawness, and pain during urination.
- Borax is helpful for those with diarrhea and bleeding oral mucosa, rash in the area, and the discharge is sticky and runny with consistency of egg whites.
- Belladonna is a remedy for bright red, painful inflamed skin that is not raw or oozing. Person is irritable.
- Chamomilla can be helpful for irritability and a diaper rash.
- Arsenicum album is indicated for itchy, burning rashes and those who have anxiety.

Acupressure

- SP9, LI4, LV3

Aromatherapy

Essential oils can help to act as an antifungal. Examples include oregano, clove, myrrh, melaleuca, and thyme. Lavender oil can help to inhibit growth of candida. Peppermint oil can help to relieve intestinal cramping. Others are cedarwood, eucalyptus globules, geranium, helichrysum, lavandin, lemon, manuka, rosemary verbenone, rosewood, and tea tree.

CONSTIPATION

Constipation is a symptom of hardened feces in persons who are having difficulty emptying the bowels; it is important to get to the root cause. Causes may be related to lifestyle, dehydration, gut problems, poor bathroom and sleep habits, and magnesium deficiency and medications (antidepressents, antacids, blood pressure meds, painkillers); it can also be associated with conditions like diabetes, thyroid disease, hormonal problems, and other chronic illnesses, older age, poor sleep, jet lag, and traveling. Diagnosed by history and physical.

Additional Integrative Modalities

Supplements

- Cod liver oil.
- Psyllium (5 g psyllium husk twice daily).
- Flax seed oil or flax seeds (1–2 tbsp daily).
- Pectin.
- Aloe vera juice.
- Others: Senna (one to four pills per day), Cascara sagrada (250 mg or 2.5 ml of tincture two to three times daily for acute constipation), triphala.
- *Children:* magnesium (100–250 mg daily), probiotics, castor oil rubbed clockwise on the abdomen, zinc (20–40 mg daily).

Homeopathy

- Nux vomica is useful in those with constipation with a great urge to defecate but nothing is passed or incomplete defecation. This works really well for those who are studying hard or who are sedentary, elderly, and addicted to laxatives. They are cold, irritable, and overstressed.
- Bryonia is indicated for those who have large burned, dry, and hard stools accompanied with headaches, congestion, burning in the rectum after passing a stool; patient is thirsty and irritable. Bryonia works well if patient is elderly.
- Alumina is a remedy in those who have no desire to defecate, and passes when the rectum is completely full. The stools may feel as if they accumulate under the left rib area and may be covered with mucus; even soft stools are difficult to pass; is indicated in the elderly. They may have memory issues.
- Natrum muriaticum is useful when the stools are hard and crumbly. They pass a stool every second day or longer and the rectum feels dry and painful. They strongly crave water and salt and may suffer from depression.
- Sulphur is found to be helpful when constipation alternates with diarrhea and stools can be passed every two to four days when the person is constipated. Stools are dark, hard, and large with feeling of incomplete defecation and symptoms of hemorrhoids and anal fissure. Rectum feels as if it is burning, and there is a strong thirst for ice cold drinks.
- Silicea is a remedy for when stools are small and hard, covered with mucus accompanied with symptoms or a sore anus, head sweats, and

the feeling of the stool sliding back in when defecating. Patients feel cold and are thin.

- Opium is best for those with no desire to defecate for days accompanied with a poor appetite; person alert to the slightest noise that keeps the person wakeful at night and drowsy during the day.
- Graphites are helpful for anyone with an anal fissure or hemorrhoids, no desire to pass a stool for days, then when the urge arrives, it presents as colicky pain and then passing of stool covered in white mucus. Bowels may ache after stooling.
- Aesculus is a remedy for those with sensations of fullness, sensation of crawling in the anus and the rectum feels hot and dry full of spikes; person feels as though a knife is being used to open the bowels.
- Nitric acidium is indicated for splinter-like pain that lasts for hours after stooling with a burning, tearing sensation with itching.
- Plumbum metallicum is indicated for sharp colicky pains with little outcome. Stools are hard, dry, and black.
- Lycopodium is found helpful to relieve constipation and gas, when there's no desire to pass a stool and when passed it is painful and is worse between 4:00 and 8:00 pm. This person craves sweets. Symptoms improve with warm drinks.
- Ammonium muriaticum is indicated for those with a burning sensation in the anus and rectum. After a lot of straining, they pass crumbly, hard, and dry stools.
- Magnesia muriatica helps with dry and hard stools that may crumble around the anus.
- Causticum is useful for older individuals who are prone to ankylosis with ineffectual desire to stool.
- Hydrastis canadensis is a remedy for those with constipated stools covered with mucus, with no desire to defecate. Very effective in pregnant women, children, and those on chronic laxatives.
- Raphanus niger helps with belly distension and gas at the left upper side of the abdomen. The distended belly is painful, and the condition is improved by passing gas.
- Calcarea carbonica is used for those who feel overwhelmed, chronically constipated, and their hands and feet feel cold and clammy.
- Sepia is used for digestive issues and constipation associated with hormonal issues and is accompanied with a heavy sensation in the rectum and the lower abdomen.

Acupressure

- LV3, LI4, LI11, ST36, CV12

Aromatherapy

Carrot seed, orange, and fennel help to soothe the effects of the digestive system. Spearmint can help to soothe the digestive system and optimize digestion. Others that can be used are black pepper, marjoram, grapefruit, ginger, mandarin, bergamot, rosemary cineole, jasmine, lavender, rose, pine, sandalwood, and ylang-ylang.

Other Recommendations

Never repress the urge to defecate. When you hold back, you are actually training your bowels to misbehave. The result is often chronic—even lifelong—constipation.

It is possible to retrain your bowels, if necessary. Sit on the toilet at the same time every day, even if you don't have an urge. Early morning or directly after exercise are usually good times. Do not strain—you'll only create hemorrhoids or varicose veins. Instead, breathe deeply, using your abdominal muscles, and try to relax.

DIARRHEA

Diarrhea can increase the frequency, volume, and wateriness, though it may be due to a virus or infection; chronic diarrhea (more than four weeks) can be a sign of another bowel issue like inflammatory bowel disease or irritable bowel syndrome. Other causes of diarrhea can be reactions to medications, sensitivities to foods or artificial sweeteners, thyroid problems, diabetes, and other chronic illnesses. Other symptoms include bloating, nausea, vomiting, and urgent need to pass a bowel movement. Diagnosis can be made by a history and physical.

Additional Integrative Modalities

Supplements

- Healing the gut supplements: probiotics, digestive enzymes, glutamine, and aloe vera juice (½ cup three times).
- Raw sprouted fiber from flax and chia seeds (3 tbsp daily).
- Others: ginger (500 mg in capsule), goldenseal (300 mg capsule four times per day), oregano oil (500 mg of capsule four times per day) as an antimicrobial, and astragalus (500–1,000 mg two to three times per day, not to be taken with a fever).

- *Children:* probiotics, zinc (10–20 mg daily), glutamine (0.3 g/kg daily), calcium (200–500 mg daily), fiber (5–15 g three times per day with plenty of water), berberine (400 mg daily), digestive enzymes, colostrums, lauricidin (¼ tsp three times daily and increase as needed to get some normal stool consistency), echinacea, aloe extracts, fatty acids.

Homeopathy

- Aconite is useful for diarrhea that occurs suddenly after a cold wind, shock, or overheating in the summer. This person has a distended abdomen and feels better after passing a stool.
- Aloe socotrina is helpful for those with morning violent diarrhea associated with rumbling in the abdomen, then gushing stools after anger outburst, exposure to food sensitivities. Stools are yellowish green and mucus filled. Symptoms worsen after meals, with excessive gas.
- Arsenicum album is a remedy for exhausting diarrhea, abdominal pain, and vomiting. Diarrhea is scant, no odor, may have blood present and burn the anus skin with passage. Symptoms improve with sips of hot drinks and worsen with cold drinks and foods and overripe fruit.
- Podophyllum is found to be helpful with diarrhea that is offensive, with a batter consistency, and is the color of pea soup. Gas is present with urgency in the morning.
- Phosphoric acidium is indicated for those with perfuse, painless watery stools with bits of food present and occurs after emotional shock or eating certain foods in excess. Feels better after defecation.
- Sulphur is a remedy for burning, explosive, and foul smelling diarrhea that forces a person out of bed at 5:00 am and who may have hemorrhoids present. Anus may be red and excoriated. Patient craves cold liquids.
- Veratum is helpful for profuse, painful diarrhea that looks like rice water that is accompanied with vomiting, cold sweats, and craving for ice water.
- China is a remedy for stools that look like a chopped egg, excessive gas, chronic spasms, exhaustion, and weakness that follows diarrhea. This person is very irritable, and symptoms worsen by the summer chills or by eating fruit.
- Colocynth is indicated for those whose excessive diarrhea, which could have been brought on by anger, is accompanied with gripping pain that forces them to double up as the pressure helps to lessen the pain along with heat. The stools are yellowish, thin, and frothy.

- Dulcamara is found to be helpful for slimy, green, or yellow stool that may have blood in it and presents itself with damp weather or getting cold after exertion.
- Pulsatilla is useful for those with stools that don't look similar and are worse at night, warm room, by cold drinks, onions, and rich fatty foods. Symptoms improve in the open air.
- Argenticum nitricum is a remedy for painless emotional or nervous diarrhea accompanied with bloating and gastric burning and can also result after sugar ingestion.
- Chamomilla helps with yellow green diarrhea in teething infants.
- Ipecacuanha is a remedy for nausea associated with diarrhea.
- Mercuris solublis is indicated for spasmodic burning or bloody diarrhea accompanied with extreme sweating.
- Phosphorus is for diarrhea present in anxious people who crave cold liquids.
- Antimonium crudum is for stools that are partly solid and partly liquid; patients have a thick, white-coated tongue and are overweight, with impetigo and hyperkeratosis.
- Natrum sulphuricum helps violent, watery diarrhea after meals with a yellow/greenish coated tongue. Patient is overweight, can have depression, and is cold sensitive.
- Paratyphoidinum can be helpful for chronic diarrhea.

Acupressure

- LI4, LI11, ST36, SP6, SP4, SP16 (abdominal cramps)
- CV6 (if with gas)
- Others: SP15, SP4, LV3

Aromatherapy

Essential oils can help to relieve abdominal cramps as they may have antispasmodic properties. Neroli, mandarin, cypress, eucalyptus, fennel, chamomile, peppermint, black pepper, and ginger are helpful.

Others that can be used are lemon balm, lavender, cedarwood, cinnamon, clove (bud), geranium, ginger, marjoram, niaouli, nutmeg, sandalwood, and spearmint.

DIVERTICULOSIS

Diverticulosis is a condition in which small bulging pouches develop in the digestive tract; it is common in those over forty. This condition is asymptomatic unless the diverticula become inflamed and infected (diverticulitis), which can cause abdominal pain, nausea, alternating diarrhea and constipation, and fever. Diagnosis is made with lab tests or imaging.

Additional Integrative Modalities

Supplements

- Gut healing supplements are important like probiotics, digestive enzymes, slippery elm (500 mg three times per day), aloe vera juice or powder (during an attack take 12–16 oz. of aloe juice per day), licorice root (100–300 mg per day), and psyllium fiber to prevent constipation.
- Others: Colloidal silver (1 tsp four times daily) and boswellia (500 mg three times per day).

Homeopathy

- Nitricum acidum is beneficial for diverticulosis in the rectosigmoid area.
- Belladonna is for those with sudden abdominal pain and cramping accompanied with constipation, worse with motion and feels better with firm pressure.
- Bryonia is useful for left-sided sharp abdominal pain that is worse with movement and relieved with heat. It is accompanied with constipation and vomiting.
- Colocynthis is for cramping, sharp pain that improves with pressure and accompanied with diarrhea and restlessness.
- Arsenicum album is for burning pain, feeling anxious and restless, relieved by warm environment.
- Ignatia amara helps with digestive spasms associated with emotional stress.
- Magnesia phosphorica helps with abdominal cramping that worsens with pressure and is relieved by warmth.
- Nux vomica can be used for cramping pain, especially when the person is cold sensitive and irritable.

Acupressure

- CV4, SP4, P6, ST36, CV6 (gas and diarrhea)
- SP16 (abdominal cramps)
- LI11 (overall gut health)

Aromatherapy

Essential oils can have an antispasmodic effect on the digestive tract to help to relax the abdomen. Examples include German chamomile, lavender, geranium, ginger, juniper (berry), Melissa, myrrh, niaouli, bitter orange, peppermint, rosemary, and marjoram.

GALLSTONES

Gallstones are tiny pieces of solid matter found in the gallbladder that are formed when cholesterol, calcium, and other particles found in bile bind to each other. Symptoms depend on where the gallstone is located and vary person to person; but when an attack occurs, it can lead to symptoms of pain, nausea, upper-right-sided abdominal pain leading to pain under the right shoulder blade or within the back by the right shoulder blade. Diagnosis can be made by imaging like ultrasound or CT and even more specialized imaging tests.

Additional Integrative Modalities

Supplements

- Supplements can improve liver health and regulate the production and use of cholesterol.
- Turmeric, milk thistle (150 mg twice daily), dandelion root (500 mg with meals) as discussed in the liver detoxification section.
- Others: Activated charcoal helps to bind and remove toxins; vitamin C (1–3 g daily) can decrease gallstone formation; vitamin E (200–400 IU per day), lipase enzymes (two capsules with meals that help improve fat digestion); bile salts or ox bile (500–1,000 mg with meals) to improve the breakdown of fats and optimize gallbladder function; phosphatidylcholine (PC) (100 mg two or three times per day) can help to make the bile smooth, decreasing stone formation; and barberry can help to cleanse the gallbladder and liver, l-methionine [1g per day]).

Homeopathy

- Berberis 6C.
- China is a remedy for when the person is oversensitive and always cold.

Acupressure

- Gallbladder health: LV3
- Others: GB34, P6, LI4, LV14, CV14, ST36 and Zhigou or TH6

Aromatherapy

Rosemary oil can help to reduce inflammation and can be massaged over gallbladder area twice daily.

GASTROESOPHAGEAL REFLUX DISEASE

Gastroesophageal reflux disease (GERD) and acid reflux symptoms include heartburn, dry mouth, bitter taste in mouth, regurgitation of acid or foods, bad breath, gum irritation, belching after meals, bloating one to two hours after meals, getting full easily, low appetite, difficulty swallowing, chronic constipation, undigested food in stool, rectal itching, anemia, waking up choking in the middle of the night, nausea, hiccups, discomfort when lying down or bending over, hoarseness, chronic throat irritation, dryness and peeling nails, sour taste in mouth, coughing at night, and soreness. As it continues to progress it can lead to blood vomit, black stools, and unexpected weight loss.

Acid reflux can be due to not enough acid, drugs like NSAIDs, birth control pills, muscle relaxers, nitroglycerine, steroids, tight clothing, pregnancy, being overweight or obese, hiatal hernia (when part of your stomach protrudes above the diaphragm), stress, large meals, food sensitivities, excessive exercise, and not enough acid.

Additional Integrative Modalities

Supplements

- Focus on gut-healing supplements like probiotics, digestive enzymes, and HCL with pepsin, L glutamine, and so on.
- Others that can help soothe the gut lining: Licorice root (DGL) (one or two 400 mg tablets twenty minutes before each meal).
- Aloe vera juice (½ cup twice a day). Helps to soothe internal inflammation.

- D-limonene (1000 mg per day for 10 doses as needed).
- Slippery elm (300 mg daily or 1 tsp or 3 ml tincture three times per day).
- Others include: chamomile tea, melatonin (6 mg at bedtime), orange peel extract (one capsule that contains 98.5% extract of D limonene every other day for twenty-one days), vitamin C, peppermint oil, capsaicin, meadowsweet (1 cup of tea with 1–2 tsp).
- *For Barrett's esophagus:* the above can also be used, along with quercetin (500–6,000 mg daily) to protect esophageal tissues, antioxidants like vitamin C (1,000 mg daily), vitamin E, selenium (200–400 mg per day), NAC (1,000–2,000 mg) and lipoic acid, other gut healing herbs like marshmallow, gamma oryzanol, and/or turmeric.
- *Children:* apple cider vinegar (¼ tsp before meals), DGL (300 mg three times daily).

Homeopathy

- Carbo vegetabilis is a remedy that can be used for those with bloating and belching/gas after eating food with light burning sensation in stomach that goes to the back. People are cold and pale, crave fresh air, and feel better with cool things.
- Nux vomica is indicated for people with heartburn that occurs about one-half hour after eating accompanied by constipation. Attacks can be brought on by excessive food, alcohol, and stress/work. Person is irritable and oversensitive to stimuli.
- Pulsatilla helps those with heartburn that is worse after eating food that is rich and fatty and while in a warm room and is better with fresh air. Attack begins two hours after eating and can be characterized by a pressure under the breastbone, bad taste in the mouth, nausea that may or may not be accompanied by vomiting, weepiness, a desire for comfort, and headaches around the eyes.
- Arsenicum album is a remedy for those with heartburn after eating, and the attack is characterized by a stone weight that is present in the stomach; the person is anxious and restless, vomits, and or retches until he/she is exhausted. Symptoms are improved with sipping on warm water and sitting up and worse in the morning hours.
- Bryonia is indicated for those with the feeling of heartburn that comes on after eating, feeling like a heavy stone is on the stomach, accompanied with nausea, faintness, and the mouth filling with bitter-tasting fluid. Symptoms are relieved by lying on the back and gets worse with pressure or slightest movement.
- China helps those with a stomach full of air; person is sluggish and apathetic and feels worse at night; symptoms aren't relieved by belching

and feel worse at night; recent loss of bodily fluids like blood, sweat, and semen; chopped egg appearance of stool.

- Anacardium helps those with indigestion that comes on one to two hours after meals. The attack is characterized by a foul taste in mouth, stomach feels blocked, and the attack can be improved if they eat again and worsen by cold drinks. Person tends to be forgetful. Anacardium can be used if you suspect a peptic ulcer.
- Argenticum nitricum is a remedy for indigestion after sweet foods, accompanied with alternating constipation and diarrhea, belching, and fluttery feeling in stomach. Can be used for suspected peptic ulcer.
- Sepia is indicated for those with heartburn that can be improved by lying on the right side and by eating. They have a sudden empty feeling in the stomach, they have a sour taste in the mouth and a lot of bloating, tenderness over the liver, and they become nauseous by seeing or smelling foods. They crave pickles.
- Lycopodium is for gas and bloating, when the person feels full quickly as the foods lead to instant gas, and the symptoms are not improved with belching. They also have symptoms of anxiety, lack of confidence, constipation, and feel worse when they wear tight clothes, in the late afternoon and evening, and improve with drinking warm fluids. Can also be used for suspected peptic ulcer.
- Phosphorus can be used for the burning sensations in the chest, which feel better from ice-cold water, but then accompanied with vomiting and nausea, soon after drinking. Can be used for likely peptic ulcer.
- Graphites can be used for those with burning hunger pains that are relieved by food or hot drinks like milk. Attack is characterized by nausea after eating sweet things. Graphites can be used for peptic ulcers.
- Kali bichromium can be used for feelings of nausea and vomiting after drinking beer. Persons complain of pain in a particular spot, so it can be used for peptic ulcers. They feel as if their stomach is distended and feel cessation of their digestive processes.
- Sulphur is indicated for those with diarrhea, burning pain, and belching that is improved from drinking ice cold drinks.
- Natrum carbonicum can be helpful for people with trouble digesting most foods.
- Antimonium crudum can help with pains in the pit of the stomach with overeating; white, thick, milky tongue with hyperkarotosis; and impetigo eruptions.
- Others that can be used are: robinia (especially with those with too much acid, worse at night, and frontal and temporal headache),

sulphuricum acidum (pain in the stomach after the consumption of alcohol and from a hiatal hernia, and ulcerative stomatitis), asa foetida (for aerophagia), nux moschata (for extreme flatulence), chelidonium majus (pain in the hepatobiliary region that radiates into the inferior angle of the right scapula), hydrastis canadensis (pain in the hepatobiliary area but the person is thin, tired, and constipated), ignatia (symptoms of paradoxical cramps and burning sensations that worsen around 11:00 am and are improved by entertainment), lachesis (when heartburn is accompanied with PMS, hemorrhoids, hot flashes, and rectal bleeding, symptoms after excessive alcohol and also during menopause), and thuja occidentalis (gas; distention of colon worse two to three hours after meals; relieved by heat; overweight and cold-sensitive, phobia-prone individuals).

Acupressure

- HP6, ST36, CV12, SP4
- Gastritis: ST21, ST36, SP4, B21, CV12

Aromatherapy

Peppermint and a ginger massage can be helpful to relieve symptoms of reflux when massaged by combining sunflower oil, peppermint essential oil, ginger essential oil, and dill oil. They can also help indigestion as some are antispasmodic, calming and warming like cardamom, coriander, and mandarin to relieve indigestion. Others include: cedarwood, roman chamomile, lemon, sandalwood, anise, basil linalool, bergamot, fennel, lavender, lemon, mandarin, marjoram, rosemary cineole, spearmint, thyme linalool. Use aromatherapy two hours between eating and exercise.

Other Recommendations

- Drink more water but not with meals, staying upright after meals.
- Stay upright after large meal and elevate the head of the bed by six inches.
- Avoid tight-fitting clothing around the middle.
- Heel drops can help to set your hiatal hernia. Standing, take a gulp of water and then come up on your tiptoes; as you swallow, drop your heels to the ground.

HEMORRHOIDS

Hemorrhoids are rectal or anal veins that become painful and swollen. There are two types of hemorrhoids: internal (those that are inside the anus or lower rectum) and external (those that are outside the opening to the anus). Symptoms include anal pain and itching; painful bowel movements; bright red blood on stool, toilet paper, or in the bowel; and a feeling of harder and tender lumps near the anus. Diagnosis can occur with a history and physical exam. To look inside the anal canal, the doctor may use an anoscope or sigmoidoscope.

Additional Integrative Modalities

Supplements

- Fiber, like psyllium husk.
- Pycnogenol (100 mg twice daily) for acute hemorrhoids.
- Horse chestnut (100 mg daily) can help to improve circulation and vascular tone.
- Witch hazel can help to reduce inflammation and pain.
- Others: Butcher's broom helps to treat chronic venous insufficiency; diosmin (1,000–3,000 mg per day in divided doses for one week for current issues, and 1,000 mg per day in divided doses for at least two to three months) to reduce symptoms of chronic or recurrent hemorrhoids); collinsonia (500 mg three times a day) to reduce swelling; bioflavonoid complex (1,000 mg two or three times daily) to reduce swelling and prevent bleeding; bilberry; vitamin E (400–800 IU of alpha tocopherol and mixed tocopherol daily).
- For temporary relief of pain and itching, use any of the following as a topical lotion: cocoa butter, zinc oxide, olive oil, or calendula gel. Salves: spread vitamin E oil, comfrey, calendula ointment, or goldenseal salve gently on anus with fingers; witch hazel is also soothing.

Homeopathy

- Aesculus is for those with large, painful internal hemorrhoids that may cause a dry spiky sensation in the rectum. Lumpy stools cause stabbing and tearing when passed, pain extends to the back. Anus feels dry, hot, and itchy.
- Aloe is best for large and painful hemorrhoids that look like a small bluish cluster of grapes that are painful, accompanied with diarrhea, sense of rectal fullness and burning, or needle-like pain in the rectum.

The pain feels better with cold applications. Mucous membranes are dry and excoriated, with sphincter problems.

- Collinsonia is found to help relieve bleeding, constipation, itching, and the desire to defecate.
- Hamamelis is a remedy for bleeding hemorrhoids accompanied with feeling bruised and sore, aggravated by heat and the slightest touch.
- Nitric acid is indicated in the presence of an anal fissure with cutting, burning pain during the entire process of defecation.
- Nux vomica is used for those with large painful hemorrhoids that burn and sting with incomplete emptying, with frequent urge to defecate, improved by cold baths; it is best for patients who live sedentary lives. The hemorrhoids are a result of constipation and excessive straining. Patients are irritable and tend to overuse drugs, meds, or alcohol.
- Pulsatilla is useful for hemorrhoids that bleed easily (dark bleeding); pain and discomfort is worse when lying down, in heat and warm stuffy rooms, better in cool air. This can be associated with constipation, aversion to fats, and weakness.
- Sulphur helps with large, itching and burning hemorrhoids when the skin around the anus is sore, inflamed, and red; symptoms worsen with warmth and at night. Flatulence has a terrible odor.
- Ammonium carbonicum is a remedy for extremely painful hemorrhoids that are worse with menses and when lying down.
- Capsicum is indicated for burning, protruding piles.
- Causticum is beneficial for sore hemorrhoids with inability to pass stool even when straining.
- Calcarea fluorica is useful for bleeding and itching hemorrhoids. Constipation, back pain, and flatulence may be present.
- Ignatia amara helps with rectal spasms, stabbing pain that is worse from being emotionally upset.
- Ratahia is helpful for cutting pain after a bowel movement with fissures and itching, relieved by cold or very hot water, may be associated with burning diarrhea.
- Arnica montana can ease the bruising sensations, which worsen with touch.
- Carduus marianus is indicated for bloody hemorrhoids that may be accompanied with constipation, liver problems, and/or varicosities.
- Graphites can help hemorrhoids with painful and itchy fissures with no tenesmus.
- Kali carbonicum is a remedy for protruding, painful, bleeding hemorrhoids improved by cold or sitting on a hard surface, associated with weakness, paleness, respiratory disorders, and flatulent indigestion.

- Nitricum acidum is best for fissures that bleed easily and are clean, sharp, and can be found radiating around the anus; they lead to sharp pain worsened by hard or soft stools, and the pain lasts after defecation.
- Sepia can be used for hemorrhoids that ooze and with prolapsed anorectal.
- Others for chronic symptomatic treatments (usually used in lower potency daily): Collinsonia canadensis can help with bloody hemorrhoids with constipation, best in pregnant women; paeonia helps hemorrhoids that burn and ooze copiously with pain before and after stooling with anal fissures and thick honey yellow oozing; Hora brasiliensis helps with anal or perianal eruptions with rectal affections, constipation that alternates with diarrhea and sensation of anal constriction; Fluoricum acidum is indicated for hemorrhoids with itching aggravated by heat and improved by cold.

Acupressure

- GV1, GV20, B30, SP6, LU3, CV4, B31, K7, B31, B32, B57
- Others: CV6, B60, SP8, LU9, LI12

Aromatherapy

Cypress oil can help to stop excess blood flow and reduce anxiety. It can be applied topically by adding three to four drops to a cotton ball and applying to the area of concern. Helichrysum oil, lavender oil, and turmeric oil can be used as an anti-inflammatory agent when applied topically. Lemon and geranium oils can act to detoxify. Juniper has an astringent action that can help to shrink varicose veins and hemorrhoids. Others that can help are neat, frankincense, cajuput, cedarwood, Roman chamomile, clary sage, cypress, niaouli, patchouli, sandalwood, spikenard, and tea tree oil.

INFLAMMATORY BOWEL DISEASE

Inflammatory bowel disease is chronic inflammation of all or part of your digestive tract; types include Crohn's disease and ulcerative colitis. Symptoms include pain, fatigue, diarrhea, weight loss, fatigue, fever, nausea and vomiting, floating stools, anemia, and even rectal bleeding and joint pains. Ulcerative colitis causes open sores or ulcers in the innermost layer of the large intestine and rectum, and Crohn's disease can happen anywhere in the digestive tract, often in patches surrounded by healthy tissue. Diagnosis can be made by blood tests, colonoscopy and sigmoidoscopy with possible biopsy, barium enema, and other imaging.

Additional Integrative Modalities

Supplements

- Focus on gut healing supplements and calcium, and multivitamin with antioxidants, zinc, vitamin C (500 mg), vitamin E (400 IU of mixed tocopherol and tocotrienols), curcumin, bromelin (2,000–3,000 mg per day), and slippery elm.
- Others can be aloe vera, DGL (300 mg two minutes before meals), enzymes (one to two capsules with each meal), glutamine (1–3 g three times daily on an empty stomach), phosphatidylcholine and IgA supplements, marshmallow, cat's claw (250 mg per day), and boswellia (can help in Crohn's, not to take more than eight weeks straight).
- *Children:* Crohn's disease: Fish oil (EPA/DHA 3 g daily), probiotics, vitamin D (1,000–5,000 IU daily), NAC (3–6 g daily), glutamine (5,000 mg daily), bromelain (250–1,000 mg daily), butyrate (4 g daily), fiber, L-carnitine (500–2,000 mg daily), turmeric standardized extract (400–600 mg daily).
- Ulcerative colitis: probiotics, fish oil (3 g EPA/DHA daily), vitamin D (1,000–4,000 IU daily), bromelain (250–1,000 mg daily), butyrate (500–1,000 mg daily), vitamin C (500–2,000 mg daily), curcumin (500–1,000 mg daily).

Homeopathy

Homeopathics can be taken every two hours for up to ten doses during an acute attack. Look for a constitutional remedy (see Appendix).

- Mercuris can be used for abdominal pain that is unrelieved with passing of stools; the offensive smelling stools have blood and mucus on them and are extremely painful when passing.
- Arsenicum is best for those with burning abdominal pain worse after midnight that is accompanied with vomiting, anxiety, and restlessness. Person feels cold and prefers warm drinks frequently.
- Phosphorus is for those whose pain improves after passing bloody stools, but the anus feels wide open afterward.
- Arsenicum album is for burning pains in the abdomen that are made better in a warm environment or with warm drinks. The person feels anxious and restless.

- China can be used for a suspected obstruction.
- Belladonna is indicated for abdominal pain that stops and starts abruptly, with a tender abdomen very sensitive to light vibrations or jolts, symptoms worsen with motion. Person's face is red and hot, and there is fever that has a throbbing or burning pain.
- Bryonia is for those that have stomachaches that feel like their abdomen is about to burst, worse with pressure and so severe that the person can't talk or move.
- Chamomilla is best for those with cutting pain that makes the person double up and cry. Attacks may follow anger, and abdomen is bloated.
- Colocynth is a remedy for those with sharp, colicky, twisting pain just below the navel that is improved with passing gas, pressure on the abdomen, or bending forward.
- Magnesia phosphoric is best with cramping pain that makes the person cry out and improves with pressure on abdomen, warmth, and friction.
- Nux vomica is for cramping, digestive pain; persons are irritable and always cold.
- Ignatia can be used for emotional stresses that can lead to spasms of the digestive tract.
- Pulsatilla is a remedy for diarrhea due to fatty foods, worse at night.
- Sulphur is indicated for burning pain, improved with cold drinks; also for explosive and urgent diarrhea that can wake you up at night. Person craves alcohol and spicy foods.
- Cambogia is indicated for chronic colitis.
- Podophyllum is for painless, explosive diarrhea that is worse after eating or drinking, followed by exhaustion; person has painful cramps in the lower legs and feet.
- Veratrum album is found useful for those with a bloating abdomen, cramping, exhaustion, chills, and vomiting with perfuse watery diarrhea that worsens after eating fruits; person craves cold liquids.
- Anal fistula: Calcarea sulph is recommended for those with a painful abscess. Silicea can be indicated for those with post-cleaning discharge, and Lachesis can be used for pain that travels up the rectum and is made worse by coughing or sneezing.

Acupressure

- SP6, ST25, B25, SP4, ST37, ST36
- ST39, CV4, LI11, SP16 (for painful cramps)
- SP15, CV12, CV9, CV6

Aromatherapy

Essential oils may improve digestive health; these include frankincense, which also improves circulation. To relieve pain, chamomile, lavender, and lemongrass oils can help. Ginger, peppermint, and fennel can help to relieve inflammation.

IRRITABLE BOWEL SYNDROME

Irritable bowel syndrome leads to diarrhea, constipation and pain after bowel movements, mucus in your stool, immediate need to go to the bathroom when you wake up and during or after meals, feeling of incomplete emptying due to the effects of changes in contractions either faster or slower.

Additional Integrative Modalities

Supplements

- Focus on gut healing supplements: probiotics, digestive enzymes, L-glutamine, fish oil (EPA/DHA 1,000 mg daily), aloe vera (half a cup three times per day), fiber 10–15 g per day, zinc.
- Others that can be used: Slippery elm, ginger (500 mg per day), and licorice root. Diamine oxidase (DAO) (one to two capsules within fifteen minutes) can help to reduce histamine levels; vitamin C, magnesium and gentian root (300 mg before meals), peppermint oil (450–1,100 mg per day before meals for all types of IBS).
- *Children:* digestive enzymes, probiotics, fiber, melatonin (3 g daily), tryptophan (1–5 g daily), peppermint oil (one enteric coated capsule three times daily), artichoke leaf extract with 13–18% caffeoylquinic acid (200–500 mg daily).

Homeopathy

- Argentum nitricum can be used for bloating pain in the upper left abdomen; nervousness; constipation alternating with diarrhea, which come on after eating sweets; tense feeling in the stomach.
- Cantharis is for nausea, vomiting, cystitis, with burning pains in the abdomen.
- Colchicum is indicated for those with nausea and watery stools made worse by the smell of food and is accompanied by tearing pains.

- Colocynth is a remedy for those with violent, spasmodic, cutting abdominal pain that is relieved by doubling over or pressure on the abdomen. Symptoms can occur after eating fruit, during diarrhea, or with anger.
- Arsenicum album is for those who feel cold and prefer warm drinks. They complain of diarrhea, restlessness, anxiety, and pains that worsen from 12:00 am to 2:00 am.
- Lycopodium can be used for those with abdominal pain and gurgling noises, bloating constipation, hemorrhoids; low self-confidence and irritability. Their symptoms are worse between 4:00 and 8:00 pm and symptoms feel better with warm drinks.
- Magnesia phosphorica is for those with spasms and cramping that is better with warmth and no nervous causes.
- Nux vomica is useful for those who have bowel problems associated with poor diet and stress. These individuals crave spicy food, alcohol, and other stimulants. Other symptoms are constipation, spasms, tenesmus, heartburn, and the feeling as if they have never completed a bowel movement. Symptoms worsen with anger or excitement and improve after a short nap.
- Ignatia is indicated for spasms, constipation with pain in the right iliac region, sensation of a ball in the throat, spasmodic hiccough worse with worries and improvement with entertainment. Patients are anxious.
- Natrum carbonicum is for people with multiple food allergies, who experience indigestion and heartburn. They crave milk, potatoes, and sweets but experience irritable bowels when ingesting them. They desire to be left alone.
- Sulphur is indicated for those who are awakened by diarrhea, with constipation that may be also present and an irritated rectum. The gas is foul smelling like rotten eggs. Persons crave sweets, alcohol, and spicy foods.
- Iris tenax is used for colicky pain in the appendicular area.
- Thuja occidentalis is a remedy for those with abdominal pain with rumbling noises/flatulence, with spasmodic diarrhea or constipation. The patient has obsessions and/or phobias.

Acupressure

- CV12 (prevents indigestion, so use before meal)
- CV6 (soothes abdominal pain, constipation and gas)
- P6 (calming effect)
- ST37, ST25, B25, B20, B21, SP6 (associated with menses)
- Abdominal pain: LI4, LI11, LV3

Aromatherapy

Peppermint, fennel, and ginger can be used to improve symptoms of IBS. Others can be chamomile, lavender, neroli, catnip, majoram, and sage. Black pepper can help to relieve constipation.

PARASITES

A parasite is an organism that can live on and in a host and lead to disease and illness. Parasites can enter into your system from contaminated food or water, and those with leaky gut or a weakened immune system are more prone to parasites. Symptoms can come in waves, but never go away. These include night sweats, fatigue, allergies, digestive issues, anal itching, unexpected high white blood cell count, skin rashes (eczema, psoriasis, or rosacea, hives or an unexplained rash), trouble falling asleep, waking up multiple times during the night, grinding teeth, muscle aches or pains, never feeling satisfied after eating, and iron deficiency anemia. Suspect parasites when your symptoms worsen after any camping trip or travel, where you may have drunk some sort of contaminated water. Testing with a comprehensive stool test can help detect parasites, but a negative test isn't always definitive.

Additional Integrative Modalities

Supplements

- Before you start a parasite cleansing program, you must have daily regular bowel movements.
- Black walnut (250 mg three times daily).
- Wormwood (200 mg three times daily).
- Oregano oil (500 mg four times daily) has antiparasitic effects.
- Grapefruit seed extract (as directed).
- Clove oil (500 mg four times daily).
- Ginger root (500 mg four times daily).
- Others include: Coptis (gold thread) (200 mg three times daily), a Chinese antiparasitic herb, and Goldenseal (300 mg four times daily) helps to fight gut and digestive tract infections.
- Other herbs: aloe, anise, barberry, cashew, curled mint, Oregon grape, papaya, pomegranate, pumpkin, sweet basil, thyme, turmeric.

Homeopathy

- Cina is indicated for pinworms or threadworms. The patient is irritable, doesn't want to be touched, grinds teeth at night; the child patient picks at its nose, has jerking movment of feet and hands; may be pale and has dark circles around the eyes.
- Caladium is helpful for worms in the vagina that can have the tendency to excite masturbation.
- Teucrium is a remedy for pinworms, round worms, and thread worms; patient has a crawling sensation in the rectum and nose accompanied with itching, nervousness, and irritabilities.
- Spigelia can help with worms and those with colicky pain around the navel and an itchy rectum, accompanied with bad breath, pale face, blue rings around the eyes, and nausea.
- Indigo helps with ascarides or thread worms that lead to convulsions and intense pain in the umbilical region.
- Sabadilla is a remedy for tapeworms or pinworms that lead to vomiting, colic, nausea, and itching of the nose or ears alternating with itching of the rectum.
- Stannum helps those with worms with pale face, dark circles under the eyes, fatigue, and a passive fever; they prefer to lie on stomach.
- Natrum phosphoricum helps to treat all types of worms. These patients often have a creamy/yellow colored coating on the tongue and symptoms of heartburn and belching.
- Filix mas helps with tapeworms. The patient is irritable and anxious, has dark circles around the eyes and an itchy nose with swollen gland.
- Cuprum nigrum helps to remove all kinds of worms, trichinosis, and even tapeworm; use small doses (1X). It can be used in alternation with Nux vomica. It can be used to treat tapeworms for four to six weeks four to five times per day.
- Others: calcarea.

Acupressure

- ST36, SP6, LU7, LI11, LU5, K27

Aromatherapy

The essential oils that help to eliminate parasites are oregano, thyme, fennel, tea tree, bergamot, peppermint, lavender, Roman chamomile, and clove.

PEPTIC ULCERS

Peptic ulcers are sores that have developed on the lining of the esophagus, stomach, or small intestine. Symptoms include pain that can be felt anywhere, worse when stomach is empty, and it flairs up at night. The pain can temporarily be relieved by food or acid blocking medication. Diagnosis is made via lab and imaging tests. About 70 percent of the ulcers are due to an overgrowth of H. pylori; others are due to NSAIDs that can damage the digestive system lining.

Additional Integrative Modalities

Supplements

- These can be done in conjunction with pharmaceutical therapy.
- Continue to focus on gut healing supplements, like probiotics and L-glutamine.
- Chamomile (1 cup four times daily) helps to sooth the nerves and heal ulcers.
- Vitamin E (400 IU of mixed tocopherols daily) can help to protect against and destroy H. pylori.
- Grapefruit seed extract (ten drops three times daily) has strong antimicrobial action.
- Zinc (75 mg twice daily) to heal lining and fight bacteria.
- Additional help for H. pylori: Vitamin C (500 mg twice daily) helps to eradicate the infections and heal tissue. Licorice root (500 mg before meals) may help stop H. pylori and heal the gut lining. Aloe vera (500 mg two to three times daily) helps to fight H. pylori. Also use mastic gum (500 mg two to three times per day for sixty days); and S. boulardii (5 billion–5 billion CFUs two to four times per day for sixty days). Supportive treatment with cabbage juice 4 oz daily for twenty-eight days. Others are citrus seed extract, goldenseal, activated charcoal, and Gamma oryzanol. Sano-Gastril, comfrey, and calendula have also been shown to heal ulcers.
- *Children:* juiced cabbage daily (may interact with cancer therapies), glutamine (500 mg twice daily).

Homeopathy

- Nux vomica is indicated for people with heartburn that occurs about one-half hour after eating accompanied by constipation and the attacks can be brought on by excessive food, alcohol, stress/work. Person is irritable and oversensitive to stimuli.

- Pulsatilla helps those with heartburn that is worse after food that is rich and fatty, in a warm room and better with fresh air. Attack begins two hours after eating and can be characterized by a pressure under the breastbone, bad taste in the mouth, nausea that may or may not be accompanied by vomiting, weepiness, a desire for comfort, and headaches around the eyes.
- Arsenicum album is a remedy for those with heartburn after food, and the attack is characterized by a stone weight that is present in the stomach, person is anxious and restless, vomits and/or retches until he/she is exhausted. Symptoms are improved with sipping on warm water, sitting up, and worse in the morning hours.
- Anacardium helps those with indigestion that comes on one to two hours after meals and the attack is characterized by a foul taste in mouth, stomach feels blocked, and the attack can be improved if they eat again and worsened by cold drinks. Person tends to be forgetful. Anacardium can be used if peptic ulcer is suspected.
- Argenticum nitricum is a remedy for indigestion after sweet foods, accompanied with altering constipation and diarrhea, belching, and fluttery feeling in stomach; can be used for suspected peptic ulcer.
- Lycopodium is for gas and bloating, when the person feels full quickly as the foods lead to instant gas and the symptoms are not improved by belching. They also have symptoms of anxiety, lack of confidence, constipation, and they feel worse when wearing tight clothes and in the late afternoon and evening, and symptoms are relieved with drinking warm fluids. Lycopodium can be used for suspected peptic ulcer.
- Phosphorus can be used for the burning sensations in the chest that feel better from ice-cold water, but then accompanied with vomiting and nausea, soon after drinking; can be used for likely peptic ulcer with "coffee ground" or bright red vomit.
- Graphites can be used for those with burning hunger pains that are relieved by food or hot drinks like milk. Attack is characterized by nausea after eating sweet things. Graphites can be used for peptic ulcers.
- Kali bichromium can be used for feelings of nausea and vomiting after drinking beer. Complaint is of pain in a particular spot, so it can be used for peptic ulcers. Patients feel as if their stomach is distended and feel cessation of their digestive processes.
- Sulphur is indicated for those with diarrhea, burning pain, and belching that is improved from ice cold drinks.
- Others for ulcers: Nitricum acidum (when fibroscopy shows a crack or a fissure; pain is itching, burning, and cramping; worse with fatty food

and better with heat; fissures are located where the mucous membranes merge with skin) and Iris versicolor (best for dumping syndrome, intense pain with burning vomiting, oily diarrhea, and migraines).
- If nervous symptoms present with the ulcer: Argentum nitricum and Arsenicum album.

Acupressure

- The earlier-mentioned points for GERD are also beneficial for ulcers, specifically ST36, SP6, SP4.
- Others: B21 and CV21.

Aromatherapy

Peppermint and frankincense can help with ulcers, and can be directly added to your water twice daily. Others that can help are ginger, clary sage, and lavender for an upset stomach. Essential oils like ylang-ylang, neroli, orange, lavender, rose, vetiver, and sandalwood are relaxing.

SMALL INTESTINAL BACTERIAL OVERGROWTH

Small intestinal bacterial overgrowth, or SIBO, is a condition where the bacteria grows in the wrong place, as normally the colon has more bacteria than the small intestine. When bacteria overgrow in your small intestine, it can promote intestinal permeability. Symptoms include difficulty to digest meals, gas, bloating, and distension of abdomen especially after meals or most of the time, odorous loose stools, abdominal pain, signs of leaky gut or chronic disease, or when patients have been diagnosed with a B12 and iron deficiency. Causes can include antibiotic use, acid suppressing medication, food poisoning, low stomach acid, and others. You can confirm SIBO with a lactulose hydrogen and methane breath test that looks for excessive gas generations by the overgrowing bacteria when they ferment sugar and starches in the diet. Retest with another breath test within two weeks of finishing SIBO treatment.

Additional Integrative Modalities

Supplements

- Wormwood.
- Berberine containing botanicals (like Berberis vulgaris).
- Caprylic acid.

- Grapefruit and other citrus seed extracts.
- Black walnut.
- Oil of oregano (150 mg, two capsules, three times per day for sixty days).
- For methane-producing bacteria add garlic extract (two capsules, three times per day for sixty days).
- Others: goldenseal.
- Supportive treatment: Peppermint tea (two to three cups per day).
- If regrowth occurs: prophylactic use of betaine with pepsin, low dose naltraxone, low dose erythromycin; bifidobactrium lactis and lactrobacillus rhamnosus can help to prevent recurrences.

Homeopathy, acupressure, and aromatherapy (oregano, thyme, and sage) are similar remedies for bloating or other specific symptoms.

• 12 •

Gynecology

A woman's body is the most magnificent stage for the majestic miracle that can form within her womb, a stage that is set for the future engineer, movie star, integrative doctor (just sayn'), or even the next president. After months of becoming perfect, inside and out, it slides (ha, I wish it was that easy!) down onto the red carpet, bedazzled in vernix and amniotic fluid—wowing the world with its presence! Let's keep the magnificent stage magnificent, and put out the blaze before it wreaks havoc on the auditorium and destroys the building.

D & D: SPECIAL CONSIDERATIONS

If inflamed, a woman's reproductive system is the first to show signs that the body is off balance; if imbalanced, girls start to show signs like abnormal periods and pelvic pains. Managing glucose effectively, healing the gut, taming the toxins will lower gynecological problems, and balance hormone levels. With symptoms of heavy or irregular bleeding, focusing on high-iron foods is important, along with vitamin C, which increases its absorption and triggers ovulation. Other foods that optimize reproductive health are rich in vitamin E (critical for many endocrine hormones and proper functioning), folate, and zinc.

THE FOUR BIG S's: SPECIAL CONSIDERATIONS

Paying attention to the Four Big S's by staying away from stress, getting good sleep, having healthy social relationships, and cultivating a spiritual practice all will help lower cortisol and balance hormones.

DYSMENORRHEA (PAINFUL PERIODS)

Painful periods can occur due to numerous issues, including hormonal imbalances and endometriosis. Diagnosis can be investigated via history and examination, along with imaging like ultrasound or even more invasive techniques. Endometriosis is when the uterine tissue lands on the pelvic tissue, leading to dysmenorrhea, painful stools, and painful sexual intercourse.

Additional Integrative Modalities

Supplements

- Vitex (Chasteberry) (400 mg twice daily) balances hormones; don't take with oral contraceptive pills.
- Fish oil (1,000 mg daily). Gamma linoleic acid from evening primrose oil or borage oil (300 mg) can be helpful.
- B complex (50 mg daily).
- Natural progesterone cream (¼ tsp days 6 through 26 of cycle, stopping after the third month of pregnancy or the week of your menses); balances out estrogen.
- Milk thistle (150 mg twice daily).
- Others: Indole 3 carbinol (300 mg daily) helps the liver in estrogen detoxification, dandelion root (300–500 mg with each meal) helps with liver detoxification, vitamin E (400 IU twice daily) helps with inflammation and estrogen metabolism, and D glucarate (500 mg daily) assists liver in estrogen breakdown. Vitamin C (6–10 g per day), B carotene (50,000 IU per day), selenium (200–400 mcg per day), lipotropics (1,000 mg choline and 1,000 mg methionine or cysteine three times per day) can also be tried.

Homeopathy

- Arnica montana is for a deep, bruising pain.
- Belladonna is for women who experience pain worse before period, like a dragging or aching sensation, skin feels hot and flushed. Blood is bright red, and symptoms are worse with lying down.
- Borax helps with pain that is accompanied with nausea and muffled buzzing in the ears; pain extends into the thighs.
- Caulophyllum helps with pain accompanied with cervical spasms.
- Chamomilla is for severe pelvic cramping; the person is angry and restless.

- Calcarea phosphorica helps tall women with scant, heavy periods with pelvic pains extending to the lumbar regions.
- Cimicifuga racemosa will help with strong contractions of the uterus (like labor pains) that get worse as the flow increases and radiate across the pelvis and into the thighs and headaches leading up to the period.
- Colocynthis will help to improve the cramping that feels better with lying with the knees up and with pressure on the abdomen.
- Dioscorea villosa helps women who experience uterine pain that forces the woman to arch her back; she feels worse with lying down and better when standing up.
- Gelsemium is great for women with scanty late periods; her uterus feels heavy with sharp pains that are soothed by heat.
- Ignatia helps those women who are anxious, stressed, and full of worry and sadness.
- Lachesis women are jealous; their menstrual cramps are accompanied with large purple clots and frequent PMS.
- Lilium tigrinum women have hypersensitivity of the vulva.
- Magnesia phosphorica is for spasmodic pelvic pain, cramping, and bloating that is soothed with heat, pressure, and movement. Patient feels worse in the cold air. Membranes can be found in blood flow.
- Murex helps with painful, heavy periods accompanied with clots.
- Nux vomica is for those women who have prolonged periods that are early and accompanied with constipation, irritability, chilliness, and feeling of exhaustion. Pain is spasmodic.
- Pulsatilla (Pulsatillapratensis) is for menstrual pain accompanied with nausea, vomiting, and weeping, better when comforted. Patient has a strong craving for sweets.
- Sepia is for hormone imbalance; patient feels irritable and craves sweets, salt, and sour foods. She has pain with intercourse and experiences pelvic heaviness.
- Staphysagria is for painful periods that worsen with repressed anger or indignation.
- Viburnum helps women with late, scanty periods with spasmodic pain extending into the front of the thighs, the loins, and to the pubis and is accompanied by feeling faint. Patients can easily faint during periods and are nervous and agitated.

Hormonal dysfunction

- Folliculinum (30C on days 8 and 20 of the cycle), cimicifuga (9C), and Lac caninum (9C five pellets once to twice a day)

Acupressure

- CV4, LV3, SP6, LI4 (pain anywhere)
- Others: SP10, GB31, ST36

Aromatherapy

Certain essential oils help to relax the effects on the mind and on the muscles. Cooling blend oils are ideal for hot flashes and general irritability.

Hot flashes: blend of bergamot, Roman chamomile (calms and soothes), rose, and geranium (increases well-being).

Moods swings: clary sage, lavender, ylang-ylang.

Dysmenorrhea: clary sage helps to balance hormones and has been shown to reduce symptoms of endometriosis. Others that can help are angelica, chamomile, fennel, ginger, lavender, frankincense and sandalwood, which can help to reduce inflammation and support healing.

For increased bleeding: cypress, frankincense, and geranium can be tried.

Scant bleeding: basil, clary sage, and juniper berry.

FIBROIDS

Fibroids are uterine growths of connective tissues that can lead to heavy, prolonged periods and even pain in women. Assessment is via history and examination/pelvic exam, and imaging (ultrasound, MRI, hysterosalpingography and/or hysteroscopy). Healing the underlying root cause and balancing hormones are key to improving symptoms.

Additional Integrative Modalities

Supplements

- B complex (50 mg daily) as B vitamins are involved in estrogen metabolism.
- Milk thistle (150 mg twice daily) helps to balance hormones and detox the liver.
- Vitex (Chasteberry) (400 mg twice daily) balances the estrogen/progesterone ratio. Do not use Vitex if you are currently taking a birth control pill.
- Others: Natural progesterone cream (¼ tsp, days 6–26 of cycle; if pregnant, stop after third month of pregnancy), as it helps to balance out low progesterone; antioxidants, N-acetylcysteine and other supplements for detoxification (1,200 mg/day), like Indole-3-carbinol (300 mg daily),

Dandelion root (Taraxacum officinale) (300–500 mg with meals three times a day), and D glucarate (500 mg daily). Vitamin E (400 IU twice daily) can help with estrogen metabolism and inflammation. Other herbal therapies: Scudder's, Fraxinus ceanothus, Turska's, and specific herbal therapies for specific symptoms (menorrhagia, dysmenorrhea, etc.). Warm castor oil packs can be effective to shrink fibroids and relieve pain when placed on the stomach, along with ginger compresses.

- Fibroid symptoms of heavy bleeding can be controlled with uterine toning herbs like black cohosh, red raspberry, false unicorn root or astringent herbs like cinnamon, yarrow, beth root, or lady's mantle, or oxytonic herbs like shepherd's purse. These can be found in combinations. The tonic herbs and astringent herbs can be used twice a day for two weeks before period, then add the shepherd's purse when the bleeding begins. A combination of all three herbs can be taken every thirty minutes for up to six doses.
- The pain and cramps associated with the fibroid can be helped with herbs like black cohosh, boswellia, ginger, turmeric, cayenne, cramp bark, mitchella repens, and enzymes like neprinol, bromelain, and wobenzym.

Homeopathy

Homeopathy has little action on sclerotic fibroids, and large fibroids that cause compression problems or bleeding should be dealt with conventionally.

- Aurum muriaticum natronatum (6C) is for painful spasmodic vaginal contractions and when the uterus feels swollen.
- Calcarea carbonica is for women who crave eggs and sweets and are easily overwhelmed, fatigued, and struggle with anxiety. Uterine hemorrhage is present in these women.
- Fraxinus americanus is a specific remedy for uterine fibroids for those women with watery brown discharge from the vagina, painful period cramps, and swollen uterus making you feel as if you need to bear down.
- Phosphorus is for those who have bright red blood and clotting and crave ice-cold drinks.
- Lachesis is for those women who feel anger and are often suspicious of others. They experience surges of heat, and their symptoms are aggravated from heat. These patients have short scanty periods as menopause approaches, and their abdominal/uterine pain improves once menstrual flow starts. Their abdomen is sensitive to tight clothing.
- Sabina is for women with lower back pain and sacral pain that reaches to the pubic bones. It is also accompanied with heavy uterine bleeding with clots.

- Silicea is for bleeding in between periods and menstrual flow heavier than usual. Patient is constantly cold.
- Sepia is for women who feel irritable and want to be left alone. They crave salty, sour, and sweet foods. Their uterus feels like it will fall out and creates a bearing down feeling.
- Sulphur is for fibroids in women who get overheated easily. They desire a cool environment. There is a strong craving for ice-cold drinks.
- Kali iodatum is for when the uterus feels as if it is being squeezed during periods.
- Calcarea iodatum is for small fibroids with yellow profuse discharge from the vagina.
- Thlaspi is for continuous bleeding.

Acupressure

- SP10, GB31, ST36, SP6, LI4 (benefiting fibroid associated pain)

Aromatherapy

Frankincense, thyme, and clary sage can help improve symptoms. Two drops of frankincense oil, twice daily, on the roof of your mouth and rubbing two drops of the other oils over your lower abdomen a couple times a day can help balance hormones naturally. Others like black pepper, rosemary, and marjoram can improve pain and increase blood flow.

INFERTILITY

If you have been having unprotected sex for at least one year and can't get pregnant, you or your partner may be infertile (primary) or have secondary infertility (inability to become pregnant or carry a pregnancy to term following the birth of one or more biological child). Causes include a broad range, from poor nutrition, environmental toxin exposure, to hormonal issues or other medical issues.

Additional Integrative Modalities

Supplements

Female Infertility Supplements

- Vitex agnus-castus (Chasteberry) (160–240 mg daily) helps to stimulate the ovaries and balance estrogen and progesterone ratios.

- Vitamin B complex (50 mg daily) is important in estrogen metabolism.
- Vitamin E (400 IU daily).
- Evening primrose oil (1,500 mg once or twice daily from day 1 to day 14 of your menstrual cycle) supports fertility efforts.
- Natural progesterone cream (20 mg to the skin daily). Start using after you ovulate and should be used under guidance of a doctor.
- Others: Black cohash, Shataviri (600 mg of the root three times a day) is an Ayurvedic medicine that helps promote reproductive health. Tribulus (should contain at least 100 mg of the key active compound; can take three times daily on days 5 through 14 of the menstrual cycle); Rhodiola (contains 4.5 mg of rosavins and 1.5 mg of salidroside per dose, about two to three tablets per day) for those with anxiety and mental stress, ginger (ten to twenty drops in warm cup of tea), and Dong quai (tablet form 1 g of root equivalent twice per day).

Male infertility supplements that improve sperm count, motility, and quality:

- L-arginine (2,000 mg twice daily on an empty stomach).
- Panax ginseng (300 mg), zinc (30 mg twice daily) along with copper (3–5 mg).
- Vitamin C (500 mg twice daily).
- Multivitamin.
- CoQ10 (200–300 mg per day).
- Vitamin C (500–1,000 mg per day).
- NAC (600 mg per day).
- L-carnitine (2,000–3,000 mg per day).

Homeopathy

- Sepia 30C for those women who are often irritable, weepy, feel cold often, with an aversion to sex. They have irregular periods, and the womb feels as if is about to drop out of the vagina.
- Sabina 30C for those women who have had previous miscarriages before twelve weeks.
- Conium 30C for women who have the desire for sex but it has been suppressed for some reason, along with breast tenderness, with areas of hard swelling.
- Lycopodium 30C is for women with a dry vagina and tenderness in the lower abdomen over the right ovary.
- Agnus 6C is best for those women when a pituitary problem is diagnosed. Take up to three times per day for three weeks for regular periods and stop when your period starts.

Acupressure

- ST29, SP6, CV4, SP8, CV4 (Improve circulation and implantation)
- B44, LV14 (improves sex drive and libido)
- CV14 (improves secretion of cervical mucus)
- K16 (autoimmune-related infertility)
- CV6 (boosts libido and improves energy, relieves stress and menses pain, and helps sleep)
- B15 (corrects cycle and hormonal imbalances)
- B23 (controls pain and improves discharge)
- B47, GV4
- Others: ST36 (to stimulate absorption), LU1 to relieve tension, Face Epang II

Aromatherapy

Essential oils that may improve fertility are ylang-ylang, thyme, and Roman chamomile. Rose oil is said to improve sperm motility.

IRREGULAR PERIODS

The woman's menstrual cycle involves a normal functioning ovary releasing an egg every twenty-five to twenty-eight days. A woman's uterus anticipates implantation and so builds the uterine tissue. When that doesn't occur, the uterus sheds the lining, known as menstruation. When your body is working properly, you are having regular, moderately pain-free periods each month; this is a sign that your hormones are balanced. Irregular periods, missed periods, or very painful and intense PMS symptoms are signs that one or more of your hormones are imbalanced. Diagnosis can be made after a detailed history, exam, labs, and diagnostic tests. There are multiple causes of irregular periods:

- High stress levels
- Poor diet, low in antioxidants and probiotic foods, high in sugar and hydrogenated fats, pesticides, or artificial additives or preservatives
- Extreme weight loss and weight gain
- Over exercising
- Thyroid disorders
- PCOS
- Stopping the birth control pill
- Food sensitivities or allergies

Balancing hormones is key to balancing irregular periods. Other signs of hormonal imbalances are infertility, weight gain or weight loss, depression and anxiety, sleep issues, low libido, fatigue, digestive issues, and hair loss and hair thinning. Specific problems that may be associated with hormonal imbalances are estrogen dominance, PCOS, low estrogen, thyroid issues, diabetes, and adrenal fatigue.

Additional Integrative Modalities

Supplements

Excessive menstrual bleeding

- Vitamin C (500–1,000 mg three times per day).
- Fish oil.
- Chasteberry extract.
- Bioflavonoids (1,000 mg per day).
- Others: Chlorophyll (25 mg per day), iron (30 mg twice a day with meals) and chasteberry.
- *Adolescents*: first two weeks of menstrual cycle: 1 tbsp of flax and 1 tbsp of pumpkin seeds. Second two weeks of menstrual cycle: 1 tbspn sesame seeds, 1 tbsp sunflower seeds, fish oil (2–4 g EPA/DHA per day), pycnogenol (50 mg daily), chasteberry (5% vitexin, 20–40 mg daily).

Homeopathy

Amenorrhea (temporary or permanent absence of periods).

- Can be taken every twelve hours for up to fourteen days.
- Aconite can be used for periods that have stopped due to exposure to dry cold or periods that stop suddenly due to an emotional event.
- Calcarea is helpful for those women with fatigue, feelings of legs being heavy, swollen and painful breasts, and anxiety.
- Dulcamara is great for women whose periods stop after extraneous exercise that causes them to be cold.
- Natrum muriaticum is for women who experience constipation, irritability, headaches, thinning hair, and recent emotional shock.
- Ignatia is for those women whose periods have stopped because of loss or grief.
- Sepia is for women who feel weak, irritable, and weepy with abnormal vaginal discharge.

- Lycopodium helps those women with lower abdominal pain, headaches, feeling of sadness, and dry vagina. Slight emotional upsets disrupt the menstruation cycle.
- Ferrum is for women whose periods have stopped and are weak, tired, face is usually pale. Their symptoms are also accompanied with occasional hot flashes, and they want to sit down all the time.

Abnormal Bleeding

- China is for women with intermittent bleeding with abdominal cramps, faintness, paleness in the face, giddiness, dark clots of blood.
- Sabina is indicated for women with blood that is dark, bad labor-like pains in the back, difficulty controlling weight, with or without clots, emotional upsets, and increased blood loss.
- Belladonna helps those women who have regular periods with bright red blood; throbbing headache in the face, is hot and flushed.
- Ipecac is best for those with perfuse bright red bleeding with nausea.
- Calcarea helps women with cramping abdominal pain and back pain, head congestion, weight problems, and general paleness.
- Ferrum is indicated for those with abnormal periods with dark, watery blood with a pale face, improved with walking around.
- Crocus helps women who have a sensation of movement inside the uterus and feel sick, worried, and weak and expel blackish clots of blood.
- Kali carbonica helps those with the general feeling of exhaustion, cold extremities, and bleeding is thin and watery without clots. These women have a feeling of dying, and warmth aggravates the symptoms.
- Borax is for perfuse bleeding with nausea and pelvic/abdominal cramps especially in the first day or two of the period; symptoms are worse at night.

Acupressure

- LI4 (pain and inflammation)
- SP10, SP6

Aromatherapy

Basil can improve delayed menstruation and scanty periods. Cypress can relieve stagnation associated with heavy bleeding or midcycle bleeding. Geranium can have an overall balancing effect on female hormones.

MENOPAUSE

Menopause is a time in a woman's life when her sex hormones start to decline due to the degeneration of her ovaries. Women can experience a wide variety of symptoms from irregular periods, hot flashes, night sweats, mood swings, irritability, depression, anxiety, vaginal dryness, increased abdominal fat, and thinning hair.

With these hormonal changes, there is increasing loss of ovarian follicles and a decreased amount of estrogen produced; this begins about six to twelve months before menopause and in the late thirties and forties and continues throughout the menopause process.

Additional Integrative Modalities

Supplements

- Black cohosh (80 mg one or two times daily) improves hormonal imbalances.
- Natural progesterone cream (about 20 mg applied to skin of wrists and forearms two to three times per day from days 14 to 25, if menopausal 20 mg three to four weeks of the month, and postmenopausal 10 mg three weeks of the month) helps with fibroids and vaginal dryness.
- Vitex (160–240 mg) regulates hormones, but don't take it with oral contraceptive pills.
- American ginseng (600–1,200 mg daily).
- Red clover lowers risk of heart complications and loss of bone density. It improves hot flashes, weight issues, and sleep troubles.
- Others include: Hops (250 mg two to three times per day) for anxiety with mild hormone balancing properties; the Chinese herb Rehmania (25–100 mg daily) reduces heart palpitations, hot flashes, and night sweats. Evening primrose, licorice root, red raspberry leaves, wild yams, sarsaparilla, and chaste tree, Dim (Diihdolylmethane) (75–300 mg per day), omega 3, calcium D glucarate, probiotics, plant phyto estrogens, reversitol, Black cohosh, melatonin, and SAMe can also be used.
- Chondroitin sulfate can be used for incontinence.
- Hot flashes: Sage (three cups of tea per day), black cohosh (20 mg can be tried for twelve weeks), omega 3, flaxseed, vitamin E (400 mg per day).
- Heavy periods: Yarrow (two droppers of tincture per thirty minutes until bleeding slows).
- Fatigue: Ashwagandha (500 mg twice daily).
- Vaginal dryness: kudzu.

- Low sex drive: Peruvian maca root (500–1,000 mg per day), arginMax for women (ginseng, ginko, MV, mineral), L-arginine (amino acid that improves circulation).
- Mood issues: St. John's wort.
- Adaptogenic herb: Maca root (1,000–2,000 mg daily) helps to improve stress, decrease cortisol, reduce hot flashes, energy and improved libido, ashwagandha, medicinal mushrooms, holy basil, and rhodiola.
- Herbs help to balance properties that can help you ease into this transition period. These include evening primrose, ginseng, licorice root, wild yams, St. John's wort, chaste tree, red raspberry, red clover, and sarsaparilla.

Homeopathy

- Amylium nitrosum is indicated for sudden onset of hot flashes and then a sensation of coolness in the body.
- Belladonna can be used in women who experience throbbing symptoms in the head or other areas with sudden onset of flushing, perfuse sweating, and other symptoms like restlessness, heat, palpitations, and headaches that occur on the right side.
- Bryonia can help those with constipation and for stools that look blackish or burned. Vagina is dry and thin.
- Calcarea carbonica is for women who feel overwhelmed, anxious, and fatigued. Other symptoms include night sweats/hot flashes and feelings of cold, leg cramps, and menses are heavy. Patients also tend to gain weight as they transition into menopause.
- Kali carbonica is great for women with loss of appetite, hot flashes, palpitations, nervousness, and backaches that worsen around 3:00 am.
- Graphites is for those women who experience hot flashes, especially on face, with cutting pains in the abdomen, scanty periods, weight gain, and nosebleeds.
- Lachesis helps those women who have hot flashes, anxiety, headaches upon waking, dizziness and flooding during periods, sleep issues, memory and concentration problems, and heart palpitations that are worse from lying on the left side. They are incredibly talkative, suspicious, jealous, and angry. They feel constricted around the abdomen and must avoid tight clothing around the neck.
- Natrum muriaticum is best for hot flashes and vaginal dryness. These women cry easily, are depressed, crave salt and cold drinks, and experience migraines and backaches. Symptoms worsen in the sun.

- Oophorinum is a specific remedy for hot flashes in women who have had their ovaries removed.
- Pulsatilla is for women with hot flashes, hemorrhoids, and varicosities. Use especially if the woman is fair haired, often feels cold, cries easily, and prefers an open air, as her symptoms worsen in a warm room. She craves chocolate and sweets.
- Sanguinaria canadensis is best for hot flashes that cause the cheeks to become red and ears feel like they are burning, so primarily in the neck and face, with the burning sensation radiating to the palms of hands and soles of feet.
- Sepia is great for heavy menstrual periods, backache, sinking feeling in the pit of the stomach, anxiety and pain during intercourse, and can even help with prolapsed uterus, incontinence, and vaginal dryness. Patient is exhausted, irritable, tearful, and craves sweets/chocolate or sour foods.
- Sulphur is great for hot flashes that are worse after exercise and at night. Patient easily sweats and craves ice-cold drinks.

In conjuction with the above remedies, Lachesis, Sulphur, and Sepia, which have just been mentioned as constitutional remedies, have hot flushes in their pathogeneses.

- Bone and joint disorders: Will discuss further in the Rheumatology section, but if associated with menopause and joint/bone issues: Kali carbonicum and Natrum sulphuricum.
- Osteoporosis: Silicea and Calcarea carbonica.
- Nervous disorder: Lachesis, Sepia, Sulphur, Thuja, Ignatia, Nux vomica, Aurum muriaticum.
- Vaginal dryness during menopause can be helped with Sepia and Lycopodium depending on symptoms.

Acupressure

- LI4, GV 24.5 (improve headaches and hot flashes)
- GV20 (for headaches and clearing the mind)
- CV17 (improve sleep and hot flashes)
- P6, B60, GB20 (irritability, dizziness, stress, and hot flashes)
- LI11 (hot flashes)
- H6 (night sweats, anxiety)
- LV3 (headaches, insomnia, mood changes)

- K3 (night sweats and mood disorders)
- SP6 (balance)
- CV6, CV17 (helps hot flashes and mood disorders)

Aromatherapy

Rub three drops of the chosen oil on the tops of the feet and back of the neck one to three times per day.

For hot flashes, clary sage, peppermint, geranium, cypress, and lime. Thyme oil can help to balance hormones.

For depressionassociated with menopause, one can use bergamot, clary sage, cypress, geranium, grapefruit, jasmine, lavender, marjoram, neroli, niaouli, sweet orange, petitgrain, rose, or ylang-ylang.

Mood swings and anxiety can be helped by bergamot, cedarwood, Roman chamomile, clary sage, frankincense, geranium, jasmine, lavender, mandarin, marjoram, sandalwood, or ylang-ylang.

Stress can be helped by Roman chamomile.

POLYCYSTIC OVARY SYNDROME

PCOS, or polycystic ovary syndrome, occurs when a woman's hormones are out of balance, leading to symptoms like weight gain and trouble losing weight, acne, irregular periods, thinning of the hair in the scalp, extra hair on the face and the body, depression, and fertility issues. Diagnosis occurs via history and examination, blood tests that will demonstrate insulin resistance and elevated testosterone, and imaging like ultrasound that will demonstrate cysts in the ovaries. Untreated, it can lead to increased risk of developing diabetes, high blood pressure, high cholesterol, and heart disease.

Additional Integrative Modalities

See Insulin Resistance section found in chapter 10 (Endocrinology).

PREMENSTRUAL SYNDROME

Premenstrual syndrome, or PMS, is common in about 75 percent of menstrual women. Symptoms include breast tenderness, mood instability and emotional changes, bloating, fatigue, cramping, and skin changes. These symptoms can start seven to ten days before the menstrual flow and end shortly after. Diagnosis is via history and physical.

Additional Integrative Modalities

Supplements

- Vitex (Chasteberry) (240 mg daily) to balance hormone levels. Don't take with oral contraceptive pills.
- Calcium carbonate (500 mg twice daily) PMS prevention.
- Vitamin B6 (50–100 mg daily).
- Zinc 15–20 mg per day.
- Vitamin E 200–400 IU per day.
- Magnesium (250 mg twice daily).
- Natural progesterone cream (¼ tsp or 10 mg applied twice daily to your thin skin like wrists at the beginning of ovulation until the day before your periods).
- Indole-3-carbinol (300 mg daily) aids in estrogen metabolism.
- Dong quai *(Angelica sinensis)* (300–500 mg twice daily, on the last seven days of your cycle) helps with breast tenderness and cramps.
- Others: vitamin A (5,000 IU per day); B complex (with 50 mg of B6); evening primrose oil (500 mg twice daily); 5HTP (50–100 mg twice daily) to boost serotonin and lower anxiety; green tea or L-tyrosine (500 mg twice to three times daily); Donq quai (300–500 mg twice daily on last seven days of cycle) helps to reduce breast tenderness; ginkgo biloba (80–160 mg twice daily); hypericum perforatum (900–1800 mg per day).
- *Preteen/teen:* calcium (800–2,000 mg daily), vitamin B1 (100 mg daily), vitamin B6 (20–40 mg daily), fish oil (EPA/DHA 2–4 g daily), magnesium (100–200 mg daily), vitamin D (1,000–4,000 IU per day), fennel extract liquid (thirty drops two times daily), ginkgo biloba leaf extract (50:1 raio, 24% ginkgo heterosides, 6% terpene, lactone, 80 mg daily), saffron (60 mg daily), valerian root (0.8%), valerenic acid (250 mg daily), chasteberry (5%), vitexin (20–40 mg daily).

Homeopathy

- Take these every twelve hours for up to three days starting twenty-four hours before premenstrual symptoms.
- Calcarea carbonica is a remedy for symptoms that include fatigue, cold sweats, anxiety, and painful and swollen breasts. These women

crave eggs and sweet things. Their feet and hands are usually clammy and chilly.

- Matricaria chamomilla is a great remedy to relieve unbearable, painful menses. The woman feels irritable, angry, and very sensitive to pain. The symptoms are better with motion and worse with warm applications.
- Cimicifuga is a remedy for a painful menses that gets worse as the flow increases. The woman experiences cramping and shooting pains that go across the legs or the thighs. Headache, stiffness in the neck and the back are common.
- Causticum is used with women who feel irritable, feel pessimistic, have to urinate frequently, and have symptoms of cystitis. These women have colicky pains in their lower abdomen.
- Kali carbonicum helps women who feel exhausted and tense, especially around 3:00 am, when symptoms worsen. It works best for those women who are overweight.
- Lachesis helps women with symptoms that are worse in the morning with emotional issues (rage, jealousy, suspicion) and painful breasts and abdomen as symptoms of PMS, improving once the menses starts. Patient often feels irritated with anything touching her throat. It is a major remedy for premenstrual syndrome. Before periods, the patient presents with headaches, aggravated by heat, sunshine, and alcohol, may also occur, as well as hot flushes. Lachesis (9C) on the nineteenth day of the cycle; Lachesis (15C) on the twentieth day of the cycle; Lachesis (30C) on the twenty-first day of the cycle.
- Lilium tigrinum is a remedy for a premenstrual syndrome that's characterized by great irritability. She crosses her legs to get relief from the feeling that her internal organs will prolapse. Fresh air brings relief.
- Lycopodium helps those who feel depressed, lack self-confidence, are irritable, experience digestive problems, and crave sweets.
- Nux vomica helps women who are constipated, have frequent urination, feel chilly, irritable, angry, and crave coffee, alcohol, spicy, or fatty foods. Symptoms improve with warmth and rest.
- Pulsatilla helps hormone balance for women who experience sudden bursts into tears, irritability, and mood swings with painful breasts and irregular periods. Symptoms improve with consolation and attention. They crave sweets, especially chocolate, and feel worse in warm rooms.
- Sepia helps women who are irritable, weepy, and emotionally flat and feel as if their uterus is going to fall out, along with experiencing breast tenderness. They are turned off by the idea of sex and crave salty and sweet foods. Symptoms improve with exercise.

- Natrum muriaticum helps in women with fluid retention, swollen breasts, and when they feed irritable and sad. Symptoms include lower back pain and migraines. Patient craves salt and doesn't like being in the sun.
- Sulphur is for when the major PMS symptom is a craving for sweets.
- Nervous symptoms: ignatia, Nux vomica, moschus, Murex purpurea, and cyclamen can be used.
- Mastodynia: Lac caninum, phytolacca, Conium maculatum.
- Headaches: sanguinaria, Lac caninum.
- Venous disorders: Hamamelis, Vipera, Aesculus hippocastanum.
- ENT symptoms: Magnesia carbonica, Lac caninum.
- Skin issues: herpes: Rhus toxicodendron, borax, croton.
- Acne: Kali bromatum, Eugenia jambosa, Natrum muriaticum, sepia, sulphur, Calcarea carbonica.
- Water retention: Natrum muriaticum, Thuja occidentalis, Natrum sulphuricum.
- Hormone balance: Folliculinum (30C on the seventh or eighth day of the cycle).

Acupressure

- LV3, SP4, SP6, GB34, ST29, B47, CV6 (improve pain)
- HP6
- To relieve digestive complaints like diarrhea and constipation: CV6
- For lower back pain: B25, B31, and B40
- To ease tension and stress: LV3

Aromatherapy

For abdominal cramps: Black pepper and rosemary. To balance female hormones: Geranium and rose oils. To reduce stress: Geranium, rose oil, lavender, bergamot, or jasmine. Increase sexual desire: Patchouli and ylang-ylang. Fluid retention: Juniper compress.

YEAST INFECTION

Yeast infection is a candidal infection of the vagina. Yeast infections can occur in areas where yeast and fungus can thrive, in moist conditions like the mouth, throat, and genitals. When the yeast overpopulates in the vagina, symptoms can include vaginal discharge, usually thick, white, clumpy (cottage cheese like) and odorless discharge, along with irritated skin around the opening to the vagina, painful intercourse or pain when urinating or during menses. Diagnosis can be confirmed via examination and culture collection.

Additional Integrative Modalities

See Candidal infections found in chapter 11 (Gastroenterology).

• 13 •

Hematology and Oncology

Our blood is our everything—our lifeline, our family, our freedom, what supports us, and what breaks us. What runs through your blood determines who you are and who you are meant to be. Keep the fire out of the veins to revive the body with hope, healing and the ability to triumph.

ANEMIA

Anemia is a condition when your blood doesn't have enough red blood cells that can carry around oxygen to your organs. Because of this, your body isn't getting enough oxygen. There are different kinds of anemia, like anemia associated with a vitamin deficiency (vitamin B12 or lack of folic acid) or chronic disease (cancer, Crohn's disease, or kidney failure), aplastic anemia (bone marrow can't make all three types of blood cells), hemolytic anemia (red blood cells are destroyed faster than the bone marrow can replace), and sickle cell anemia (makes the red blood cells form crescent or sickle shape that can block blood flow resulting in pain). Symptoms may be fatigue, pale skin, shortness of breath, feeling cold, irritability, chest pain, dizziness/lightheadedness, and palpitations or rapid heartbeat or headache. Severe anemia can cause damage to your organs. The most common anemia is iron deficiency anemia. Diagnosis can be made by history, physical, blood tests, and occasionally biopsy.

D & D: SPECIAL CONSIDERATIONS

Healing the gut is important for appropriate digestion and absorption of nutrients that the body needs for appropriate function, like B12, zinc, and magnesium. Work on nourishing the spleen, as it is responsible for red blood cell production. Focus on foods like squash, green leafy vegetables, and bitters like Romaine and arugula. Consume iron-rich foods (beef/chicken liver, organic grass-fed meats, leafy greens, and beets) and remove processed foods and junk foods from your diet, balancing insulin levels. Foods rich in vitamin C will help your body absorb and retain iron. Other foods that help are black strap molasses, leeks, figs, eggs, cherries, strawberries, cashews, and brewer's yeast (rich in iron, folic acid, and B12). Cook in a cast-iron pot or pans, as the foods will absorb the minerals from the cookware. Sometimes, juicing will allow your body to digest foods appropriately.

THE FOUR BIG S's: SPECIAL CONSIDERATIONS

Stress and worry can deplete your spleen and liver.

Additional Integrative Modalities

Supplements

- Iron (50–100 mg of well-absorbed iron like ferrous fumerate, glycerate, or citrate): Take with vitamin C to help with absorbtion.
- B12 (1,000–2,000 mcg daily in the methylcobalamine form sublingual) and folic acid (800–1,200 mcg daily sublingual) if your doctor has diagnosed a deficiency.
- Vitamin C (250–500 mg with each dose of iron).
- Green superfood powder: Spirulina (2,000 mg daily or one heaping teaspoon daily) stimulates RBC production. Choose one that contains spirulina, vitamin B12, dandelion, and folic acid.
- Others include alfalfa, dandelion, burdock, yellowdock (one capsule or twenty drops of tincture) and gentian; these improve iron absorption have been shown to clean blood and improve iron absorption and have been shown to treat anemia by stimulating the digestive system to easily absorb iron and other nutrients. Don't use with chronic pain or frequent urination; may cause your blood pressure to drop.

Homeopathy

- Ferrum phosphoricum can be used for iron deficiency and by persons with a pale face bur that flushes easily, a generally robust appearance, and oversensitivity.

- Calcarea phosphorica is for those with anemia during growth spurts (first two years of life or during adolescence) or chronic anemia in adults. Anemia is accompanied by poor digestion and irritability.
- China officinalis will help anemia due to blood loss or illness. Patient is usually cold, overly sensitive, and exhausted.
- Natrum muriaticum is for anemia that's accompanied by dull or muddy complexion, dry mouth and lips, headaches, and tendency to cold sores and constipation.
- Picric acidum helps anemia that is coupled with mental overload.
- Arsenicum helps those with B12 deficiency.

Acupressure

- SP6, ST36 (support circulation)
- LI4 (headache)
- CV4, SP10, LI6 (stress, headaches, or neck/facial pain)

Aromatherapy

Essential oils like ginger oil and citrus oils can improve anemia symptoms as they may improve iron absorption. Cinnamon oil supports blood sugar balance; ginger, eucalyptus, and black pepper can improve poor circulation. For liver cleansing or support, ledum can be tried. Others that can help improve symptoms are lemon, thyme, chamomile, peppermint, and spikenard.

CANCER

Cancer is a scary word that no one EVER wants to hear. Cancer refers to diseases that can be characterized by the growth of abnormal cells in the body that divide without control and can potentially invade and destroy other normal tissues. Tumors are formed when these abnormal cells form masses, but some cancers, like leukemia, don't form solid tumors.

By receiving this diagnosis, most are left with a deep sense of hopelessness, but it can also be accompanied with a new revival of your inner self. The immune system plays an extremely important role in helping us defend and remove cancer. Learning to lower the inflammation in your body will allow you to give your body a fighting chance, instead of fighting an uphill battle. It will help build a stronger, healthier you, with a body strong enough to combat symptoms and side effects associated with cancer treatments and lessen the risks of relapse or recurrence, lowering the chance of developing a second cancer. Cancer changes your life and the lives around you—let's make it for the better! Let's get your body the nutrition it needs to heal! You got this!!!

D & D: SPECIAL CONSIDERATIONS

Maintaining an acid/alkaline balance by drinking alkaline water (add lemon or lime juice and/or hydrogen peroxide), increasing your intake of raw veggies, and removing grains and dairy will all optimize detoxification. Increase omega 3 fatty acids, calcium, vitamin D like cod liver oil, blue green algae, conjugated linoleic acid, mushrooms, folic acid (effective against breast, pancreatic, and colorectal cancer), melatonin, vitamin B pyridoxine, and vitamin C. Low-carbohydrate diets with intermittent fasting help to stabilize insulin, which improves estrogen dominance.

Tumor cells overexpress insulin receptors, allowing more glucose in to feed the tumor, so it's important to manage any insulin resistance. Fiber is best to lower the amount of estrogen and estrogen metabolites, which are available to stimulate the breast tissue and lower insulin and glucose levels that feed the tumor cells. Incorporate anticancer foods like cruciferous vegetables, pomegranate, turmeric, garlic, green tea, oolong tea, olive oil, bean sprouts, strawberries, figs, olives, selenium, tomatoes, dietary fiber, ginger, onions, and quercetin (can be found in capers, cocoa, hot chili peppers). For postmenopausal women, calcium and selenium are vital. It is important to keep your body mass index (BMI) below 25. Intermittent fasting can help to lower the risk of cancer, but always talk to your doctor, as fasting should be avoided in those who are in the course of treatment or are weak. Men should avoid beta carotene, so take as little vitamin E and calcium as possible. Also avoid vitamin E, alcohol, grilling or cooking in a wok, and blood in meat.

THE FOUR BIG S's: SPECIAL CONSIDERATIONS

Like environmental toxins, stress is a carcinogen. Reducing stress will improve quality of life and also has an inhibiting effect on tumor growth. To optimize emotional health, releasing suppressed emotions is very important, as caging in any suppressed emotions can lead to illness. Replace these emotions with positive ones. Strong social support is very important, along with connecting to your inner intuition. Follow your calling and recognize your reason for living. You seriously are amazing, inside and out, an inspiration to those around you!

Additional Integrative Modalities

Supplements

Though it is best to get most of your nutrition from foods, there are some situations where you can add a dietary supplement. Several supplements have been shown to reduce the risk of developing cancer.

- Probiotics can optimize your immune system.
- Vitamin D has been shown to have a preventive effect on recurrence of malignancies and can support healthy bones.
- Vitamin C has an antioxidant activity.
- Calcium/magnesium can support bone health.
- Omega 3 fatty acids: Studies suggest that patients with breast, prostate, and non-small lung cell cancer may derive biochemical and clinical benefits from omega 3.
- Mushroom supplements are beneficial.
- Turmeric has antitumor activity.
- Coenzyme Q10 is an antioxidant and can help in malignancies, especially in people who receive cardiotoxic chemotherapy.

Supplements that can be taken during and after cancer:

- For stress, fatigue, and depression: levocarnitine, ginseng, royal jelly, brewer's yeast, maca powder, wheat germ, camu camu, zinc, and magnesium.
- Hair growth: brewer's yeast, B1, and B6.
- Weight loss: green tea, caffeine, common ash, and meadow sweet.
- Erectile dysfunction: vitamin D, L-arginine (2–5 g daily), pycnogenol (40 mg twice daily to three times per day).

Be careful with what you choose, and always check with your doctor about supplement-pharmaceutical interactions, as botanicals can decrease the concentration and efficacy of the cancer treatment (like Echinacea, grapeseed, kava, St. John's wort, and possibly garlic). Gingko can lead to increased toxicity of the chemotherapeutic interventions.

Homeopathy

The homeopathic view is that cancer represents a profound breakdown at every level, and home prescribing is not really appropriate in such circumstances. For acute symptoms, take a 30C potency four times daily.

- Cadmium sulphuratum can help with symptoms of vomiting, hair loss, and fatigue.
- Nux vomica works best for those who complain of GI symptoms, like indigestion, nausea, or constipation.
- Ipecacuanha can be used for patients with persistent vomiting and nausea, especially when the vomiting doesn't relieve any symptoms.
- Arsenicum can help with restlessness, burning pains, anxiety, and nausea.
- Radium bromatum is specific for radiation poisoning, especially when it is followed by arthritic complaints.
- Arnica montana helps any bruised or restlessness sensations.
- Eupatorium can help for aching bone pain that is worse with motion and is often accompanied by stiffness and chills.

Acupressure

- P6, LI4 (reduces pain)
- extra 1 acupoint (anxiety)
- LV4 (helps with abdominal distention or pain)
- Others to improve your immune system and the liver are B23, B47, CV6, K27, and ST36

Aromatherapy

Herbs can strengthen your immune system. Combine bergamot, chamomile, and lavender in aromatherapy applications. Or place several drops in a warm bath or for massage.

Others that can help with specific symptoms are:

- Fatigue: rose, jasmine, or geranium.
- Anxiety or stress: lavender and Melissa.
- Pain: black pepper, rosemary, and ginger.
- Antibacterial/antifungal/antiviral: tea tree oil.
- Digestive issues and nausea: peppermint or ginger oils.
- Juniper can break down toxins; others are cedarwood, frankincense, mandarin, sweet orange, and rose.

Nutritional Protocols

Supplemental nutritional programs include the Gerson Therapy and Juicing, Budwig protocol, Proteolytic Enzyme Therapy, Vitamin C Chelation, Frankincense Essential Oil Therapy, and Oxygen Therapy.

• 14 •

Nephrology

Put out the fire and keep the pee pee train running smoothly! You'll be glad you did, I promise! Let's hear it for going #1! Yay!

D & D: SPECIAL CONSIDERATIONS

Optimize kidney health by lowering inflammation, healing the gut, and optimizing glucose control. Drinking enough water will keep your kidneys working effectively and lower the risk of getting kidney stones. Eating a nutrient-dense diet can help balance the body's pH; these foods include fresh fruits and vegetables and vitamin E–rich foods (avocados, olive oil, berries, almonds, and butternut squash), which can help balance oxalate levels and prevent mucous membrane damage. You can also balance pH with lemon or apple cider vinegar. Consuming foods with magnesium and potassium can help to balance calcium levels in the body (leafy green veggies, bananas, avocado, and melons). For kidney disease, follow your doctor's recommendations depending on your specific condition.

For stone prevention: Avoid regular unsprouted grains and foods high in oxalic acid (spinach, tomatoes, collards, eggplant, beets, celery, sweet potatoes, almonds, blueberries, blackberries, strawberries, parsley, and cocoa); these can increase oxalate in people prone to kidney stones. Elevated zinc can increase the odds of stones in those prone to it. Avoid too much vitamin C (more than 4 g per day) as it may worsen kidney stones. Caffeine and alcohol can make stones worse as both are dehydrating. For uric acid stones, don't overindulge on meat and limit dairy. For cysteine stones, avoid methionine-rich foods like soy, wheat, and dairy.

THE FOUR BIG S's: SPECIAL CONSIDERATIONS

Regular stress management will lower inflammation. Exercise is great, whereas being sedentary can cause bones to release more calcium into the blood.

KIDNEY STONES

Kidney stones are stones that are present in the urinary tract. Stones grow slowly over several months or years and are made of minerals like oxalate, uric acid, and calcium. Symptoms of kidney stones are abdominal pain, nausea, vomiting, fever, chills, excruciating pain in the buttock area with constant movement to relieve pain, and pain in the genital area as the stone moves. Your doctor may confirm diagnosis with a CT scan, ultrasound, and/or X rays.

Additional Integrative Modalities

Supplements

Use these for prevention of calcium oxalate stones:

- B vitamins like B6 (50 mg daily). Vitamin B6 helps to reduce calcium and oxalate levels.
- Magnesium (250 mg once or twice daily with meals); prevents calcium-oxalate crystals.
- Calcium 300–1,000 mg per day.
- Vitamin E (400 IU daily) can be in an antioxidant or multivitamin.
- Aloe vera juice/gel (¼ cup daily) decreases urinary crystals.
- Inositol hexaphosphate (120 mg daily).
- Cranberry extract (400 mg twice daily of a standardized extract or as directed on the container) helps to prevents UTIs.
- Turmeric and ginger.
- Vitamin A (5,000 IU daily) prevents kidney stone formation.
- Others: R. tincture and R. crispus.
- Uric acid stones: folic acid (5 mg per day).
- Magnesium-ammonium-phosphate stones: acidify with ammonium chloride (100–200 mg three times per day).
- Bushite and struvite stones: acidify urine with cranberry juice.

Homeopathy

These should be given as often as necessary for up to ten doses while waiting for help. A higher potency is selected when the characteristics of the sensitive type are present.

Remedies that prevent relapsing are discussed next.

- Calcarea carbonica is effective both as a remedy in renal colic and as a remedy of the chronic reactional mode.
- Belladonna is used for right-sided, sudden, excruciating pain worse with any jarring and accompanied with a flushed face and high fever.
- Berberis vulgaris is a remedy for sharp stitching pain that is felt between the hip bone and lower ribs and radiates to the ureters, bladder, thighs, and testes. Pain is worse by slightest movement and is relieved by lying on the painful side.
- Cantheris is for a pain that feels like knives stabbing in all directions, leading to burning sensation in the bladder. The person is thirsty; the thought of food is nauseating, and the person has an intolerable urge to urinate.
- Dioscorea helps when pain forces you to stretch or arch the back backwards for pain relief.
- Lachesis is for left-sided kidney pain that may cause hemorrhaging.
- Lycopodium is for right-sided pain that stops at the bladder; pain in the back is improved by urinating, urine is clear with red sediment in it, symptoms are worse between 4:00 and 8:00 pm.
- Nux vomica is a remedy for right-sided pain that stabs toward genitals and down the right leg, accompanied by nausea, vomiting, or right-sided pain that can shoot to the rectum, leading to bladder urgency. The person is very irritable and cold sensitive.
- Tabacum is for renal stones that cause pain that radiates and darts down the ureter, causing a cold sweat and nausea.
- Calcarea phosphoric is a remedy for phosphate stones, and the person feels short of breath and fatigued.
- Pareira brava helps those with urogenital pain and helps to prevent recurrent pain.
- Sepia is indicated in those with enuresis and who have a tendency to superinfections.
- Lithium carbonicum is best for uric acid stones and can be accompanied with Lycopodium and Calcarea carbonica.

- Solidago virga aurea helps with pain in the lumbo-costal angles.
- Sarsaparilla helps those with stones and skin disorders.
- Benzoicum acidum is a remedy indicated in uric acid stones for patients when they have a tendency for recurring UTIs and the urine smells strongly of ammonia.

Acupressure

- B23, GB34, K3, LI4

Aromatherapy

Essential oils can help to detoxify. Those that are beneficial are lime, lemon, orange, grapefruit, and helichrysum essential oils. To relieve abdominal pain: chamomile, lavender, and marjoram. These can be combined with a carrier oil and massaged into the lower abdomen twice daily or can be added to a bath.

• 15 •

Neurology

> You have brains in your head. You have feet in your shoes. You can steer yourself in any direction you choose.
>
> —Dr. Seuss

But if the brain is on fire, it will likely steer you in the direction you don't wish to go. So extinguish the flames and take back control!

D & D: SPECIAL CONSIDERATIONS

As we talked about earlier, the connection between gut and brain is very intimate. To lower inflammation in the brain, we must lower inflammation in the gut and control insulin resistance. Brain derived neurotrophic factors (BDNF) allows growth of neurons. If low, it can increase risk of Alzheimer's. Raise BDNF with turmeric, DHA omega 3, coffee, and coffee fruit extract. Other foods great for the brain are grass fed butter (high in butyrate and raises BDNF) and other healthy fats, probiotic and prebiotic foods like garlic, leeks, onions, and acacia gum.

THE FOUR BIG S's: SPECIAL CONSIDERATIONS

Emotional stress and anxiety can lead to inflammation and the release of certain chemicals in the brain that can provoke vascular changes and symptoms like migraines. So relaxation strategies and aerobic exercise are very important for optimal brain health.

DEMENTIA

Dementia, including Alzheimer's (now referred to by some as diabetes type 3), causes problems with memory, behavior, and thinking; symptoms get worse over time and can start to interfere with day-to-day living. Doctors diagnose Alzheimer's and other forms of dementia based on a detailed history, exam, and laboratory tests.

Additional Integrative Modalities

Supplements

- Reversatrol (100 mg twice daily).
- Turmeric (350 mg twice daily).
- Alpha lipoic acid (600 mg per day).
- Coconut oil (1–2 tbsp daily).
- Others: Vitamn E (2000 IU per day), CoQ10 (200 mg daily), Gingko biloba (120 mg daily); Phosphatidylserine (300 mg daily); astaxanthin (2–4 g twice daily); Huperzine extract (0.2 mg of huperzine A daily); Bocopa monnieri (150–450 mg per day); acetyl L carnitine (1,000 mg three times daily) helps to improve brain cell communication and memory; vitamin B12 (800–1,600 mcg daily); DMAE, L glutamine (500 mg three times daily); magnesium; NAC (500 mg three times per day); Nicotinamide adenine dinucleotide or coenzyme Q10; potassium (500 mg per day); SAMe (400–600 mg), vitamin C (500–1,000 mg in three divided doses); Phosphatidylserine (300 mg daily) improves brain cell communication and memory and has shown benefits for early-stage Alzheimer's disease; melatonin; increased doses of B; turmeric (1,500 mg daily of a standardized turmeric extract); and jellyfish extract (10–20 mg daily of standardized extract of jellyfish).

Homeopathy

- Alumina is indicated with sudden worsening of confusion with reduced memory impairment and constipation. 30C daily for three or four days.
- Lycopodium helps for those that have trouble recalling words and are fearful. Take 30C two times daily for two weeks.
- Calcarea is indicated in those who can't remember most words, and exhibit childish behavior and wandering attention.
- Plumbum helps those who are colicky, suffering from a nervous complaint, have difficulty finding words, and are anemic.

- Anacardium is helpful for those with problems in memory related to names, are absent-minded, and have two different personalities at conflict.
- Sulphur is a remedy for those who have difficulty remembering names and words.

Acupressure

- K1, H7 (improves memory)
- L7, P6, LU1, GV24.5, and ST36

Aromatherapy

Rosemary and frankincense can help to support brain function. Others that can help with symptoms of dementia by providing a calming effect are lavender, ylang-ylang, orange, sandalwood, and rose. To help with concentration and focus, peppermint, basil, thyme, and cardamom can be used.

HEADACHES

Headaches are a pain that can occur anywhere in the region of the head or neck. Different types of headaches are tension headaches, cluster headaches, and migraines. Symptoms include throbbing, pulsating, and pounding pain that can begin on one side of the head and may spread to both or stay on one side; they can last anywhere from 4 to 72 hours and may be accompanied by symptoms of nausea, vomiting, irritability, loss of appetite, fatigue, parts of your body feeling numb, and light, noise, or movement may worsen the pain. Diagnosis can occur with a detailed history and physical and possibly some imaging.

Additional Integrative Modalities

Supplements

- Magnesium (200–600 mg per day).
- Butterbur (50 mg two to three times per day with meal).
- B-complex vitamin combination of B2 (400 mg daily), folic acid (2 mg), B6 (25–75 mg), and B12 (400 mcg per day).
- B12.
- 5HTP (50–100 mg three times per day).
- Coenzyme Q10 (100 mg three times daily).
- Alpha lipoic acid.

- Others: Feverfew (250–500 mcg of parthenolides daily), ginger root (fresh, about 10 g per day or dried 500 mg four times per day, extract standardized to contain 20% gingerol), and shogaol (100–200 mg three times a day for prevention; 200 mg every two hours, up to six times a day, for acute migraine), medicinal mushrooms, Capsaicin cream, kudzu, and melatonin.
- *Children*—tension: magnesium (200–400 mg daily), melatonin (3 mg daily); migraines: CoQ10 (100–300 mg daily), fish oil (EPA/DHA 2–4 g daily), vitamin B2 (40 mg daily), butterbur extract (15% petasins 50–150 mg daily), feverfew (20–100 mg daily), magnesium (400 mg per day).

Homeopathy

- Aconite is indicated for sudden onset of headaches that feel as if there were a tight band around the head and accompanied by apprehension; worsens in cold or drafty surroundings.
- Arnica helps those with a headache that feels sharp (occasionally), bruised, achy, aggravated by stooping.
- Apis is a remedy for a stabbing burning or stinging headache where the rest of the body feels tender and bruised, and aggravated in hot and stuffy environments.
- Belladonna is indicated for right-sided throbbing of congestive headaches that begin in the back of the head and extend to the right eye or forehead. The headache is accompanied by dilated pupils, sensitivity to light, hot skin, and a flushed face; aggravated by the hot sun, noise, and jolts and improved by lying down in a dark quiet room.
- Bryonia helps those with left-sided pain especially in the eye or the forehead, extending to the whole head, accompanied by constipation, nausea, irritability, wanting to be alone, and the person is thirsty; symptoms are worse with movement and improved with rest and pressure.
- Calcarea phosphorica is a remedy for irritable school children with digestive aches and chronic headaches; pain is intense in the back of the head, and they crave smoked meats.
- Cimicifuga is a remedy where the headache is accompanied with neck stiffness associated with hormonal changes either during menopause or during the menstrual cycle.
- Gelsemium helps those with tight-band-like-feeling headaches, mostly occipital, with back of the neck pain, eyes feel bruised, feels as if face is purple and congested, limbs are weak and shaky, fatigued, dizzy, blurred vision, and pupils are dilated. Urinating and raising the

head improves symptoms, and symptoms can be preceded by visual disturbances or double vision.

- Glonoinum helps with violent, congestive, pounding headaches made worse with movement of the head, stooping, and heat; improved with cold applications.
- Hypericum is indicated with a bursting or aching headache with a hypersensitive scalp, aggravated by foggy and damp weather.
- Ignatia is a remedy for a headache that most describe as a tight band across the forehead or a nail on the side of the head. The headache is associated with neck/back spasms and can begin after trauma or emotional grief. Symptoms are improved by entertainment and caused by the slightest emotion or effort.
- Iris is a remedy for a constricted migraine headache associated with the symptoms of nausea, vomiting (mostly bile), and blurred vision; improved with movement. The headaches occur during days off or at the beginning of vacations and are accompanied by burning sensations throughout the digestive tract with vomiting.
- Lachesis helps left-sided pulsating, burning headaches that the person can wake up with. Associated with a flushed face, and is improved by the open air and aggravated by heat and touch.
- Lycopodium is for right-sided temple or forehead headaches worse between 4:00 pm and 8:00 pm, aggravated from being hungry, from overheating and trying to concentrate, accompanied with dizziness.
- Magnesia phosphorica is indicated to help relax tight muscles and tension headaches.
- Natrum muriaticum helps those with blinding, throbbing headaches that are triggered by sunlight, grief, and stress and improved by lying down in a dark and cool room. Tingling may be present in the lip, tongue, and nose.
- Natrum sulphuricum helps those with headaches that may have been triggered by a head injury.
- Nux vomica is indicated for bruising headaches that can be triggered by food sensitivities, constipation, being overworked, and stress; worse first thing in the morning and with noise and lights; better when the person gets up or with cold applications. Person is irritable, has a stomachache, nausea, and is dizzy.
- Pulsatilla helps when headaches feel as if the head is about to burst; worse in the evening, around period; aggravated by rich, fatty food; occur around men; and patient easily bursts into tears.
- Ruta helps those with a pressing headache aggravated by reading and improved by rest. Symptoms are associated with fatigue.

- Sanguinaria canadensis helps with congestive headaches that throb and burn, starting in the morning and peeking in the midday, improving in the afternoon, associated with redness of the cheeks. Pain begins in the back and spreads to the top of the head and settles over the right eye. Symptoms are improved by sleeping, releasing gas, or lying down and are aggravated by motion, light, noise, or odors.
- Silicea helps headaches that begin at the back of the head and are located above the eye; patients are prone to head sweats, and symptoms improve with head being warm.
- Spigelia helps those with a sharp, darting pain over left eye, made worse from stooping or moving suddenly.
- Thuja is indicated for those with left-sided headaches, like a piercing nail.

Headaches associated with digestive symptoms:

- Lac defloratum is for headaches associated with constipation; pain starts in the front of the head and moves to the back.
- Lac canium is indicated when the headache changes sides.
- Kali bichromium helps in those with supraorbital migraines with pain on one spot on the right side associated with yellow; it involves nausea and vomiting, gastritis, and visual problems. Symptoms are improved with pressure and aggravated with drinking beer.
- Venus merceneria is indicated with headaches that are associated with constipation, increased gas, and coated tongue.
- Others: Iris.

Headaches associated with emotions:

- Kali phosphoricum is indicated for those with headaches associated with being overworked and fatigued and with an increase in sexual desire.
- Phosphoricum acidum is indicated for headaches with a sensation of heaviness in the head and pressure, made worse by motion and noise and improved by rest and lying down; accompanied by the inability to think or concentrate, fatigue, and weakened memory.
- Zincum metallicum is indicated for headaches that are made worse with any intellectual effort, nervous fatigue, pale individuals who are intolerant to wine or alcohol with decreased vision.
- Anacardium orientate is indicated for headaches, irritability, feeling of a split personality, and for overworked individuals; symptoms improve with eating.

- Cyclamen is indicated when headaches are related to menstruation and proceeded by visual disturbances or dizziness, made worse by coffee or open air.
- Actaea racemosa is indicated for headaches that are proportional to the menstrual flow with painful periods.

Acupressure

- Cluster: GB14, GB20, hold B2 with B10, fan fingers over GB6–11, end with LI4
- Migraine: B10, TW16, GB12, GB6–11, GB14, LI4
- Tension: GB21, GB20, GB12, GB6–11, B 3–9, LI4
- Sinus: GB20, GB17, SI8, LI20, ST1, B1, B2, GB14, LI4

Aromatherapy

Essential oils that may be beneficial: peppermint, lavender, eucalyptus, frankincense, rosemary, rosewood, grapefruit, coriander, lemongrass, bay laurel, lemon balm, marjoram, ginger, sandalwood, wintergreen, anise, basil, linalool, and Roman chamomile.

NERVE PAIN

Nerve pain causes a person to feel pins and needles, electric shocks, and tingling in the affected extremity due to nerve damage. Causes include diabetes or prediabetes, other chronic illnesses, trauma, medication, toxins, autoimmunity, cancers, deficiencies (like B12), or even infections, like Lyme disease or herpes zoster. Diagnosis is made via a detailed history, physical, laboratory testing, imaging, and nerve conduction studies.

Additional Integrative Modalities

Supplements

- Alpha lipoic acid (300 mg twice daily) protects against nerve damage and lowers insulin resistance.
- Capsaicin cream (0.075%) applied up to four times daily.
- Evening primrose (360 mg daily) lowers pain sensations.
- Chromium (600 mcg daily) improves insulin sensitivity.
- Cinnamon (1–2 tsp to a meal daily).

- Vitamin B12 (500–5,000 mcg per day depending on lab value), B6 (30 mg per day).
- Others: Energy revitalizing system multinutrient powder, acetyl l-carnitine (500–1,500 mg twice daily) generates energy to heal the nerve cells; Neuro-Eze (phase 1 to 2 neuropathy), rub into area two to three times per day, most effective early phases of small fiber neuropathy; and magnesium.

Homeopathy

- Mezerum is indicated for nerve pain that is worse with warmth and at night; best for ciliary neuralgia and pain associated with tooth decay.
- Hypericum perforatum helps with shooting pain along with numbness, tingling, burning sensations.
- Lachesis helps with pain that is worse after falling asleep.
- Aconite is used for those who feel the affected part is congested and numb; flair occurs after exposure to cold.
- Arsenicum is helpful for an attack that is characterized by searing, hot-needle-like, burning pain that can be triggered by cold and accompanied with exhaustion, restlessness, and the feelings of being cold.
- Colocynth is for lacerating pain improved with heat and can be triggered by cold or damp, especially in cases of facial neuralgia.
- Magnesia phosphorica is best for intermittent and darting pain, sudden in onset, that can be improved by pressure or heat and aggravated by cold and bending forward, especially involving side of the head and neck.
- Ranunculus is for pain right above the eye or the rib cage.
- Spigelia is beneficial for pain above the left eye aggravated with any type of motion.
- Pulsatilla is best for acute facial neuralgias, rheumatic in origin.
- Verbascum is helpful for pressure/crushing pain in the zygomatic bones aggravated by talking and sneezing, chewing, cold air, or pressure.
- Platinum helps constrictive, cramping pain with numbness and tingling, worse at night and at rest, and profuse, thick, and exhausting menses.
- Belladonna helps with infraorbital neuralgic pain radiating toward the temples, ears, and back of the neck, worse around midnight, from noise, motion, chewing, or cold air and relieved with rest.
- Chamomilla is a remedy for violent pain with numbness, improved with heat.
- Kalmia latifolia is for pain that follows the course of the nerve; worse with movement and during the first part of the night.

- Aranea diadema helps with nerve pain that occurs after cold and damp weather exposure; numbness of the arm may wake patient up from sleep; feels as if the upper limb is swollen, worse at night.
- Others that can help are: Allium sativum, Arsenicum album, Capsicum annuum, Carbolicum acidum, Dioscorea villosa, Dolichos pruriens, Gnaphalium polysephalum, Iris veriscolor, leusinum, Mercuric solubilis, Phytolacca decandra, Sanguinaria canadensis, Selenium metallicum, Stannum metallicum, Staphylococcinum, Tallium metallicum, and Thuja occidentalis. Peripheral: Coffea cruda.

Acupressure

- SI18, LI4
- Lower extremity: K6, B62, GB30, GB34, GB39, SP6
- Hands: LU10, LI4, SJ5, LI11, LI15, baxie points
- Trigeminal neuralgia: LI4, ST25, ST44, TB17, GB20

Aromatherapy

Lavender, peppermint, and frankincense can help to lower inflammation and dull pain. Others that can help nerve pain are cajuput, chamomile, citronella, clove, geranium, marjoram, nutmeg, peppermint, rosemary cineole, sandalwood, yarrow, and St. John's wort–infused oil.

PARKINSON'S DISEASE

Parkinson's disease is a chronic degenerative condition of the nervous system that is caused by nerve cells in the brain. A chemical called dopamine starts to break down and die, leading to movement impairment, as dopamine is a neurotransmitter that messages the parts of the brain that control movement. Symptoms include tremor, loss of balance, stiffness and rigidity, poor posture, slow blinking and movement, memory loss, mood disorders, dementia, and digestive and speech issues. Diagnosis is made via history, physical, and imaging.

Additional Integrative Modalities

Supplements

- Coenzyme Q10 (1,200 mg daily).
- Vitamin C (750 mg four times daily).

- Vitamin E (400 IU per day).
- Green superfood formula with spirulina, chlorella, and wheatgrass.
- Others: Inosine monophosphate (500–3,000 mg/day depending on uric acid levels), Carnitine monohydrate (20 g for five days, then 4–10 g per day), caffeine pills (50–200 mg twice daily max or one to two cups of coffee), Nicotinamide adenine dinucleotide (NADH; 5 mg twice daily), N-acetylcysteine (NAC; 500 mg three times daily), melatonin (300 mcg–1 mg per night), Proanthcyanides (increase daily dose from 80 mg to 380 mg taken in three divided doses; don't exceed daily dose of 380 mg), vitamin B6 (increase daily dose from 75 to 150 mg; don't exceed a daily dose of 150 mg), contraindicated with levodopa, zinc (30 mg per day; large doses can interfere with body's absorption of essential minerals, impair blood cell function, and depress immune function). Iron and manganese should be avoided.

Homeopathy

- Argenticum nitricum is indicated for those with movement issues (like uncoordinated movements and imbalances) and tremors of the hand.
- Causticum is helpful for those with hand tremors that are worsened with writing accompanied by a slow paralysis mostly on the right side.
- Helleborus is indicated for those with brain fog and slow speech.
- Mercurius is best for those with trembling hands and stammered speech that is accompanied by excessive sweat, patchy memory and concentration, loss of willpower, overproduction of saliva, and a sweet metallic taste in the mouth. Symptoms are aggravated by perspiration; and patients are sensitive to heat and cold.
- Natrum muriaticum is a remedy for hand tremors, constant nodding of the head, and dropping things.
- Plumbum is a remedy that helps progressive paralysis, cramping, and muscle wasting.
- Hyoscyamus is indicated for those who behave obscenely, are full of jealousy and suspicion, and are restless. Every muscle twitches.
- Agaricus helps those who feel their spine is extremely sensitive, with stiffness of the extremities that can jerk and tremble.
- Rhus tox helps stiffness or cramping that is improved by movement and aggravated by dampness or immobility. Moving is difficult on first attempt. Little tremor.
- Gelsemium helps those with staggering gait, tremors, and weakness that affects the eyes, tongue, and when trying to swallow.
- Manganum can be used when there is no other effective remedy.

Acupressure

- B18, B23, GB20, GB34, GV14
- Others: GV14, K3, LV3, SP6, LV2, GV20, GV21, CV23, ST36

Aromatherapy

Frankincense oil can reduce inflammation, and vetiver oil can reduce tremors. Essential oils for muscle aches and pains can help; these include myrrh (promotes mental balance), lavender, cardamom, tea tree, clove, nutmeg, fennel, and peppermint.

RESTLESS LEG SYNDROME

Restless leg syndrome is a chronic neurological disorder that causes unpleasant sensations in the legs and an uncontrollable urge to move them. Symptoms may occur typically in the evening, disturbing sleep; your legs feel like they are tingling, cramping, burning, throbbing, or creeping, forcing you to move them. Diagnosis can be made by a detailed history, physical, and laboratory tests. Primary RLS can have no apparent cause; secondary RLS can be associated with conditions like neurological disorders like Parkinson's disease, peripheral neuropathy, diabetes, thyroid disease, fibromyalgia, anemia or iron deficiency, ADHD, nutrient deficiency (like magnesium or folate), varicose veins, chronic medical conditions, and pregnancy.

Additional Integrative Modalities

Supplements

- Iron (30–60 mg) and calcium (100 mg) on an empty stomach to bring ferritin level to more than 60 ml.
- Magnesium, vitamin D (400 mg), folic acid, and 5HTP.
- Amino acid L-tryptophan.
- Sufficient iron, B vitamins, omega 3 fatty acids, magnesium, calcium, and trace minerals.
- Finally, boost your brain's ability to make gamma-aminobutyric acid (GABA); in addition to taurine supplements, compounds that boost your brain's ability to make GABA include N-acetylcysteine (NAC, 500 mg–2 g) and lipoic acid (600 mg).

Homeopathy

- Arsenicum album is recommended for those who feel chilly, have general feelings of restlessness and anxiety, and always want to move their legs.
- Phosphorus is a remedy indicated for those who take catnaps that seem to help steady the limbs, where the twitching is worse when lying on the right side, especially in elderly persons.
- Zinc is indicated for those with twitching, restless, and trembling lower extremities, even while asleep.
- Agaricus is beneficial for legs that twitch, tingle, tremble, and itch that cause the person to wake up, feeling worse in cold weather or an early sleep.
- Belladonna is indicated for legs that spasm and feel hot despite the cold; this is worse when trying to go to sleep.
- Ignatia is indicated for those who have jerky legs that come on after emotional trauma with insomnia and despair of ever sleeping again.
- Kali carb help with the jerking movements that occur mostly between 2:00 and 4:00 am.
- Sepia is a remedy for restless legs that are worse during the day but improved with exercise.
- Tarentula is helpful for the feeling of the legs twitching and the irresistible urge to move them all the time and jerking movements with yawning.

Acupressure

- CV6, ST38, GV20, GV26, B20, LV3, LV5, CV17, ST36

Aromatherapy

Essential oils like cypress, rosemary, black pepper, ginger, lavender, marjoram, nutmeg, and cedar wood can help to improve symptoms, as they have antispasmodic qualities. Others that can help are frankincense and chamomile.

SEIZURE DISORDER

A seizure happens when there is abnormal electrical activity in the brain that may come on suddenly, varying in duration and severity. Recurrent seizures are known as epilepsy. There are several types of seizures, including generalized (subtypes in adults are tonic clonic and absence and in children febrile and infantile spasms) and partial seizures. Symptoms range from twitching of the muscles to having brief loss of consciousness. Causes can be due to strokes, brain tumors or injuries, electrolyte imbalances, cancer, medications, or infections. Diagnosis can be made via history, neurological exam, and several tests, including EEG.

Additional Integrative Modalities

Supplements

- B6 (50 mg three times per day).
- Folic acid (0.4–4 mg per day).
- Zinc (25 mg per day).
- Bacopa leaf (200–400 mg per day in two to three divided doses of an extract standardized to 20% bacosides).
- Others: Sedative herbs that can help are chamomile, kava, valerian, and passionflower; manganese (10 mg three times per day), selenium (100 mcg per day), taurine (500 mg three times per day), ubiquinone (100 mg per day).
- Don't take gingko biloba and Panax ginseng, St. John's wort (interacts with seizure medications), or white willow.
- *Children:* Fish oil (2–4 g of EPA/DHA per day), taurine (500 mg three times daily), GABA (750–1,500 mg daily), B6 and B12, melatonin (3 mg per day).

Homeopathy

- Aconite helps with those with seizures that are brought on by a fever or by a scare.
- Aethusa helps those with episodes that can be described as teeth clenching and thumbs that are clenched inside their fists and drowsy spells after vomiting or passing stool; pupils are dilated and the seizure usually follows digestive symptoms or gastroenteritis.
- Belladonna helps those who have eyes wide and staring; the person is red and hot, and symptoms are made worse by excessive movement or jolting; useful for seizures with a high fever.
- Chamomilla helps those who have thumbs clenched inside their palms, one cheek is red and the other one is white, and patient has green/yellowish watery diarrhea. Episodes can be triggered by outbursts of anger or by teething.

- Cuprum metallicum helps those with a violent attack triggered by vomiting and menstruation and who can be characterized with blue face and clenched lips and fists, accompanied by mental dullness.
- Glonoinum helps those who have a seizure episode triggered by heat or exposure to sun; their fingers and toes are spread wide and they have a hot head with congestion.
- Ignatia helps those with twitching that begins in the face, which is pale. The seizure can be triggered by emotional trauma or upset.
- Zinc helps those who are bad tempered before an attack, head rolls from side to side with fidgety movements of the lower extremities, and a pre-rash stage of infectious illness.
- Causticum is helpful for seizures that may be triggered by emotional shock, and patients tend to feel hopeless and fearful.
- Cicuta is indicated with status postseizure that occur after a head injury.

Acupressure

- GV20, GV26, CV14, SI3, SP4, B15, LV1, B60, K6, LV3, ST40

Aromatherapy

Essential oils with a calming and relaxing effect can help to relieve symptoms due to stress; these include jasmine, ylang-ylang, chamomile, lavender, and clary sage. Frankincense oil is helpful for decreasing seizures.

Don't use rosemary, fennel, sage, eucalyptus, hyssops, pennyroyal, tansy, thuja, wormwood, or spike lavender.

Other Recommendations

Hyperbaric oxygen chamber

• *16* •

Ophthalmology

Your eyes are the window to your outer and internal world. The orchestra of inflammation that may be silent in your body can be visualized literally from deep within your eye, allowing your doctor a glimpse into your body. Optimize your health by lowering inflammation for a clearer window to the world!

D & D: SPECIAL CONSIDERATIONS

Some of the best food for your eyes are dark greens, carrots, green beans, red peppers, peas, nuts/seeds, berries, egg yolks, and wild-caught fish, as these contain antioxidants; eye vitamins like A, E, C; and zinc with carotenoids like lutein and zeaxanthin that protect the eyes by lowering free radicals and relieving inflammation. Blueberries and cherries contain anthocyanin, which helps to fight free radicals that can damage your eyes and keeps the collagen around the eye flexible. Chromium (present in brewer's yeast) and magnesium both have beneficial effects on the eye.

THE FOUR BIG S's: SPECIAL CONSIDERATIONS

Relieving stress, improving sleep, and optimizing social and spiritual health are important to healing the overall inflammation in chronic eye conditions. Avoid tanning beds, and protect your eyes from heat when taking a sauna. Use eye exercises and acupressure to keep them feeling comfortable. Massage your temporomandibular joint (TMJ), temples, and neck three times a day. Other precautions to protect your eyes are to wear sunglasses and a hat for UV light protection.

CATARACTS

Cataracts are clumps of protein that collect on the lens of the eyes and are the most common cause of vision loss in people over forty. Most cataracts develop over time. Symptoms of cataracts depend on their maturity and location of the cataract (cortical/posterior/subcaspular/nuclear). When they first start to develop, they may only change vision in a small area of your eyes. Symptoms are blurred or double vision, halos around lights, fading or yellowing of colors, frequent changes in eyeglasses or contact lens prescription, brown spots in the visual fields, and increasing difficulty with night vision. Diagnosis can be made via a history and detailed eye examination.

Additional Integrative Modalities

Some professionals believe that cataracts can be prevented and delayed.

Supplements

- Multivitamin (one or two daily) with B complex vitamin (50–100 mg daily) vitamins B2 and B3 are protective; vitamin C (1,000 mg three times daily, if tolerated); and vitamin E (400–800 IU daily with a meal) helps with healing after laser eye surgery.
- Vitamin A (10,000 IU daily with a meal) an antioxidant.
- Others include: riboflavin (3–5 mg per day), selenium, and bilberry (an anthrocyanside; 80 mg two to three times daily) decrease free radicals.

Homeopathy

For temporary treatment, choose the appropriate following remedy and take 6C three times a day for one week and then twice daily up to one month. If you notice an improvement, and your vision continues to improve, take a two-day break, then take the remedy twice a day for another month. Ideally, you will need to find a constitutional remedy with the following (see Appendix).

- Calcarea can be taken as soon as the circular lines are visible on the lens and your doctor tells you that you have early stages of cataracts.

Once you start to experience symptoms, you can switch to a different remedy.

- Phosphorus helps to improve the sensation of a mist or veil before the eyes or if you feel that something is being pulled tightly over your eyes.
- Silicea can help those with later stages of cataracts that begin to interfere severely with sight.
- Ruta graveolens helps those with red, hot eyes with dimmed vision.
- Digitalis purpurea can be used for symptoms of dim and double vision. Lid margins may be red, swollen, and agglutinated in the morning.
- Secale cornutum can be used for hard or soft cataract that is accompanied with headaches, roaring in the ears, and vertigo.
- Naphthalinum can be used for a cortical cataract.

Acupressure

- UB1 and UB2 (at early stages of cataracts)
- Yuyao, SJ23, GB1, Qiuhou, ST1, LI3 (improve circulation)
- LI4

Aromatherapy

Essential oils should never be put in the eye or on the eyelids. Clove oil is the most powerful antioxidant that taken internally can prevent and slow cataracts. Lavender can also be helpful.

DIABETIC RETINOPATHY

Diabetic retinopathy is a complication of diabetes that is caused by damage to the blood vessels of the light-sensitive tissues in the retina. Initially it may cause no symptoms, but then may lead to blindness. Diagnosis is made via a dilated eye exam.

Additional Integrative Modalities

Supplements

- A multivitamin with a B complex (50–100 mg daily) with B12 (1–2 mg daily (if tolerated), vitamin C (1,000 mg three times per day), and vitamin D.
- Vitamin E (400–800 IU daily at mealtime).
- Vitamin A (5,000 IU per day).

- Magnesium (500–1,000 mg at bedtime).
- Zinc (30 mg daily for several months).
- Essential fatty acids (500 mg twice daily).
- Alpha-lipoic acid (200 mg twice daily).
- Lutein (6–10 mg daily).
- Zeaxanthin (0.5–1.0 mg daily).
- Chromium (50–200 mcg daily).
- Copper (2 mg daily while taking zinc).
- Bilberry (100 mg twice daily).
- Garlic (one odorless pill daily).
- Alpha-lipoic acid (200 mg twice daily).
- Others: Quercetin (1,000 mg daily), Vanadyl sulfate (20 mg daily for two weeks, then 2 mg daily), Phosphatidylinositol (PI), Gymnema sylvestri (50 mg per day) and fenugreek (15 mg per day).

Homeopathy

- Arnica can be used as soon as floaters in the eye are seen.
- Conium can be used if arnica doesn't stabilize condition within twelve hours.
- Lachesis can be used to help prevent further leakage of blood vessels in the retina, after the condition has been stabilized (can take every four hours for up to six doses).

Acupressure

Similar to eye health acupressure points and diabetic acupressure points.

Aromatherapy

Cinnamon oil and coriander oil can help relieve diabetes by supporting the pancreas, improve weight loss, and help in general management of diabetes prevention. Coriander oil helps by enhancing the secretion of insulin from the pancreas and exhibiting insulin-like activity at the cellular level.

DRY EYE

Dry eye is a condition that occurs when a person doesn't have adequate tears to lubricate and nourish the eyes. Dry eye can occur when there is an imbalance of production and drainage. There are multiple causes of dry eye, such as hormonal changes, medications, and medical conditions like rheumatoid arthritis, sjogren's, diabetes, and even thyroid and inflammation of the eyelids. Environmental conditions like smoke, dry and windy climates, and even LASIK surgery can contribute to drying eyes. An eye exam with a complete history can help to diagnose dry eye, along with measuring the volume of your tears and production using the Schirmer's test.

Additional Integrative Modalities

Supplements

- Fatty acids (1,000 mg DHA and 500 mg EPA once or twice a day) and fat-soluble vitamins like A (20,000 IU daily for the first month, then 10,000 IU daily) and E (400–800 IU daily with a meal).
- Magnesium (500 mg at bedtime).
- B-complex vitamin (50–100 mg daily) with B12.
- Vitamin C (1,000 mg three times daily, if tolerated).
- B-complex vitamin (50–100 mg daily).
- Calcium (750 mg daily, at a different time from magnesium).
- Zinc (30 mg daily for several months).
- Copper (2 mg daily while taking zinc).
- Chondroitin and glucosamine sulfate (100–500 mg daily).

Homeopathy

- Alumina can relieve dry eye when objects look yellow and eyes feel cold.
- Belladonna helps dry eye that presents as a very hot, red, or swollen eye; pupils are dilated.
- Bryonia alba relieves dryness associated with eye pain.
- Nux moschata can help dry eye when objects look larger, look very distant, or vanish; the patient is unable to open eyes.

Acupressure

- UB1, ST1, GB1

Aromatherapy

- Castor oil and flaxseed oil can help with dry eye.

GLAUCOMA

Glaucoma is a slow-progressing chronic disease that causes a build-up of fluid in the eye that can lead to optic nerve, retinal, and lens damage. It is the second leading cause of blindness. There are no early symptoms, but as the disease progresses, you can lose side vision followed by central vision loss. Other symptoms can be blurry vision, rainbow-colored halos around lights, red eye, headache, nausea, vomiting, and pain. Diagnosis can be made at your eye care professional's office with visual acuity, visual field, pupil dilation, and tonometry tests.

Additional Integrative Modalities

Supplements

- B-complex vitamin (50–100 mg daily) with B12.
- Fish oil (600 mg of EPA and 400 mg of DHA daily) helps relieve intraocular pressure.
- Magnesium (500–1,000 mg daily) helps to relax the blood vessel wall and improve blood flow.
- Vitamins A and D (unless in multivitamin).
- Vitamin C (1,000 mg three times daily).
- Vitamin E (400–800 IU daily, taken with a meal).
- Zinc (30 mg daily for several months).
- Copper (2 mg daily while taking zinc).
- Alpha-lipoic acid (200 mg daily) antioxidant has been shown to improve vision for some people with this disease.
- Lutein (6–10 mg daily).
- Garlic (one odorless pill daily).
- Others: Bilberry (160 mg twice daily); Astaxanthin (2 mg per day); CoQ10 (300 mg daily), which can help prevent free radical damage; Ginkgo biloba extract to improve circulation (fifteen drops twice daily), Coleus forskohlii; Trifola.

Homeopathy

- Physostigma venenosum can be used for open angle glaucoma with muscle spasms and neurological problems.
- Phosphorus can help those with glaucoma with vertigo.
- Spigelia helps with sharp pains.
- Belladona is useful for glaucoma associated with blurred vision and pain in one eye that is made worse by bright light (30C).

Acupressure

These points are especially helpful for people who use their eyes a great deal and suffer from eyestrain:

- ST3 (relieves pressure on the eyes)
- UB10 (sooths tired eyes and headaches)
- LI3, LI4, Cuan Zhu, and B1

Aromatherapy

To improve eyesight, frankincense and helichrysum oil can be used. Cypress oil improves circulation, which can relieve glaucoma. Lavender, rose, sandalwood or ylang-ylang, bergamot, and jasmine can help to reduce anxiety and tension.

Other Recommendations

Avoid eyestrain for long periods of time, don't watch TV in the dark, and avoid drugs that jeopardize the eye.

MACULAR DEGENERATION

Macular degeneration is an age-related chronic illness that is the leading cause of vision loss in people over sixty in the United States. This condition affects the tissues in your retina, which is in charge of central vision, the macula. This leads to blurred vision, a blind spot in the center of your vision, and can interfere with reading and being able to perform everyday tasks. It can affect one or both eyes. The first symptom you may notice is when you need more light to see up close. There are two types of macular degeneration, wet and dry. Dry AMD (age-related macular degeneration, the more common type) is degeneration of the macula and causes gradual loss of central vision; wet AMD is characterized by blood vessels that grow under the retina in the back of the eye, leaking fluid and blood, and it involves a sudden loss of central vision.

Symptoms of dry AMD are blurring of print when reading, haziness of vision, and a blurred spot in the center field of vision, which may get larger and darker. Symptoms of wet AMD are loss of central vision, sudden blind spot, object appearing farther away or smaller than usual, and straight lines that appear wavy.

Diagnosis is via a vision field test, and testing with an Amsler grid that involves covering one eye and staring at the black dot in the center of the checkerboard-like grid. If the straight lines in the pattern look wavy or lines are missing, that can point to macular degeneration. Other tests that can diagnose macular degeneration are fluorescein angiography and optical coherence tomography.

Additional Integrative Modalities

Supplements

- Multivitamin: one or two capsules as directed with meal with vitamin A (10,000 IU per day) and D, magnesium (500 mg daily), fish oil DHA (500 mg two times per day), selenium (50–200 mcg daily), taurine (200 mg daily), B complex (50–100 mg per day), B12 (1–2 mg per day), chromium (200 mcg daily), zinc (30 mg or less daily), vitamin E (400–800 IU daily with meals).
- Digestive enzymes as required.
- Vitamin C (1,000 mg, once to three times daily, if tolerated).
- Garlic (one odorless pill daily, 1,000 mg).
- CoQ10 (60–120 mg daily).
- Ginkgo biloba extract (fifteen drops once or twice daily).
- Beta-carotene (5,000–10,000 IU daily).
- Lutein (6–20 mg daily with a meal), an antioxidant that protects the eyes and the skin and prevents oxidative damage of the macula.
- Zeaxanthin (.5–1.0 mg daily with a meal) helps to protect the eye tissues (lens and macula) for clear vision; prevents oxidative damage and prevents glare, light sensitivities, and other eye disorders.
- Bilberry (100 mg twice daily) an antioxidant.
- Copper (2 mg daily, while using zinc).
- Others: Astaxanthin (2 mg daily) can help to prevent retinal damage.

Homeopathy

Homeopathy may be helpful for macular degeneration. A constitutional remedy can help with symptoms, so seeing a licensed homeopath is important.

Acupressure

- ST36 (improve digestion and nutrition absorption)
- GB37 (improve vision and relieve watery eyes)
- GB39, LI3, LI4, UB1, GB20, Tai yang, P6, LV2, SP6

Aromatherapy

Frankincense oil has been shown to improve eyesight; cypress oil can improve circulation; and helichrysum can improve vision and support nerve tissue function. Three drops can be applied twice daily on the lateral area of the eye, but not directly into the eyes.

Other Recommendations

- Test yourself regularly with the Amsler grid.
- Eliminate unnecessary medication, as some medications may deplete essential nutrients, vitamins, and minerals and accelerate macular degeneration.
- Optical devices that enlarge visual images and other low-vision aids are available as you need them.

• 17 •

Pediatrics

Nature has given us an amazing gift—children—with the responsibilities to protect them in every way we know. One of a parent's worst nightmares is to look into their child's eyes and see the light that was once brightly shining now consumed by a chronic health condition. Sadly, chronic disease is now the "normal" for children, when what really should be normal are children full of fun and excitement, engaged, with the energy to keep up with those around them; they have eyes that are clear and bright with no dark circles, swelling, or redness; they can fall asleep in less than thirty minutes; they are eating a variety of foods including vegetables and fruit; they have little to no gas, bellyaches, and should have snake-like poops. Let's protect these little gifts by keeping the fire out of their little bodies, to prevent any such nightmare.

D & D: SPECIAL CONSIDERATIONS

Educating our children from the very beginning is important for their overall health. I teach my children exactly what is going on when they eat food and the importance of taking care of the little "pets/friends in their bellies." They know that eating chemicals, sugar, and other toxins will kill the pets that are protecting them and keeping them healthy. Children are constantly growing and need high-nutrient foods to sustain all the energy and growth. Teach them to "go down the list" every time they want to eat, as veggies, clean protein, and healthy fat are critical for growing strong brains and bodies.

Breast milk is the most perfect food for babies as it supports a healthy gut microbiome, making them smarter and preventing disease. If they don't seem to tolerate breast milk, look for food sensitivities that can lead to colic, gas, reflux, and other symptoms. If you can't breast-feed, it is best to find a natural organic formula and supplement with fish oil and probiotics. Follow the weaning schedule listed in the appendix. Limit juice as it displaces nutrient-rich foods, lowering immunity. But most importantly, limit screen time and get them to play outside, as the microbes that live in the soil can increase their biodiversity for optimal health and happiness.

Pay attention to subtle signs that your child's health may be becoming imbalanced. If your child is having any symptoms of colic, gas, spitting up, indigestion, congestion, rash or hives, cough, difficulty breathing, abdomen digestion, constipation or other digestive issues, chronic ear infections, cradle cap, projectile vomiting, fits/tics, sinus issues, or adenoids, these may be risk factors for developing bigger health problems down the road like autism, autoimmune disease, or mood disorders. If you notice these symptoms, remove one or two of the problematic foods at a time, starting from the food that your child eats the most, following the Gut Rx. Breast-feeding mothers can follow the same protocol, eliminating and watching symptoms in their baby. Though there is no standard protocol, for those with serious issues—like colitis, autoimmunity, seizures, or autism—a gut healing diet like GAPS (Gut and Psychology Syndrome Diet) along with avoiding their food sensitivities and following my foundations of good health (section one) is a great starting point. Supplements should be added slowly and gradually, as some children with autism may regress with certain supplements like B12 or GABA/glutamate. Those children with folate deficiency should not have ANY kind of dairy, including camel's milk.

Clean up your child's surroundings. Pesticides and other environmental toxins can lead to neurodevelopemental damage while disrupting the endocrine system. Heavy metal detoxification is very important for improving autism, helping the body maximize glutathione. Optimizing gut health and limiting the daily toxin exposure will help protect against any adverse effects of vaccines. Homeopathics can also be used to prevent or limit vaccine side effects.

THE FOUR BIG S's: SPECIAL CONSIDERATIONS

Managing stress is essential in any healing and disease-prevention program, as our thoughts, feelings, and emotions directly affect our children's physical health. Parenting can directly affect the child's brain chemicals. Developing bonds of love, respect, and honor and being involved in a child's life can help to activate a sensory nerve in the child's brain that releases oxytocin and natural opioids, which decrease stress response systems and provide the child with feelings of well-being and help the brain develop. Help them with their big feelings, help them use their words, and take time to understand their painful feelings. It's important to get down and cuddle, play, look them in the eyes when they talk, laugh, read to them, and provide them with imaginative explorative activities. Place order in their lives by establishing family rules and clear boundaries; this will actually lower everyone's stress and help your children feel secure. Offer them an encouraging, safe, serene, well-structured environment, keeping the lines of communication with your child open, being careful not to judge or negate your child's feelings, and disciplining in ways to preserve his or her dignity can all deepen the emotional bond between you and your child.

Older children can learn to reduce the effects of stress by practicing abdominal breathing or mindfulness techniques such as meditation, prayer, yoga, and tai chi. Establish proper bedtimes so that the adrenal glands don't go into overtime and cause undue stress. Focus on gratitude to build the child's sense of humor, optimism, and resilience; I sing the grateful song with my children daily, where we each sing what we are thankful for—most of the time we end up laughing so hard because my little one will be thankful for his poop. Be aware and honest about your own stressors and emotions as children are like sponges and can sense and absorb even subtle changes in your mood or behavior.

Additional Integrative Modalities

Supplements

Most children should be taking fish oil, vitamin D, or cod liver oil and probiotics to optimize health and prevent illness, especially if they aren't obtaining it from their diets. Botanical medicines not to be used for infants and toddlers: aloe vera (under ten years of age), buckthorn bark, cajeput oil, camphor, eucalyptus, fennel oil, horseradish, mint and peppermint oils (external application), nasturtium, rhubarb root, senna, and watercress.

- *Colic*: probiotics, fennel tea (¼ tsp three times daily) or chamomile tea (¼ cup three times daily).
- *Failure to thrive*: glutamine (250 mg/kg) and probiotics.
- *Picky eating*: if you eliminate dairy, replace with calcium (900–1,000 mg, split into two doses) and add a new food every two weeks and 15 mg of zinc if your child is more than three years old; multivitamin, vitamin C (100 mg), vitamin D, vitamin A (2,500 IU or less), selenium, chromium, vitamin D (800–1,000 IU per day).
- *Dyspraxia*: fish oil, vitamin D complex, phosphatidylcholine.

Homeopathy

Homeopathy is an excellent and effective choice for children. Use the same types and dosages similar to adults.

Acupressure

The adult points can also be used for children and can be administered while massaging, bathing, dressing, or nursing. Infants respond promptly to acupressure, so only apply pressure for ten to fifteen minute-sessions, in a small circular motion with light pressure for ten to thirty seconds at a time; stretching isn't required for infants.

Colic points: L12, B47, K3, HP3, LV3
Teeth pain: TW5, LU9, LI4, LI11, ST3, SI18
Sleep: GB20, SP4, SP6, H5, HP4
Pain: LI4, LV3
Digestion and nausea: P6, ST36
Anxiety: GV20

Aromatherapy

Essential oils are very beneficial for children and are very potent, so you only need a very small amount to achieve efficacy. A child's skin is thinner, so dilute in the carrier oil before applying to the child. Aromatherapy is amazing for children, and you don't need to worry about skin reactions.

Teething: clove and grapefruit oils
Temper tantrums: ylang-ylang, rose
Colic: lavender, roman chamomile, fennel, marjoram, bergamot, ylang-ylang

Age-appropriate essential oils:

Three days to three months: Roman chamomile, lavender, and mandarin.
Three months to five years: the above plus bergamot, cedarwood, Eucalyptus smithii, frankincense, geranium, ginger, lemon, sweet marjoram, sweet orange, rose, rosemary, sandalwood, tea tree, thyme linalool, ylang-ylang.
Five years to puberty: all oils that are good for adults are considered safe for children, but use in smaller amounts.

Bodywork

Massage and chiropractic/osteopathic manipulations are very beneficial for children and are great ways to show affection and love. Touch stimulates the body to help release hormones that help the child develop appropriately; it's a great way to bond, and it improves overall circulation and healing.

Hydrotherapy

Hydrotherapy is a very healing for a child.

AUTISM

Autism is a neurobehavioral disorder that presents early in childhood, in varying degrees. Symptoms may include social challenges, communication difficulties, repetitive behaviors, sensory processing problems, sleeping problems, seizure disorders, and associated medical issues. Autism can be diagnosed via a detailed history and professional assessment by a developmental pediatrician or other qualified professional; but to get to the root causes of the symptoms, additional assessments including blood tests may be indicated.

Testing

Start with the basic testing as we discussed in chapter 4 (Adjusting the Holistic Rx for Your Condition). Common deficiencies seen in children with autism include calcium, selenium, zinc, magnesium, iron, cysteine, sulfate, taurine, B12, B6, lysine, methionine, essential fatty acids, and vitamin D, E, and A. There are many tests available to help identify other chemical or other physiological imbalances, so consider the following list of tests: minerals (like red blood cell minerals, or whole blood minerals, zinc, copper), urine organic acids, amino acids, essential fatty acids, fat-soluble vitamins, reduced glutathione, lipid peroxides, plasma cysteine, plasma sulfate, CSDA, food allergy testing, immune testing (IgA, IgM, IgG, IgG subclass levels, lymphocyte subsets natural killer cell activity, vaccine titers, viral titers), thyroid antibodies, antimyelin basic protein (MBP) antibodies, folate receptor antibody test, PANDAS profile (ASO titer, anti-DNAase B titer), provoked urine testing for heavy metals, urine, porphyrins and genetic polymorphisms, test for mold, heavy metal toxicity, chronic viral and bacterial infections (see chapter 5 [Autoimmune Disease]), start with viral IgG and IgM titers to HHV1, HHV2, HHV6, CMV, and Epstein Barr panel. Consider lyme panel, bacterial infections, ESR, hsCRP, platelets, Streptococcus markers (ASO titers and Anti-DNase antibodies), stool cultures, urine cultures, and urine organic acid testing.

Additional Integrative Modalities

Supplements

- Fish oil (1,000–3,000 mg of EPA and DHA combined).
- Probiotic.
- Cod liver oil with Vitamin D (2,000–5,000 IU daily with meals).
- Digestive enzyme (one or two capsules with each meal).
- B complex with B12 (1,000 mcg daily) and B6 (0.6 mg per kg).
- Multivitamin with zinc (10–20 mg daily), selenium (50–100 mcg, depending on weight, daily), calcium and magnesium (6 mg/kg), vitamin E (100–400 IU per day) with essential amino acid combination, vitamin C.
- Detoxification: Supplements to focus on are antioxidants like vitamin C (1,000 mg per day), vitamin A (5,000 IU per day minimum), NAC (600 mg daily), selenium (100 mcg daily), glutathione (transdermally 100–200 mg twice daily), melatonin (1 mg per day).
- Support methylation: Methyl B12 injections (check with your integrative practitioner before takine MB12), raise glutathione (IV, transdermal, and nebulized), folic acid, TMG (trimethylglycine; start with 250 mg twice daily; side effects are hyperactivity and more emotional behaviors) or DMG (dimethylglycine), NAC (can be taken orally, but in some kids can lead to yeast overgrowth, so it should be given transdermally [100–200 mg twice daily or higher to 2,000 mg per day]).
- To reduce behaviors commonly seen in autism such as sensory defensiveness, sleeplessness, eye aversion, stimming, scripting: tyrosine, TMG, GABA, NADH, Cerefolin, Deptin, tryptophan (100 mg daily), essential amino acid combination (500–2,000 mg daily), GABA (500–1,000 mg three times daily), spectrum awakening (¼ tsp three times daily).
- Treat infections with oregano oil, olive leaf extract, garlic, lauricidin, caprylic acid.
- Others that can be discussed with your physician: taurine; coenzyme Q10; iron; chromium; BH4 (tetrahydrobiopterin; 1–2 mg/kg of body weight for treatment); melatonin (1–3 mg/day with weekly increase of 1–2 mg if not effective) for treatment of sleep issues; carnosine (this amino-acid-like substance improves neurological function) (400 mg twice daily or as directed by a doctor); iron can be tried (especially if deficient; 10–80 mg of elemental iron per day); chromium (50–100 mcg daily); vitamin K; L-carnitine (250–500 mg daily); DMAE (100–500 mg per day); silymarin; 5HTP; activated charcoal; pantothenic acid (B5); phosphatidylecholine; oral gamma globulin; pycnogenol; other herbs like quercetin, curcumin, creatine (750 mg to several grams per day), carnisine, SAMe.

- Treat according to symptoms of hyperactivity, inactivity (chapter 18 [Psychiatry]), poor sleep (see insomnia), digestive issues in the respective chapters.
- To limit die off: Epsom salt baths can help with detoxification. Start one new supplement at a time, giving three to four days before adding another supplement. Start with half the target dose for one to two days to see how it is tolerated.
- Keep a diary, and look for patterns of behavior changes.

Homeopathy

Finding a constitutional remedy is key (See Appendix), so work with a licensed homeopathic practitioner for a personalized treatment plan.

- Chamomilla is indicated for those children who repeatedly bang their heads on the wall, get upset with noise, lash out when approached, and are restless and irritable.
- Silicea helps those who have head sweats at night, count things over and over on the floor, and have sweaty and smelly feet.
- Hyosyamus is indicated for children who go into fits of laughter, mutter, play with their genitals, and are suspicious of unfamiliar objects.
- Agaricus is useful for those who are fearless, mutter, and sing, talk but don't answer, move head constantly, and have double vision.
- Cuprum metallicum is great for tension and those who are aggressive, obsessive, inflexible, irritable, and tense with tics and hand banging behavior.

Acupressure

Traditional Chinese Medicine may help with behavioral problems in children with autism, as it addresses specific energy points and pathways. See a licensed practitioner for a personalized treatment plan.

Aromatherapy

Lavender oil helps for calmness, and frankincense oil helps support the brain, while vetiver essential oil can help balance brain waves. Others that can help are sandalwood and cedarwood.

Other Therapies

- Hyperbaric oxygen therapy. Before hyperbaric oxygen treatment: begin the supplement protocol and help your child detox first; beware of all the risks like fatigue, lightheadedness, ear pain, or even serious lung complications, so weigh the risks over the benefits (mostly present if the duration or pressure is too high).

- Infrared sauna.
- Chelation detox.
- Allergy desensitization.

EAR INFECTIONS

Ear infections occur when fluid becomes trapped in the middle ear, leading to earaches and thick fluid from the ear. Other symptoms are fever, loss of appetite, digestive issues, irritability, or trouble sleeping. Infections can be caused by a virus or bacteria due to swelling of the tubes from an upper respiratory infection or an allergy, leading to fluid buildup that can easily get infected. Diagnosis occurs via a detailed history and exam.

Additional Intergrative Modalities

Supplements

- Fish oil.
- Garlic oil or garlic/mullein or probiotic mixed in olive oil few drops in each ear.
- Garlic oil or garlic/mullein a few drops in each ear.
- Zinc (10 mg twice daily for those older than two years).
- Vitamin C (500 mg twice daily for children six to twelve years).
- Echinacea (2 ml four times daily for children).
- Vitamin D3 (400–2,000 IU daily for children two to twelve years).
- Others: Vitamin A (2,000–5,000 IU daily up to five days for up to six years old), goldenseal (2 ml four times daily for children), or larix (one to two tsp for infants and four times a day for older children).

Homeopathy

Read through this list and locate the symptomatic remedy that best matches your symptoms. Give 6C, 15C, or 30C once or twice daily. For acute earaches, give 30C hourly up to six doses. Children may take the remedy as long as symptoms continue and stop when they improve.

- Aconitum napellus is used for the beginning six hours of an ear infection, with bright red ears, violent pain with increased thirst that can occur after being in the cold, dry wind.
- Belladonna is a remedy for sudden onset of earache, with staring eyes, hot flushed face, fever, cold feet, unusual sensitivity to touch, excited and incoherent behavior. Right ear is more affected than left.

- Chamomilla is used for that child who is very irritable and angry, screaming/crying who wants to be carried. Ear infection usually is associated with teething. One cheek is red and the other pale.
- Hepar sulphuris is used when pus or drainage is present from the ear. Child is irritable, ears are sensitive, and the sharp pain is improved with warmth.
- Pulsatilla is used for those who are weepy, feverish, with pain that feels as if the pressure is pushing out; who have yellowish green discharge from the nose; symptoms improve with cold applications or in open air, worsen in warmth; and the child wants to be held and comforted.
- Lachesis is helpful when the left ear is infected and when it moves to the right, improved at night and with warmth.
- Lycopodium is a remedy for right-sided ear infections, in an irritable, gassy child with digestive upsets. Symptoms improve with warmth and worse between 4:00 and 8:00 pm.
- Mercuris solubilis or vivus helps with earache with smelly drainage, increased sweat, bad breath, and increased salvation; it worsens at night with a thick coating on tongue.
- Aconite is indicated for those with an attack that occurs after cold exposure. Patient is anxious and restless.
- Silicea helps with chronic ear infections and can be used for acute ear infections in thin individuals who are cold-sensitive especially to wind. It can also be used in perforations of the eardrum.
- Ferrum phosphoricum helps with those who have fever but don't act sick.

Acupuncture and Acupressure

- TW21, SI19, and GB2, TB17, K3 help to ease pain.

Aromatherapy

Tea tree oil has powerful antiseptic properties. Others that are beneficial are basil, cajeput, Roman chamomile, eucalyptus radiate, lavender, and rosemary. Massage on the outer ear.

PEDIATRIC AUTOIMMUNE NEUROPSYCHIATRIC DISORDERS ASSOCIATED WITH STREPTOCOCCUS (PANDAS)

A child can be diagnosed with PANDAS when symptoms include motor and/or vocal tics, obsessions and/or compulsions, moody or irritable behavior, separation from loved ones, and anxiety attacks that may appear following a strep infection or symptoms that worsen following a strep infection. Symptoms can appear suddenly. PANDAS usually affects children ages three to puberty. Diagnosis can occur via a history, physical, and laboratory testing (see Autism testing).

Supplements

- Vitamin D3, B12.
- Calcium.
- Magnesium.
- Zinc.
- Iodine.
- Omega 3.
- Detoxification and gut healing supplements.

Homeopathy, acupressure, and aromatherapy are similar to autism and anxiety (in psychiatry).

Tips for Picky Eaters

- **Stock up for success.** Only stock your home with appropriate and healthy foods.
- **Set a good example.** It is important to model healthy habits, as children imitate their guardians.
- **Family mealtime is key.** Set a standard of only having one meal as you are one family.
- **Involve them.** Involve your children in picking out veggies, fruit, protein, and fat sources from the grocery store and in food preparation.
- **Make it fun!** Cut their veggies into shapes and arrange in colors of the rainbow.
- **Stand your ground and be consistent**—don't give in to allowing foods that aren't healthy. Be patient with new foods—one good bite of food is better than no good bite of food, but no bites of food is better than a bite of poison. Sometimes your children might need to go to bed hungry, but they won't let themselves starve, I promise!
- **Knowledge is power!** Educate your children about the relationship between food and the body. Explain to them what happens when they eat good food versus bad food. Tell them about all the good bugs/pets in their belly that they have to feed and that they need to starve the bad guys so that the bad guys can go bye-bye and the good guys can win.
- **Swap for healthy.** Switch their favorite foods with healthier options. If your kid likes brownies, make them healing brownies (with almond flour)! It's a great treat after he finishes his veggies, protein, and fat! Yum!!!

• 18 •

Psychiatry

Without optimal psychological health, it is hard to obtain optimal physical health. So let's keep the inflammation out of our minds, allowing us to truly be who we were meant to be.

D & D: SPECIAL CONSIDERATIONS

Healing the gut, balancing insulin, and avoiding toxins are critical for appropriate neurotransmitter function and overall mental health. Following a gut healing protocol, like GAPS, and avoiding your food sensitivities can help you heal the body and the mind. Starting your day off with a high protein breakfast will optimize brain function for the rest of the day.

Eat foods high in tryptophan (like turkey, chicken, and tuna), complex carbs like butternut squash and sweet potatoes, raw milk (if tolerated from goat or sheep), magnesium (green leafy vegetables, sesame and sunflower seeds), and B vitamins (organic meat, brewer's yeast, liver, green leafy vegetables).

THE FOUR BIG S's: SPECIAL CONSIDERATIONS

Managing stress and sleep can help to lower inflammation, optimizing mental health. Cardiovascular exercise boosts dopamine and serotonin, so combine aerobic conditioning, weight training, burst training, and stretching. Exercising before work can help you concentrate on the task at hand. Connect with nature, play daily, get optimal sleep, and get enough sunlight or light therapy (thirty to sixty minutes with a 10,000-lux bulb in the morning).

ADHD

Attention deficit hyperactivity disorder (ADHD) is characterized by difficulty concentrating and being easily distracted, irritable, disorganized, unable to sit still, and impulsivity. According to Dr. Daniel Amen there are seven types of ADHD.

- Type 1 (classic ADD or ADHD) is when the person has symptoms of inattentiveness, hyperactivity, impulsivity and restlessness, distractibility, and disorganization.
- Type 2 (inattentive ADD) is when the person is not hyperactive but inattentive, disorganized, and easily distracted.
- Type 3 (overfocused ADD) is when the person frequently gets stuck in loops of negative behavior that can lead to frequent oppositional and argumentative behavior, excessive worrying, inattentiveness, obsessiveness, and inflexibility.
- Type 4 (temporal lobe ADD) presents with a short fuse, dark thoughts, irritability, easily distracted, disorganized, and mood instability; patient may struggle with learning disabilities.
- Type 5 (limbic ADD) presents with inattentiveness, easily distracted, disorganization, and pessimistic and depressive tendencies.
- Type 6 (ring-of-fire ADD) presents with cyclic moodiness that may be oppositional and overly sensitive/irritable.
- Type 7 (anxious ADD) presents with characteristic symptoms but also is nervous, predicts the worst, and has anxiety that may present with physical symptoms.

Types 3 through 7 may or may not present with hypersensitivity. Testing can be performed at the child's school or at a licensed mental health professional's office.

Additional Integrative Modalities

Supplements

- Fish oil (1,000 mg per day of EPA/DHA).
- B complex (50 mg daily).
- Multimineral supplement (500 mg calcium, 100–300 mg magnesium, especially if the person has tics, is over focused, and has sleep/anxiety issues) and 5–20 mg zinc twice daily (especially if the person has learning or memory issues).
- Probiotic.

Specifics—

- GABA (250 mg twice daily).
- Rhodiola rosea helps with focus.
- Inositol (2–6 g twice daily) if anxious, sleep issues, or overfocused; use powder.
- Pycnogenol (50–200 mg) can help if hyperactivity or impulsivity is present.
- Phosphatidylserine (200 mg can be used if learning or memory problems are present.
- Bacopa, Gotu kola, American ginseng, for those kids who are hyperactive and underfocused.
- SAM-e helps with depression and fatigue.
- L-theanine (200–400 mg) especially if the person is anxious (100–300 mg twice daily for kids).
- Ginkgo biloba (60–120 mg daily).
- DMAE (100–400 mg daily) helps with learning and attention.
- Chromium (for blood sugar issues; 400–800 mcg per day).
- Phosphatidylserine.
- L-carnitine (1–2 g daily).

Dr. Amen's Recommendations

- Type 1: Rhodiola, green tea, ginseng, L-tyrosine, zinc, grapeseed, or pine bark (abbreviated stimulating supplements)
- Type 2: stimulating supplements
- Type 3: 5-HTP plus stimulating supplements with a lower protein and higher smart carb diet
- Type 4: GABA, gingko, vinpocetine, huperzine A, ALC, PS, NAC, and ALA PLUS stimulating supplements with a higher protein, lower carb ketogenic diet
- Type 5: SAMe plus stimulating supplements
- Type 6: GABA, 5HTP plus stimulating supplements
- Type 7: L-theanine, Relora, magnesium, holy basil, plus stimulating supplements

Homeopathy

- Hyoscyamus niger is indicated for children who are very impulsive and violent, sexually precocious, and talkative.

- Stramonium is a remedy for multiple fears, anger, rage, tendency to destroy things, with night terrors.
- Sulphur helps those who are stubborn, curious, and always thirsty for cold drinks and craving spicy foods. They sweat easily and are hyperactive.
- Tarentula hispanica is for those who are impulsive, mischievous, restless, and hurried, loving dance and music.
- Coffea tosta is for extreme moodiness with a constant flow of ideas and anxiety with insomnia.
- Kali bromatum helps with the inability to sit still, constantly moving hands, and frequent night terrors.
- Luesinum helps when the nervousness prevents concentration; appears wrinkled, nervous, and unstable. Symptoms improve in the mountains.
- Hepar sulphur patients are excitable, irritable, hypersensitive to pain with recurring suppurations.
- China is a remedy for irritable, touchy individuals who have frequent insomnia and may have worms.
- Staphysagria is indicated for irritable and touchy individuals who rarely explode with anger and often masturbate.
- Moschus is a remedy for individuals with agitation and anxiety, with sexual problems. They have paradoxical symptoms.
- Medorrhinum helps those who have poor memory, are irritable, with major temper tantrums in children, violent toward other kids, inattentive, hands and feet are always moving, never finish what they start, and symptoms improve at the seaside. They crave oranges and ice.
- Chamomilla is a remedy for the irritable, anxious, agitated person who doesn't like to be talked to, as they are hypersensitive specifically to pain.
- Lachesis mutus is helpful for those who are very talkative, jealous, oversensitive, and occasionally depressed.
- Nitricum acidum helps those with fatigue, who are indifferent and sometimes depressed.

Attention and memory issues: Baryta carbonica (timid, mental fatigue, backward, and a slow learner), calcarea phosphoric (anxiety with mental and physical fatigue), natrum muriaticum (quickly discouraged, frequent headaches, craves salt, intense thirst, thin, with good appetite, indifferent), zincum metallicum (fatigue, worry a lot, can't keep still [especially feet], and poor memory), silicea (anxious, fatigue, easily discouraged, nervous, irritable, prone to respiratory infections, and sensitive to the cold; feet sweat easily; have difficulty concentrating), agaricus muscarius (slow, with tics), anacardium orientate (fatigue after the slightest effort, sensitive, poor memory, indifferent, symptoms improve with eating, cruel to animals and people, low self-esteem, and antisocial).

Inattention with fatigue: tuberculinum (very stubborn and demanding, impatient, also have recurring viral infections like rhinopharyngitis or bronchitis, get bored easily with violent tempers, and crave milk and smoked meats), psorinum (fatigue with anxiety, fear of the future, and an inferiority complex), sepia (mental fatigue with irritability and poor memory), aurum muriaticum (lack of motivation, extreme irritability, anxiety, and depression), phosphoricum acidum (indifferent, frequent headaches, poor memory), and kali phosphoricum (frequent headaches, sleep problems, hypersensitivity, irritability, with nervous exhaustion).

Acupressure

- CV12, LI11, P6, H7, LU1, and SP6

Aromatherapy

Vetiver, cedarwood, cardamom, peppermint basil, thyme can help to improve focus and alertness. Calming oils are ylang-ylang, neroli, orange, lavender, rose and sandalwood, chamomile, and vetiver.

ANXIETY

Anxiety is normal feeling of nervous, but constant anxiety, regardless of the circumstance can lead to other chronic ailments. Types include panic disorder, social anxiety disorder, generalized anxiety disorder, and specific phobias. Symptoms include muscle tension, feelings of restlessness, fast heartbeat, stomach upset, fatigue, irritability, and/or trouble falling asleep. Diagnosis is made through a detailed history, physical, and basic labs.

Additional Integrative Modalities

Supplements

- Vitamin C (1,000 mg in the morning).
- Magnesium and calcium (500 mg calcium and 250 mg of magnesium twice daily).
- B-complex (50 mg with 1 mg of folate).
- 5HTP (50–200 mg twice daily).
- Kava (200–250 mg three times daily).

- GABA (500 mg three times daily).
- Adaptogenic herbs like Ashwagandha and tulsi.
- Inositol (3–5 g twice or three times daily), EPA (1–2 g of EPA).
- St. John's wort (900 mg per day of quality product divided twice daily).

Obsessive Compulsive Disorder (OCD)

OCD is a mental health disorder characterized by a pattern of unreasonable fears (obsessions) leading to repetitive behaviors (compulsions) that interfere with your daily routine.

- Physical: Inositol (18 g/d), NAC (600–1,200 mg twice daily), improvements may take up to twelve weeks), milk thistle (600 mg/d), and glycine

Trauma

Trauma is an emotional reaction to an emotionally painful and traumatizing event that can leave someone feeling powerless and overwhelmed. When someone fails to recover from that event, it is called posttraumatic stress disorder (PTSD).

- Inositol (3–6 g three times daily).
- Magnesium glycinate (125–250 mg twice daily in the morning and at bedtime).
- Melatonin (0.5–1 mg) if there are sleep issues.
- *Children*—Anxiety: inositol; L-theanine; kava (if comfortable with risk); herbals like California poppy, lemon balm, valerian, and so on.
- OCD: inositol, L-theanine, and/or herbals to reduce ambient anxiety, consider NAC.
- PTSD: inositol and L-theanine and/or herbals.

Homeopathy

- Aconitum napellus can be used for acute panic attacks with sense of doom, which worsen around midnight.
- Arsenicum album is for anxiety, agitation, and insecurity with fast heart rate and disturbed appetite; obsessed about cleaning and organization.
- Calcarea carbonica helps anxiety accompanied with feelings of being overwhelmed, cold, irritable, sadness, and fatigue.
- Gelsemium is for acute anxiety from crowds; also for diarrhea and trembling.

- Kali phosphoricum can help with poor memory, general anxiety, and fatigue.
- Pulsatilla is for anxiety about being alone.
- Chamomilla is for anxiety with anger, oversensitivity to pain, and irritability.
- Ignatia is for those who are very sensitive to contradiction, moody, have a tendency to spasm (ball in throat and abdominal pain); improved by entertainment.
- Magnesia carbonica is for those with nervousness and spasmodic pain, who are prone to diarrhea with sour-smelling sweat.
- Cyclamen is indicated for those with exhausting perfectionism and feelings of abandonment, worse during menses, accompanied with migraines and vertigo.
- Magnesia muriatica is a remedy for anxiety associated with cramp-like pain, constipation, nervousness, and agitation with paresthesia.
- Nux vomica is a remedy for irritability, anger, intolerance to contradiction, and aggressiveness, with digestive symptoms. Insomnia occurs around 3:00 or 4:00 am.
- Nux moschata helps with those who are anxious, emotionally sensitive, suffering from abdominal distention, and have dry mucous membrane.
- Stamonium is a remedy for anxiety that is associated with tics, agitation, and laryngeal or esophageal spasms.
- Lycopodium is a remedy for those who have anxiety about a new situation or stage anxiety, crave sweets, and feel worse in stuffy rooms.
- Arsenicum is indicated for those who are restless, overly tidy, cold, and fatigued.
- Phosphorus is best for nervousness with extreme sensitivity to others and they love reassurance; symptoms worsen during thunderstorms.
- Calcarea is for a person who is easily forgetful, feels cold, and easily becomes overweight.
- Natrum muriaticum is for those who hate sympathy and dwell on morbid topics.
- Ignatia is for a person who has symptoms that follow an emotional trauma like the death of a loved one or a breakup.
- Tarentula is best for those whose tendency to overwork leads to anxiety; has difficulty relaxing night and day.

Hysteria

Hysteria is a disorder that converts mental stress into a physical symptom: overdramatic or attention-seeking behavior.

- Ignatia helps with lump in throat, other symptoms brought on by emotional upset, weepiness, and moodiness.
- Valeriana is indicated for sensations of floating, losing identity, and sleepiness.
- Platinum is a remedy for when a patient feels numb and cold, haughty and contemptuous.
- Moschus is for those who have palpitations, complain of difficulty breathing, are overdramatic and manipulative. Moschus is associated with hysterical emotional behavior, changes in level of sexual excitement, and hyperesthesia.
- Asafoetida is indicated for one that develops asthma, hysterical cough, nausea and vomiting with retching, as if the body is about to explode.

Phobias

Fear of Heights

- Argenticum is indicated for fear associated with the impulse to jump.
- Borax is for fear associated with the sensation of falling.
- Sulphur is for fear of heights associated with extreme giddiness.

Fear of Dark

- Stramonium is for the person who fears the dark, talking and praying continuously.
- Phosphorus is for those with serious anxiety, fearful of the future and the dark, hypersensitive to everything, feeling fatigue and agitation; symptoms improve with reassurance.

Fear of Performing in Public

- Lycopodium helps those with anxiety about performing, low confidence about eating in public, who are grouchy upon waking, who feel full after a small amount of food, and who are socially inadequate. Craves sweets with digestive upset.
- Gelsemium is for a person who feels weak at the knees for test anxiety, accompanied by trembling.
- Anarcardium anxiety leads to stomach upsets, specifically for a musician.
- Argnticum nitricum can be used for those in a rush with issues organizing time, and fear that can lead to diarrhea and gas; or for those who have no control over emotions.

Obsessions and Compulsions

- Aurum is for the person who has thoughts of dying and feels worthless.
- Anacardium is for those who feel as if the body and mind are separate and like they are being controlled by someone else.
- Silicea is used for unshakable feelings that one is not good enough; these persons feel like they need to sit on the floor and count small objects.
- Thuja is for when a person is convinced that live animals are wriggling around in the stomach, limbs are brittle and may break, and has warts.

Acupressure

- HP7, HP6, TW5, H7, H5, LU1
- TW15, B10, P3, P6 (for nervous tension)
- H7, GV24.5, CV17, LV3, GB13, K27, SP6, B23
- TFT (thought field therapy) uses acupressure point to help to break up energy patterns that can lead to symptoms.

Aromatherapy

Essential oils can provide a relaxing effect. These include lavender, rose, vetiver, ylang-ylang, bergamot, chamomile and frankincense, neroli, sandalwood, and orange.

Other calming and soothing ones are cypress, palmarosa, helichrysum, patchouli, clary sage, jasmine, lemon balm, and lime. During a panic attack, frankincense can help to improve deep breathing. Bergamot helps to restore appetite, while peppermint, melissa, lavender, and chamomile can help to improve digestive complaints like diarrhea or cramps.

Other Recommendations

- Cranial electrotherapy stimulation.
- Four step behavioral technique: Relabel (call the obsessive thought or urge what it really is), Reattribute (answer the question of "why"; attribute these feelings not to yourself but to your OCD), Refocus (learn to work around your thoughts as they occur), Revalue (give less value to your anxiety and more value to your life).

BIPOLAR DISORDER/MANIC DEPRESSION

Bipolar disorder is a mood disorder defined by depressive lows and manic high energy states. Diagnosis is made via history and physical.

Additional Integrative Modalities

Supplements

- Fish oil.
- Adaptogenic herbs like ginseng, holy basil, ashwagandha, and rhodiola.
- EFAs (0.5 for ages four to eight, 1g for ages nine to eleven and 2g for ages twelve and above 2 of EPA per day).
- Magnesium (citrate or aspartate, 150 mg up to age six, 300 mg for ages seven to eleven, 40–500 mg for ages twelve and above).
- Vitamin C (250 mg a day for ages three to five, 500 mg a day for ages six to eleven, and 1,000 mg per day for ages twelve and above).
- EMPowerplus (five capsules three times daily [loading dose] then four to fives capsules/powder twice daily as maintenance, before beginning meds).
- Inositol (3–6 g three times daily).
- Begin diet and supplements first, allowing a two-month trial before moving on to meds. **Never SAMe, SJW, 5HTP, ginseng, or gingko with bipolar depression, even if family history of bipolar.
- *Children bipolar:* fish oil (500–1,000 mg of EPA), inositol (3–6 g two to three times daily); if emotionally deregulated think of DBT, avoid St. John's wort, SAMe, ginkgo, ginseng, stimulants and antidepressents, consider EMPowerplus as a central biochemical intervention. If no current psychiatric or contraindicated medications, can increase to five capsules three times after food over a few days. If on medication, can locate a practitioner to cross taper. If manic persists, consider choline bitartrate (300–500 mg two or three times daily), NAC.

Homeopathy

- Apis aids those that feel as if they are going to die; they are very jealous and aren't thirsty.
- Hyoscyamus helps a person who has hallucinations, makes obscene remarks, and is afraid of being poisoned.
- Belladonna is a remedy for high fevers, red face, wild eyes that are staring.
- Cannabis indicated for those with exalted ideas, feeling that time is slow, and exhibiting uncontrollable laughter.
- Phosphorus helps those with rapid oscillating moods and a temper; it has a calming effect.

Acupressure

See respective sections depending on predominant symptom.

Aromatherapy

See respective sections depending on predominant symptom.

DEPRESSION

Depression involves feelings of sadness, loss, frustration, low sex drive, fatigue, helplessness, and others that can cause problems in day-to-day living. There are multiple types of depression, like major depression, dysthymia (mild depression that is long lasting), atypical depression, adjustment disorders, postpartum depression, premenstrual dysphoric disorder (one week before period), seasonal affective disorder, and bipolar disorder. Diagnosis can be made with a detailed history, physical, and basic labs.

Additional Integrative Modalities

Supplements

- Adaptogen herbs, Rhodiola and ashwagandha (1,000 mg twice daily).
- Vitamin B complex (50 mg daily); make sure it contains folate as 5-methyltetrahydrofolate or folinic acid and B12 as methylcobalamin or hydrocobalamin or adenosylcobalamin.
- Multivitamin with magnesium (400 mg per day), zinc (15–30 mg daily) with copper (1–3 mg daily), iodine (200 mcg to 3 m), Atlantic kelp, selenium (100–200 mcg per day) is ideal for anxiousness and depression and those who have low thyroid function or low T3 levels, iodine and selenium.
- St. John's wort (300–500 mg daily).
- Evening primrose (start with 500 milligrams twice daily).
- Cod liver oil from Atlantic cod for at least 2,500 IU of vitamin A and 250 IU of vitamin D per teaspoon.
- Adrenal and hypothalamus glandular.
- Digestive enzymes with protease, lipases, amylase, and betaine HCL.
- SAMe (400–1,600 mg per day); don't take if taking an antidepressant medication and levodopa, as it may lead to serotonin syndrome and rare with meperidine, pentazocine, and dextromethorphan; has not been studied in children younger than twelve but can be well tolerated in those older than fourteen; can be taken twenty to thirty minutes before meal.
- L-theanine (200 mg per day) can help to reduce anxiety and support a relaxed but focused mind-set (meditation in a capsule!).

- N-acetyl cysteine (600–1,800 mg per day).
- Rhodiola (100 mg every week up to 400 mg per day); look for 2–3% rosavin and 0.8–1% salidroside.
- Curcumin (500–1,000 mg twice daily).
- Others: Chromium picolinate (400 mg twice daily; most helpful in atypical depression characterized by excessive sleep and appetite; ginkgo biloba (60–120 mg twice daily of a standardized product containing 24% fiavone glycosides and 6% terpene lactones) improves blood flow to the brain and enhances neurotransmitter activity and can be used for slow/fatigue ridden depreesion.

Depression with agitation/anxiety

- Inositol (3–6 g two or three times daily).
- L-theanine (100 mg to 200 mg) twice daily.
- Kava needs to follow liver function tests, and use only high-quality product.
- 5HTP (50–150 mg twice daily).
- Passionflower (250 mg or 0.5 ml two to three times daily) relaxes the nerves and is gentle enough to use during the day.
- Relora (250 mg two to three times per day with food).

If Period Related

Start with maca and progress to chaste tree. Maca (use according to label), chaste tree (150–250 mg containing 30–40 mg of dried fruit extract); inositol is best for when blood sugar imbalances are at the root of the menstrual irregularity, so it improves insulin sensitivity, reduces male hormones (at doses 2–4 g daily) and has been studied for anxiety and OCD (at doses 12–18 g daily). Can combine myo-inositol and d-chiro-inositol in a 40:1 ratio for the most effective hormone balancing.

Children: B complex (50 mg with 1 mg of folate), fish oil (500–1,000 mg of EPA) and vitamin C (500–1,000 mg daily); chronic depression or fatigue, explore adrenal health and consider adaptogens like rhodiola or ashwagandha. If emotional regulation is an issue, select St. John's wort and SAMe as appropriate.

If tapering off an SSRI

Broad spectrum amino acid as well as a high-quality tryptophan or 5HTP supplement; take 500 mg a day of tryptophan taken with a simple carbohydrate on an empty stomach and work up to 3 g per day or 50 mg three times a day and work up to 200 mg three times per day, taken on an empty stomach, along with a complementary amino acid tyrosine (1,500 mg two to four times daily before meals); Inositol, pharmaGaba, or phenibut can be a helpful calming agent during this time. Amino acids are only needed during the medication taper.

Homeopathy

- Arsenicum album is indicated for those with intense fatigue, restlessness, worrying, seeing no hope for a cure, pessimistic, exhaustion, always cold, obsessessing about cleanliness. Depression causes weight loss, anxiety, and insomnia between 1:00 and 3:00 am.
- China has helped those with racing thoughts, vivid dreams, oversensitivity to stimuli like noise and light, and feeling cold.
- Aurum metallicum is for deep depression, disgusted with oneself, and even suicidal tendency. Symptoms improve by being in the sun. ***Note:*** Suicidal tendencies should always be discussed with a doctor or suicidal hotline.
- Ignatia amara aids depression that follows emotional trauma, with constant sighing and a sensation of a lump in the throat.
- Natrum muriaticum helps in those who don't show their emotions, are emotionally reserved and withdrawn, and reject sympathy due to embarrassment. They crave salt and have aversions to the sunlight.
- Pulsatilla helps those who burst into tears at the slightest provocation and want a lot of reassurance and attention; depression worsens around a cycle or menopause. Symptoms are worse in a warm environment, with improvement with crying, sweets, open air, and attention.
- Nux vomica is a remedy for those who find fault with everyone and are extremely irritable.
- Sepia is indicated for those who feel irritable, have low libido, are tearful and always cold.
- Kali phosphoricum is for depression as a result of overwork. Mental fatigue is a common symptom that this remedy helps.
- Graphites is indicated in individuals who are full of anguish, apprehensiveness, and hesitation.
- Anacardium orientate can help those with poor memory, mental cloudiness, indifference, slowness to understand, and depression. They may feel as if they have a split personality. Symptoms improve by eating.
- Kali bromatum is indicated for a patient who is agitated, distracted, and moves constantly and has blunted sensitivity to pain.
- Lachesis mutus is for depression alternating with excitement. Depression is characterized by mutism, worry, sensitivity, fear of dying, and jealousy without reason. Insomnia is usually before midnight.

- Kali carbonicum is indicated in those who are fatigued, hypersensitive, and worried about their health.
- Kali phosphoricum is indicated for fatigue, irritability, listless depression, fear of crowds; symptoms follow overwork or grief.
- Lycopodium is for exhaustion, depression, low libido during depressive phases, with poor sleep.
- Natrum carbonicum is a remedy for depression and poor memory with sensory hypersensitivity especially to noises, not tolerant to sunshine or heat that leads to headaches.
- Natrum sulphuricum is used for those with depression, who are not talkative, are worried and irritable in the morning; symptoms improve with eating, are worse in the evening and wet weather.
- Nitricum acidum is for the depressed patient worried about health, annoyed, angry, easily cries, and rejects comfort. Symptoms include insomnia with unpleasant dreams and vague pain.
- Phosphorus is helpful for those with irritability, fatigue, and agitation countered by indifference.
- Psorinum is for one who is depressed with little reaction, worries about the future, feels inferior and fears being incurable, with little reaction, and emaciated.
- Selenium is a remedy for needing to stay in bed and sleep often, with fatigue accompanied by skin disorders.
- Phosphoricum acidum is indicated with nervous exhaustion with difficulty concentrating, with headaches. Depression usually is after mental shock or worries.
- Sepia helps depression with those who are prone to easily crying, complain of memory problems, want to be alone, are irritated by consolation; symptoms worsen with menses, with craving for sweets and salty/sour foods.
- Silicea can be used for lack of energy, sensitivity to cold, tendency to suppuration, and irritability.

Acupressure

- GB20, GB21, LV3, LV5, LV14, K27, B38, B23 (accompanied by fear or fatigue)
- B47, GV24.5, K27, CV17 (relieve depression made worse by grief or anxiety)
- ST36 (depression with digestive and fatigue)
- GV19, Tai yang, P6 (ease anxiety and depression)

Aromatherapy

Essential oils have been proven to elevate mood; these include bergamot oil, lavender, Roman chamomile, and ylang-ylang. Others that can help are frankincense, cedarwood, cinnamon, neroli, mandarin, orange, lemongrass, helichrysum, jasmine, litsea, basil, geranium, tuberose, ravintsara, clary sage, benzoin, sandalwood, marjoram, and neroli.

Other Recommendations

The Fisher Wallace cranial electrical stimulator (CES) is a device that generates a low-intensity alternating current that is transmitted across the skull for twenty minutes twice daily to promote alpha wave activity and to modulate neurotransmitters, endorphins, and cortisol. Using a light box will help with sleep.

EATING DISORDERS

Eating disorders, like anorexia, bulimia, and binge eating disorders, can be caused by an obsession with food and body weight and shape and can lead to serious and fatal consequences. Symptoms may include extremely restricted eating or overeating, then trying to get rid of the food, distorted body image, fatigue, dehydration and other symptoms that can develop over time and can be fatal. A diagnosis can be made through a detailed history and physical with basic labs that can determine the specific deficiencies and root cause (according to Dr. Greenblatt MD in the book *Answers to Anorexia*). The following labs can be drawn: zinc taste test, amino acids, CBC with differential, celiac screening, cholesterol panel, CMP, copper, essential fatty acids, folate and vitamin B12, homocysteine, iron and ferritin, magnesium, methylmalonic acid, red blood cell trace minerals, thyroid, urinary organic acids, urinary peptides, vitamin D 25OH, zinc, and referenced-EEG.

Additional Integrative Modalities

Supplements

- Calcium citrate with vitamin D (250–500 mg twice daily).
- Probiotic (10–20 CFU per pill).
- Plant-based digestive enzymes with DPP IV and HCl with meals.
- Vitamin C (1,000–2,000 mg per day).
- Essential fatty acids.
- High-potency multivitamin.

- Zinc chelate (30–90 mg daily), along with 3 mg of copper. Studies have found that zinc deficiency is common in people with anorexia or bulimia. It is also required for the senses of taste and smell and for appetite.
- Magnesium glycinate.
- B-Complex (50–75 mg twice daily).
- 5-Hydroxytryptophan (5-HTP) (100 mg two or three times daily) supports serotonin levels. Do not use in combination with pharmaceutical antidepressant or antianxiety medications.
- Gentian root (ten drops in water or 300 mg fifteen minutes before each meal) improves digestion and appetite.
- St. John's wort (300 mg of a 0.3% hypericin extract two or three times daily). Do not use in combination with pharmaceutical antidepressant or antianxiety medications.

Homeopathy

- Natrum muriaticum is indicated for one that dislikes sympathy, puts weight on bottom and thighs, with a thin neck.
- Calcarea is for one who is overweight, always cold, timid, easily forgetful, craves eggs, and is apprehensive.
- Ferrum is indicated for anemic pallor, but easily flushed, weak and oversensitive.
- Pulsatilla helps those who weep easily and are timid, uncomfortable with stuffy rooms, and feel better with company and cool air.
- Argentum nitricum is for those with claustrophobia, as well as being afraid of tall buildings, enough to cause diarrhea.
- Pulsatilla is for one who weeps easily, worse in hot and stuffy rooms.
- Sulphur can be used when no other remedy is appropriate.
- Ignatia amara works for eating disorders with emotional swings, with crying easily; person does not want consolation.
- Lycopodium is useful for digestive issues like bloating stomach, also for those who get low blood sugar, who have irritability and low self-esteem.
- Natrum muriaticum is for someone with longstanding grief, depression. The person craves salty foods, has great thirst, and is averse to sun.

Acupressure

- CV12, ST36, SP6, LI4, LV3, LI11, P6, ear shenmen, SP16 (can help bring appetite back to balance)

Aromatherapy

Oils that are used for appetite loss are bergamot, buchu, galangal, dill, tarragon, cinnamon, lemon, lemongrass, fennel, wintergreen, litsea, peppermint, nutmeg, and ginger. Others for anorexia are rose, clary sage, lavender, and ylang-ylang.

Other Recommendations

- Get professional help.
- Stop the dieting mentality.
- Focus more on a happy and healthy weight.
- Support those who are struggling, try to withhold judgment and be supportive, avoid commenting on their weight, be there without trying to fix the problem, and set a good example by trying to handle stress without going toward food.

INSOMNIA

Insomnia is a common sleep disorder that can make it hard to fall asleep or stay asleep; you wake up too early, frequently waking throughout the night and then not being able to get back asleep; all these can lead to daytime sleep impairment. Diagnosis can be made by a comprehensive sleep history, a patient daily diary of nighttime sleep, daytime wakefulness, a full history also including a medical and history of psychiatric or substance abuse problems, along with ruling out adverse effects of medication.

Additional Integrative Modalities

Supplements

- Melatonin (1–3 g half an hour before bed, for a short time). Talk to your primary care provider before taking melatonin with pregnancy, breast-feeding, or cancer or before using in children under the age of six; be cautioned when taking other sleeping medications as it may intensify their effect.
- Passionflower (500 mg before bed or 1–2 ml a half hour before bedtime).
- Valerian (600 mg before bed or 2 ml a half hour before bedtime).
- Calcium and magnesium (500 mg calcium/250 mg magnesium).
- Combination: Valerian (30%), linden (20%), kava (20%), chamomile (20%), and catnip (10%) (promotes GABA release) in tea form or mix

of valerian root, wild lettuce, Jamaican dogwood, passionflower, hops, and L-theanine; patient can take one to four capsules at bedtime.

- Others: 5-HTP (100–400 mg at night), hops (Humulus lupulus; take 500 mg or 1–2 ml a half hour before bedtime; this is a nervine that relaxes the nervous system), vitamin B12 (1,500 mg in capsules or 400 mg of the sublingual tablet form daily; passionflower; reishi; St. John's wort; chamomile; catnip; skullcap; lavender; lemon balm; GABA (500–1,000 mg); magnolia (365 mg); combinations of L tryptophan and niacinamide (500–1,000 mg qhs); theanine (100 mg at night and 100 mg in the middle of the night if you wake up and can't fall back asleep); lemon balm (80–160 mg; makes it easy to stay asleep and fall asleep); D ribose (5 g BID); calcium (600 mg); ashwagandha; and phosphatidylserine.
- *Children:* 5HTP (50–100 mg before bed), melatonin (0.3–3 mg before bed), taurine (1,000 mg before bed), GABA (750 mg before bed), magnesium (65–350 mg before bed), chamomile tea and valerian tea (one cup before bed). DMSA protocol, TMG (250–500 mg once or twice a daily), magnesium (400–800 mg at bedtime), 5HTP (50–100 mg at bedtime), naltrexone transdermal (1–4 mg at bedtime). California poppy tincture (two to four droppers full as needed), catnip (one cup two to three times a day), linden tea (one cup three times per day). The above herbs can also be added to bath water (1 qt of tea to a bathtub of water).

Trouble falling asleep

- Herbs and stretching, warm bath before bed, practicing meditation and deep breathing, massage or acupuncture

Trouble staying asleep

- Associated with adrenal problems, glucose metabolism, hormonal dysfunction, or anxiety; use Eleuthero, Rehmannia, and the mushroom Reishi may be helpful.

Homeopathy

- Coffea helps when the mind can't shut off so you can't sleep and are wide awake at 3:00 am.
- Nux vomica is for those who are tired due to mental strain or after indulging in rich food or alcohol, wake up at around 3:00–4:00 am, thinking about business; then fall asleep just when they are supposed to

get up for the day, so they remain irritable and have nightmares. They are sensitive to light, noise, or sound.

- Pulsatilla helps with insomnia that is worse with rich food. The person feels too hot so takes the covers off, then feels too cold, lies with arms above head and not thirsty. The person is restless in first sleep.
- Aconite is for when insomnia is accompanied by the fear of dying, sleep problems are worse after panic or shock with nightmares and restlessness.
- Chamomilla is a remedy for the feeling of being wide awake and irritable during the first part of the night. It can be used for a child who wants to be carried around.
- Lycopodium is for the person who wakes up at 4:00 am, excessively dreams due to fear and stress, talks and laughs in sleep, and the mind is very active at bedtime. The person has poor confidence, digestive problems, and a craving for sweets.
- Cocculus is for that person who is used to being up at night; feels too tired to sleep; is giddy, weak, dizzy, with trouble thinking and irritable.
- Ignatia is a remedy for excessive yawning but can't fall asleep; for insomnia caused by emotional upsets with crying, mood swings, loss of appetite, excessive sighing, and muscle twitches.
- Arnica is indicated for when the person is overtired and fidgety. These persons dream that they are being chased by animals and have the feeling the bed is too hard.
- Opium is a remedy for sensitivity to sound; for when the bed is too hot; for when the person feels tired, but is unable to get to sleep, and if they do, they are unable to arouse, snoring heavily.
- Arsenicum is indicated when the patient wakes up between midnight and 2:00 am, is anxious and restless, apprehensive, and worried with fears and insecurities.
- Rhus tox is for one who is irritable, can't sleep, and may have discomfort.
- Aurum is for the person who has depression and dreams about problems at work, dying or hunger, and depression dominates.
- Arsenicum napellus helps those who have restlessness, panic that they may wake someone up, and have experienced a terrifying situation.
- Kali phosphoricum is for insomnia due to overwork or mental strain. Person is anxious, depressed, and sensitive.
- Sulphur is for insomnia that comes from feeling hot at night or itching, so the person kicks off covers or sticks the feet out.
- Zincum metallicum is used when the arms or legs are restless making it hard to stay still, usually from being overworked.
- Baryta carbonica helps for memory disorders.
- Gelsemium can help with emotional problems.

- Hepar sulphur aids in those with emotional oversensitivity.
- Phophurus can help those who are anxious, easily tired, and hyperactive.
- Lachesis mutans is a remedy for mental excitement, nightmares, oversensitivity, and touchiness.
- Actaea racemosa is helpful for someone who is very emotional and this is worsened by menstrual flow.
- Argentum nitricum is indicated for those with phobias, vertigo, and who are emotional.
- Phosphoricum acidum is a remedy for those who are exhausted by intellectual effort.
- Staphysagria is helpful for those obsessed by injustices. They are highly sensitive and easily indignant.
- Stramonium is indicated for those with night terrors who need a night-light to go to sleep or remain asleep.
- Hyoscyamus niger is a remedy for the one who mumbles, laughs, cries, or startles suddenly during sleep with tendency to tics.
- Kali bromatum helps night terrors with constant moving of hands and extremities with occasional sleepwalk, prone to worms.
- Cina is a remedy for agitated sleep with grinding of teeth or groaning and worse during the phases of the moon.

Acupressure

- B38, P6, H7, B10, GV16, GV20, GV24.5, CV17, K6, B62, SP6, H7
- Disturbed sleep: B5, B20, P6
- Difficulty falling asleep: B15, B23, K3
- Indigestion: SP16
- Pain relief: LI4

Aromatherapy

Essential oils can help you relax and get to sleep. Examples include yarrow, dill, neroli, petitgrain, bergamot, lemon, orange, star anise, bay laurel, lavender, Roman chamomile, nutmeg, myrtle, marjoram, allspice, tuberose, sandalwood, valerian, vetiver, ylang-ylang, jasmine, rose, angelica, bergamot, cedarwood, cistus, clary sage, jasmine, mandarin, marjoram, melissa, and spikenard.

SCHIZOPHRENIA

Schizophrenia is a chronic mental health condition that affects how a person behaves, feels, and thinks; persons with this condition interpret reality abnormally.

Symptoms may include disordered thinking and speech, hallucinations, delusions, and can be disabling as it can impair daily function. Diagnosis can be made by a trained professional with a detailed history, and tests may include imaging.

Additional Integrative Modalities

Supplements

- Niacin (3,000 mg per day).
- HTP (300–600 mg).
- Omega 3 fatty acids.
- Serine (have an amino acid test before initiating).
- Magnesium.

Homeopathy

- Lachesis is a remedy for paranoia; helps a person who feels constriction in the throat, doesn't want to wear clothes; symptoms are worse in the morning and after sleep; also for depression.
- Belladonna is for those who have wild staring eyes and are red in the face.
- Stramonium is indicated for a person who is violent, swears or prays, and hears voices and is talkative.
- Hyoscyamus helps with inappropriate language and behavior with suspicion and paranoia.
- Tarantula helps those who are always busy, bustling, bothered by music, and irritable.
- Thuja helps with strange sensations with anxiety and depression.
- Anacardium is for those who feel they have two different selves that are trying to gain control.

Hallucinations

Hallucinations are perceptions that have qualities of real perceptions without the external stimulus.

- Absinthium helps with depression, disorientation, dizziness, and hallucinations; loss of memory, giddiness, tendency to fall backward.
- Agaricus is indicated when the hallucinations transform the visual image, the person shaking and trembling.
- Belladonna aids in visual hallucinations like monsters with hideous mouths and eyes, red hot and staring eyes; person was hot.

- Cannabis helps when you feel like seconds feel like hours with uncontrollable laughter.
- Hyoscyamus is for those with marked paranoia, feeling persecuted or controlled by external forces and muttering with obscene talk and behavior. Greatly suspicious.
- Opium is for the person who is tired and lapses into heavy sleep.
- Stramonium is for someone who sees ghosts, hears voices, and says prayers. This person is very talkative.

Paranoia

Paranoia is thoughts related to conspiracy or a threat and involves severe anxiety or fearful feelings.

- Lachesis is for mild symptoms.
- Hyoscyamus is for symptoms of acute and severe nature.

Acupressure

- PC7, GV20, ST40

Aromatherapy

Essential oils are calming, so depending on the symptoms, they can help to bring relief.

SUBSTANCE ABUSE

Substance abuse is the overuse of drugs, alcohol, or tobacco, which may even begin in childhood. Causes may include a chaotic home environment, lack of nurturing and parental attachment, poor social coping skills, inability to handle stress, poor school performance, or association with the wrong peer group. Symptoms vary widely from inability to keep up with daily activities, forgetfulness, lying and other oppositional defiant traits, frequent hangovers, pressuring others to drink or use drugs, getting in trouble with the law, irritability and/or disappearing money or valuables. Abuse may lead to hallucinations, behavioral changes, dilated pupils, involuntary shaking, muscle cramping, and teeth clenching,

Additional Integrative Modalities

Supplements

- Free form amino acids (three to six capsules three times per day on empty stomach higher end if in acute withdrawal).
- Glutamine (1,000 mg three times per day).
- Pancreatic enzyme three times per day with meals.
- Ester C (1,000 mg three times per day).
- B-complex (50 mg twice daily).
- Melatonin (1–3 mg at night).
- Calcium citrate (500 mg three times per day).
- Magnesium glycinate (300 mg three times per day).
- EFA omega-3 (EPA 400 mg three times per day).
- Inositol powder (4–6 g three times per day).
- Others include: multivitamin (take as directed on the container; supplies a combination of vitamins and minerals that assists detoxification and improves your mood); milk thistle (Silybum marianum) (250 mg three times daily of a product standardized to 80–85% silymarin extract; chromium (200 meg two or three times daily), improves mood and energy levels; 5-hydroxytryptophan (5-HTP) (100 mg three times daily on an empty stomach, taken before bedtime), helps with sleep. ***Note:*** Do not take this if you are on a pharmaceutical antidepressant or anti-anxiety medication.
- *Adolescent*: substance abuse: inositol (3–6 g two or three times per day), B complex (50 mg with 1 mg of folate), fish oil (500–1,000 mg of EPA), vitamin C (500–1,000 mg of vitamin C). If true dependence, glutamine (1,000 mg or more three times daily) and calcium/magnesium (1:1) (250–500 mg twice daily).
- Add free form amino acids (should include L-tryptophan): 3–6 capsules on an empty stomach three times daily for the first few months to help with withdrawal issues with true dependence. If highly motivated or chronic, consider neurofeedback training. If severe dependence and impaired nutrition, consider IV nutritional support over the first two months of recovery.

Homeopathy

- Arsenicum helps when one has fear of being alone, anxiety, fatigue, and restlessness, with symptoms worse at 2:00 am and improved with warmth.

- Lachesis is for the person who feels persecuted, jealous, paranoid, suspicious, depressed, and talkative. Addictions get violent. Symptoms worsen with heat, and the person can't stand anything touching the throat.
- Aconite is a remedy for sudden panic, feeling cold, and a sense of dying.
- Absinthium helps with depression, disorientation, dizziness, and hallucinations.
- Hyoscyamus, for those with marked paranoia, feeling persecuted or controlled by external forces, and muttering with obscene talk and behavior.
- Ignatia amara is helpful for those who want to be left alone, with hysteria, emotional breakdowns, sensation of lump in the throat, anxiety and having twitches or spasms. They are constantly changing moods and symptoms.

Alcoholism

- Nux can help from a hangover in the morning, and those who are emotionally withdrawn with digestive symptoms, irritability, anger, with sensitivity to touch, odors, sound, and light.
- Capsicum is indicated for the stomach pain that can occur after heavy drinking.
- Lachesis is for those who are social binging, hate tight clothing, and talk too much.
- Avena is a remedy for a person more depressed and irritable than usual.
- Zinc is for those sensitive to noise, who experience fatigue, apprehension, and trembling.
- Sulphur is indicated for those who crave alcohol and go on binges, with abnormal flatulence, nervous exhaustion, and solitary drinking. They feel warm and better from cool air and drinks, and they crave spicy food.
- Kali bichromium helps with nausea and vomiting associated to alcohol with stringy catarrh.
- Lycopodium is indicated for those who have low self-esteem and are irritable, chilly, have digestive problems, and crave sweets. It can be used in alcoholism or drug addiction.

Acupressure

- ST36, SP10 will help in the detoxification process.
- LU1 will help with depression or anxiety.

- GB20 will help with fatigue.
- Addiction to nicotine: LI4, LI20, ST36, LV3, GV20.

Aromatherapy

Essential oils like peppermint, clove, cinnamon, cilantro, and grapefruit can help curb cravings; and lavender, sandalwood, orange, marjoram, and grapefruit can help improve withdrawals.

Juniper breaks up poisons and speeds their exit from the body. Using the calming essential oils and mood lifting oils can all help to improve symptoms. Others include rose oil (lifts depression), bergamot (helps to relieve anxiety, depression, and compulsive disorder), and clary sage.

Other Recommendations

Hypnotherapy is a therapeutic technique that uses hypnosis to treat the condition.

• 19 •

Pulmonology

By controlling our breath, we can control our universe from the inside out. Lower inflammation only to maximize the moments that take our breath away!

D & D: SPECIAL CONSIDERATIONS

Healing the gut and avoiding food sensitivities like dairy may lead to production of excess mucus. Detoxifying your environment is key and should be done regularly. Maintaining the health of your mucous membranes is important. Eat foods with carotenoids and vitamin A, like sweet potatoes, carrots, berries, and leafy greens. Magnesium can improve muscle spasms and promotes muscle relaxation. Quercetin, found in garlic, mustard seeds, and onions, can help to fight bacterial infections and improve overall immune health. Folate helps to protect the lungs and can be found in green leafy veggies, nuts, and lentils. Omega 3 fatty acid foods, like fish, nuts, and flaxseeds, reduce airway inflammation. Foods with vitamins like B5 and B6 can help support stress and adrenal function. Staying hydrated is important for your airways to function appropriately.

THE FOUR BIG S's: SPECIAL CONSIDERATIONS

Stress can worsen breathing issues and airway inflammation, so incorporating relaxation skills and targeting specific emotional imbalances are vital steps for optimal health and can improve airway function. Exercising in cold air can exacerbate attacks, so cover up as needed.

ASTHMA

Asthma is a chronic inflammatory condition of the lungs that leads to narrowed airways and affects breathing. Common symptoms are shortness of breath, pain and pressure in the chest, coughing, and wheezing. Asthma can be triggered by allergens, pollution and other irritants, infections, cold air, heavy physical exertion, poor digestive function, hormonal imbalances, stress, and anxiety. Asthma can be diagnosed by history and lung function tests, including other tests like blood tests, imaging of chest and sinus, and allergy tests.

Additional Integrative Modalities

Supplements

- Optimize Vitamin D, as it can support immune health and slow declining lung function.
- Magnesium can reduce asthma severity.
- Vitamin C (500–1,000 mg daily) acts like an antioxidant that reduces free radical damage and inflammation.
- B vitamins help support cognitive function and immune health. Specifically B3 and B12 lower wheezing and antihistamine. Choline (3 g daily) reduces severity and frequency of asthma attacks.
- Essential fatty acids (1–2 tbsp of flaxseed oil or 4–8 g of fish oil daily).
- Zinc can help to support adrenal health and relieve stress.
- Quercetin can reduce the release of histamine.
- Pycnogenol (1 mg per pound of body weight daily) is a natural anti-inflammatory herb. Don't take if you have diabetes or high blood pressure.
- Lycopene (130 mg daily) has been shown to be helpful for those affected by exercise-induced asthma.
- Boswellia (800 mg three times a day) improves lung function.
- Others include: Carnitine, ginkgo biloba, adrenal nutrients, N-acetyl cysteine, NAC, bromelain (500 mg three times a day on empty stomach), Astragalus (500–1,000 mg twice daily), prevent respiratory infections that can trigger asthma; do not use if you have a fever. Thymus (as directed on the label or by a functional integrative doctor) reduces asthma attacks in children.

- *Children:* for the mother throughout pregnancy (fish oil EPA/DHA 2–4 g daily), vitamin C (1,000 mg daily), magnesium (200 mg daily), vitamin D (1,000–4,000 IU daily), vitamin B6 (1–20 mg daily), Cordyceps sinesis (100–500 mg daily or 5:1 tincture thirty drops twice daily).

Homeopathy

During an asthma attack, take 30C every ten or fifteen minutes until the symptoms subside. Long-term use of the proper homeopathic remedy can reduce your susceptibility to asthmatic attacks. You can take remedies 6C every fifteen minutes for up to ten doses.

- Aconitum napellus (30C) is for attacks that come all of a sudden, especially after exposure to cold dry wind, fear of dying, and anxiety. Attacks occur at night.
- Antimonium tartaricum helps with asthma that is accompanied with exhaustion, weakness; mucus in the lungs causes a rattly breathing that can't be coughed up, skin is pale, cold, and clammy.
- Arsenicum album helps those with an attack between midnight and 2:00 am. These people feel restless, anxious, and cold, thirsty for sips of warm water; symptoms improve when sitting up.
- Carbo vegetabilis is for people who feel chilly and faint, yet better when being fanned or near a window. They may have a sensation of fullness in the upper abdomen and the chest and may feel relief from burping. They feel worse from talking, eating, or lying down.
- Chamomilla is for those who find fault in everything, want to be picked up and carried, and are irritable.
- Cuprum helps those with asthma attacks involving vomiting after each spasm of the lungs and in the rest of the body.
- Ignatia is for when an attack comes on after an emotional breakup, after grief, or other emotional upset.
- Ipecac is a remedy for those with nausea and whose chest feels heavy. It is helpful when a lot of mucus formation causes coughing, gagging, and vomiting.
- Hepar sulph is for when the asthma improves in damp conditions.
- Kali carbonicum is for asthma that is bad between 2:00 am and 4:00 am; the person sits with face on knees and leaning forward helps relieve symptoms; person is usually chilly, tired, and pale looking.
- Lachesis is a remedy for those who feel like their asthma is worse in the morning upon waking. Person sits hunched forward and feels constriction in the throat made worse by anything worn around neck.

- Medorrhinum is for chronic asthma, when the person craves fruit like oranges and is prone to respiratory infections.
- Natrum sulphuricum is a remedy for asthma that is often associated with early morning diarrhea, worse in damp and cold weather and from 4:00 am to 5:00 am.
- Nux vomica helps asthma that is bad after a digestive upset and around 4:00 am. Person feels irritable and chilly.
- Phosphorus helps those with asthma with a lot of coughing and thirst; the person feels better when comforted or held.
- Sambucus nigra is for an attack that comes on suddenly in the middle of the night; the person has blue extremities and is unable to lie down. Patient feels pain in the head and is better with sitting. Nose is completely congested.
- Pulsatilla pratensis is for asthma symptoms with yellow-greenish phlegm that is coughed up and leads to gagging. Symptoms improve with fresh air and being comforted, but worsen after eating fatty foods and in a hot and stuffy room.
- If mucus production is the major symptom: Use ipecac, Kali carb, and Blatta orientalis (acute/subacute attacks with bronchial obstruction and coarse rales heard on exam).
- If spasm or edema is the major symptom: Use Arsenicum album, Antimonium tartaricum, drosera (dry cough with hoarseness causing temporary cyanosis of face triggered by speaking or laughing), lachesis, samucus, aralia racemosa (attack with coughing occurs every night when going to bed), cuprum metallicum (coughing at night or when breathing cold air, improved after drinking cold water), and lung histamine (15C) and histaminum (7C) for histamine-dependent symptoms.
- If anxious: Use ignatia amara, gelsemium, arsenicum, or lachesis.

Acupressure

- LU1, LU6, LU9, LU10, K27, LU7, ST13, ST16, B36, CV17, B12, B13, K6, and Ding Chuan point
- Allergic Asthma: LI4 and K6

Aromatherapy

Essential oils can help manage allergies and mucus production. Make a homemade vapor rub with eucalyptus oil, lemon, and peppermint oil, which will help to open airways. Frankincense oil can be used to improve inflammation and anxiety and can be used with sandalwood and lavender especially if symptoms are due to an emotional upset. Asthma brought on by exposure to allergens will benefit from chamomile and helichrysum, which have an anti-spasmodic action. Others can be caraway, Roman chamomile, niaouli, lemon balm, marjoram, rosemary, geranium, myrtle, and clove.

Other Recommendations

Consider Nambudripad's Allergy Elimination Techniques (NAET) and salt inhalation therapy with a Himalayan salt crystal lamp.

CHRONIC OBSTRUCTIVE PULMONARY DISORDER

Chronic Obstructive Pulmonary Disorder (COPD) is a progressive disease that causes coughing, large amounts of mucus, wheezing, shortness of breath, chest tightness, and other symptoms and usually refers to emphysema and long-lasting bronchitis. These diseases lead to blockage of bronchial tubes and air sacs. Other symptoms include frequent respiratory infections, production of increased mucus, and difficulty exhaling. Your doctor can diagnose with chest X ray, CT scan to look for severity, and blood and sputum test.

Additional Integrative Modalities

Supplements

- NAC (1,200–1,800 mg daily).
- Ginseng (especially Panax ginseng) helps to decrease bacteria in the lungs.
- Magnesium.
- Others: Pelargonium sidoides for stages II and III COPD (thirty drops TID for twenty-four weeks), L-carnitine (but don't take this if you have hypothyroidism or history of seizures).

Homeopathy

- Bryonia (30C) is a remedy for painful, stabbing, dry cough with chest pain and headache that must be relieved by supporting elbows on the back of the chair. Patients are very thirsty.
- Belladonna can be used for sudden onset, flushed face, high temperature, with symptoms worse at night and when lying down with a headache.

- Kali bicromium helps those with a stringy phlegm that is difficult to cough up; the person feels worse between 4:00 am and 5:00 am.
- Causticum is a remedy for coughing that leads to involuntary passing of urine.
- Hepar sulph is indicated for those who are chilly and irritable, who have a choking cough made worse by uncovering a part of the body.
- Rumex is used for dry, tickly cough at the back of the throat, made worse by talking and by cold air, worse at night, preventing the person from sleeping. The person feels better when their head is under the blanket.
- Stannum is a remedy for a sweetish-tasting phlegm and sore, dry throat, with violent cough during the evening. The person is hardly able to talk, and symptoms worsen by talking or laughing.
- Sticta helps those with a dry hacking cough at night, made worse by bringing up phlegm.

Acupressure

- Bronchitis: LU1, LU9, K27, ST13
- COPD: LU1, LU6, LU9, K27, ST13

Aromatherapy

Eucalyptus oil can be helpful for people with COPD (not suitable around young children). Others are basil, cedarwood, peppermint, hyssops, and thyme thymol.

• 20 •

Rheumatology

Tired of being achy and breaky? Extinguish the fire in your muscles and joints!

D & D: SPECIAL CONSIDERATIONS

Food sensitivities can lead to pain, so consider elimination of nightshades along with what we talked about in the foundations of good health: incorporating anti-inflammatory herbs like boswellia, garlic, ginger, turmeric, and devil's claw. Foods high in sulfur reduce joint inflammation. Natural forms of collagen include bone broth, amino acids, chondroitin sulphates and glucosamine, and antioxidants to lower inflammation.

High-antioxidant foods and high-fiber foods are important. Include foods rich in B12, C, D, as well as folic acid and magnesium. Melatonin-rich foods are also important. Eat foods high in tryptophan (like turkey, nuts, grass-fed dairy, wild fish, free-range chicken, and sesame seeds). Sea veggies, wild-caught fish, alkaline food, and green leafy vegetables are high in minerals for bone formation and optimal health. Spasms can be due to magnesium deficiency and low potassium.

THE FOUR BIG S's: SPECIAL CONSIDERATIONS

Managing stress is key in improving immunity by combining weight-bearing activities (three times a week), along with aerobic, flexibility, and resistance and strength training to help strengthen bones and build bone mass. Yoga, lumbar stabilization exercises to improve core, tai chi, and Pilates can help to increase range of motion, improving stiffness and pain. Mindfulness-based stress reduction techniques, EFT tapping, journaling forgiveness, and properly addressing trauma can all improve overall inflammation and pain.

ARTHRITIS

Arthritis is a chronic condition characterized by inflammation of the joints. Three types are osteoarthritis, psoriatic arthritis, and rheumatoid arthritis. Osteoarthritis is a degenerative disease of the joints, occurring when the joint cartilage begins to break down leading to symptoms like swelling, redness, pain (worse with activity), morning stiffness that resolves after movement, limited range of movement, warm to touch joints, muscle weakness, growth of bone knobs near the joints of the outermost fingers, and clicking sound in the joints. Diagnosis is made via a detailed history, physical, and imaging.

Additional Integrative Modalities

Supplements

- Fish oil (1,000 mg of EPA/DHA per day).
- Turmeric (1,000 mg a day).
- Proteolytic enzymes like bromelain.
- Ginger (up to 2 g per day in divided doses).
- Glucosamine sulfate (1,500 mg daily) can be combined with chondroitin (800–1,200 mg per day). *Caution*, if severely allergic to shellfish, chondroitin is made from bovine cartilage, so vegetarians be cautioned.
- SAMe (600–1,200 mg per day).
- Capsaicin cream (0.015–0.075% up to four times per day).
- Others: Vitamin B6 (10–20 mg q day), Vitamin C (1,000 mg q day), Vitamin D, Vitamin E, Calcium, Green tea (one cup brewed at least 279 mg EGCG split into two to three doses), Silymarin (200 mg BID), Carotenoids (lutein + astaxanthin) (2–4 mg), grapeseed extract (200 mg divided in the am and pm), reversatrol (250 mg), boswellia (300 mg BID), pomegranate (250–500 mg BID), ginger (500–1,000 mg), licorice (1.5 gm), glycyrrhizic acid (400 mg) take no more than one month, then take one month off, NAC (600 mg), Methylsulfonylmethane (MSM) (2,000 to 8,000 mg daily), and collagen (40 mg daily of undenatured collagen).

Homeopathy

- Calcarea fluorica is best for those with malnutrition of the bones with enlarged hypermobile joints, bone spurs, depression, and increased urination at night. Symptoms improve with heat and warmth, but are worse with rest and changes of weather.
- Rhus tox is indicated for those with symptoms of stiffness worse in the morning that improves with movement and warmth; aggravated by cold, damp, and immobility.
- Bryonia is a remedy for severe pain that is improved with cold and rest and worse with heat and movement. Associated symptoms are swollen hot joints and irritability.
- Pulsatilla helps those with joint pain that is aggravated by heat and warmth; symptoms improve with coolness; pain wanders from joint to joint. Patient is weepy.
- Calcarea phosphorica is for those who have joint pain, bone pain, and spurs (mostly in the neck) that feel numb, painful, stiff and cold; aggravated by cold, weather changes. They experience weakness when climbing the stairs.
- Ledum is a remedy for painful, swollen, warm joints that seem to progress up the body; it can be used for the aftereffects of steroid injections or for small joints like the toes. Pain is aggravated at night by the warmth of the bed and relieved by cold applications and rest. Ledum can be used in gouty arthritis, particularly if the person is craving alcohol.
- Arnica is a remedy for bruising joint pain that can be triggered or made worse by an injury.
- Aconite can be used for severe sudden flare-ups in the cold or dry weather. General feelings of anxiety and restlessness may be present.
- Apis is indicated for joints that are painful to touch, hot, or swollen; display pinkish edema, with improvement by cold and aggravated by pressure or touch.
- Belladonna can be used in those joints that are red, hot, and burning with swelling. Symptoms may come on suddenly and feel worse with motion.
- Dulcamara can be indicated in joint pain that is aggravated by cold, damp weather, after being overheated, and after rest and that improves with movement. Digestive symptoms may be present, like diarrhea.
- Mercurius is for aches and pains that are worse at night, with heat and cold, and that are accompanied by offensive sweats.
- Ruta graveolens is indicated for articular pain that may be due to trauma, improved with movement, and aggravated by rest.

- Radium bromatum is a remedy that can be used for pain in the knees and lumbosacral region. Joints feel as if they are going to give way. Symptoms are improved by heat or movement and aggravated by prolonged rest and at night.
- Rhododendron can be used in erratic/searing pain that is aggravated by stormy weather and improves as soon as the storm breaks out.
- Kali brochromium can be used for sudden onset of well-localized pain improved with motion. It can be used for sciatica, on the left side, and for coccydynia that is aggravated with sitting.
- Calcarea carbonica is for joint pain made worse from coldness and dampness in an overweight and cold-sensitive individual.
- Sulphur is a remedy for burning pains improved with cold.
- Nux vomica can be used for spasmodic pain, particularly in the back and the loins, forcing the patient to sit up in bed in order to turn over. Symptoms are aggravated by cold, movement, or lying down on the side that hurts. Pain is improved by heat and rest. Symptoms may be associated with digestive disorders like hemorrhoids or dyspepsia, nervousness, hypersensitivity to pain, and restlessness.
- Colchicum is indicated for pain and stiffness that are worse during the winter and at night.

Infective arthritis (homeopathics should be used with antibiotics)

- Hepar sulph is indicated when joints are swollen with pus and are sensitive to the slightest pressure and a draft.
- Belladonna can be used with those with red face, staring eyes, high fever, and delirium. Symptoms worsen with the slightest movement.
- Aconite is indicated when the infection comes on suddenly, associated with pain, fever, and apprehension.
- Bryonia is a remedy for painful and swollen joints that are sensitive to the slightest touch and movement.

Knee pain

- Benzoic acid is indicated for painful swollen knee joints that make a cracking sound with the skin over the joint being very dry.
- Causticum is indicated for knees that crack upon walking. It can also be used for pain in the neck and jaw that improves with warmth or wet weather.
- Berberis as indicated in knees that feel stiff and sore.
- Agnus helps with knees that feel cold.

Shoulder pain

- Sanguinaria is indicated for pain in the right shoulder that is worse with movement or pressure and wears off during sleep.
- Chelidonium is indicated for pain in the right shoulder and around the angle of the shoulder blade accompanied with headaches.
- Ferrum is a remedy for pain in the shoulder that is worse around midnight and the person was cold, being overheated, or sitting still. Symptoms are improved with walking.
- Rhus tox is indicated for burning pain in the shoulder, with pains that wear off with gentle exercise and worsen in cold damp weather and after sleep or rest.
- Sulphur is indicated for pain in the shoulder with the tendency to bring the shoulder forward and the shoulder feels heavy and dead.
- Solarium malacoxylon is a remedy to help cure calcification of the shoulder.

Small joints of the hand: Actaea spicata (when pain is located to proximal interphalangeal joints with bouchard's nodes), Polygonum aviculare (when the pain is located in the distal interphalangeal joint with Herberden's nodes), 3X of each (>60 ml of each) twenty drops daily, in some water, to be held in the mouth before swallowing. Caulophyllum (intermittent pain in the small joints that wander from one to the other). Viola odorata helps to relieve pain in the wrist and metacarpals, pain radiating to the arm and worse in the morning and improved after getting up.

Heel pain: Hekla lava can be used, especially when calcaneal spurs are present (5C twice daily along with medorrhinum 15C twice monthly).

Acupressure

- K3, K6, ST41, B60, B62, and LI11 (reduce pain in elbows and shoulders)
- TW5, LI4 (pain in the upper extremity and neck)
- SP5 and K3 (ankle pain)
- GB20 and ST36
- Others: Ba Feng, Ba Xie, and yang lin qian

Aromatherapy

Essential oils can help to reduce stress, relaxing tight muscles and improving pains and well-being. Frankincense can help to reduce inflammation.

Lavender is a mild analgesic and antispasmodic. Marjoram helps to relieve pain from arthritis. Black pepper, eucalyptus, and ginger stimulate circulation and also have analgesic, anti-inflammatory properties. Nutmeg, peppermint, and yarrow oils also decrease inflammation. Lemongrass along with the anti-inflammatory properties of rosemary can help to improve pain. Other essential oils that can help with arthritis are myrrh, turmeric, orange, yarrow, lemon verbena, mugwort, birch leaf, cedarwood, cypress, wintergreen, helichrysum, star anise, juniper, nutmeg, marjoram, parsley, benzoin, plai, jasmine, rose, chamomile, angelica, Canadian balsam, bay laurel, bergamot, benzoin, silver fir, and rosemary. Knee pain can be helped with peppermint and eucalyptus.

CHRONIC PAIN

Pain can come on suddenly and can last six weeks (acute) or can last more than three months (chronic). Back pain is a shooting, stabbing, or aching pain in the back that may radiate down the leg, limiting range of motion. Causes may be due to muscle or ligament strain, bulging/prolapsed/ruptured disk, osteoporosis, skeletal irregularities, and/or arthritis. A diagnosis can be made after a detailed history, physical, and imaging that may include xrays, MRI/CT, bone scan, nerve studies, and blood work, looking for the root cause.

Additional Integrative Modalities

Supplements

Back Pain

- Fish oil (2,000 mg daily).
- Turmeric (1,000 mg daily).
- Proteolytic enzymes and bromelain (500 mg three times a day in between meals) and papain (500 mg three times per day).
- MSM (2,000–8,000 mg daily).
- Magnesium (400–500 mg daily) and calcium (500 mg).
- Others: Devil's Claw (50–100 mg harpagoside), white willow (240 mg of salicin daily or 5 ml of the tincture form three times daily), collagen (40 mg daily of undenatured collagen to reduce back pain caused by osteoarthritis), ginger (1,000 mg/day), turmeric (300 mg TID).

Chronic Pain

- Vitamin C for chronic regional pain syndrome (500 mg of vitamin C) on day of fracture and for fifty days thereafter to prevent chronic regional pain syndrome.

- Antioxidants and vitamins.
- Bromelain (2,000 mg in two divided doses and 500 mg of quercetin twice daily) (contraindication: pregnancy, bleeding disorders, uncontrollable BP).
- Topical: Castor oil, charcoal poultices, hot ginger tea, salt packs, cold mashed tofu, topricin, homeopathic cream, mustard foot baths.
- SAMe, MSM, DLPA (don't use with MAO drugs).
- Enzyme supplementation (1 cap three times a day) with meals.
- B vitamins.
- Carnosine, alpha lipoic acid, acetyl carnitine, and chromium.
- Omega 3, vitamin A, C, E, Ca, and Magnesium.
- Antioxidants: CoQ10, DMAE, mineral manganese.
- Arctic Root, Ashwagandha, ginseng, astragalus, cordyceps, dong quai, eleuthro, maitake, milk thistle, reishi.
- Glucosamin and chondroitin (Glucosamine 1,500 mg/day).
- Turmeric.
- Reservatrol.
- melatonin.

Homeopathy

For acute back pain, take a 30C potency four times daily. For chronic back pain, take twice daily for two weeks to see if there are any positive improvements.

Cervical spondylosis (wear and tear of spinal disks)

- Argentum nitricum can be used for headaches behind the forehead associated with flatulence and numbing of the limbs.
- Agaricus is indicated for tendinitis of the back of the neck associated with weakness, shaking, and chest constriction.
- Picric acid is indicated by shooting burning pains up the spine into the head.

Coccydynia (pain in coccyx)

- Hypericum is indicated for pain in the coccyx that is brought on by a fall.
- Causticum is for when the coccyx feels achy bruised and is improved with wet and damp weather.
- Silicea is indicated for pain and constipation that is increased with pressure and a draft.

- Antimonium tartariam is indicated for when the coccyx feels heavy.
- Cicuta is a remedy for jerking, tearing, recurrent pain.
- Kali brochromium is indicated when the pain gets worse with walking or sitting.

Back pain

- Aconite is a remedy for sharp pain that is worse with drafts and cold dry weather.
- Arnica is a remedy that is used for pain after injury. The area feels bruised and sore.
- Rhus tox helps with those that have lower back pain that feels bruised. Improves with movment, and worsens with damp cold weather and rest. It is best for sprained muscles or ligaments.
- Byronia helps lower back pain and stiffness that comes on in dry cold weather and is made worse by the slightest movement. The spot feels sensitive to touch and is bruised. The area feels better when it is rubbed.
- Aesculus helps with lower back pain or sacral pain that radiates to the right hip, which worsens with sitting, walking, or stooping.
- Antimonium tartarium is indicated for those with a continuous pain associated with nausea, vomiting, fatigue, and cold sweats. Aggravated by cold and eating and improve with standing up and moving around.
- Sulphur is a remedy for violent stitching pain that is made worse with movement and the heat of the bed.
- Cimicifuga is a remedy for lower back pain, stiffness, and aching muscles that feel bruised. Pain prevents sleep and causes restlessness, and is improved with warmth.
- Ignatia helps those with cramping and back spasms following emotional stress.
- Magnesia phosphorica helps with back spasms improved with warmth
- Calcarea carbonica is indicated for chronic lower back pain and weakness aggravated by damp coldness. Associated with heavyweight individuals who are cold sensitive.
- Dulcamara helps with pain that is made worse with exertion, cold, and stooping.
- Rhododendron is for back pain that is worse in cold weather or before a thunderstorm.
- Nux vomica is for pain that is aggravated by cold or movement. The pain may be accompanied with irritability, cold sensitivity, and constipation. Symptoms improve with warmth and or aggravated by cold.

- Ruta graveolens is used for pain of the neck and lower back. It is best for sprains or strains. Pain is worse at night.

Neck pain

- Cimicifuga is indicated for neck stiffness accompanied with sensitivity of the whole cervical and upper thoracic spine.
- Lacnanthes is helpful for pain in the upper arm, elbow, and right side of the neck. Symptoms accompanied with perspiration. Symptoms aggravated by movement.
- Dulcamara is for neck pain located at the top of the nape. Aggravated by cold and improved by heat.
- Bryonia is best for those with pain that is worse with movement and the slightest touch.
- Causticum is indicated for pain at the top of the nape of the neck stiffness between the shoulder blades, and improves with the wet weather.
- Actaea racemosa is best for cervical pain in those who work in a bent forward sitting position. Pain is aggravated by cold and during menses and pain is improved by heat.
- Lachnantes is indicated in those with a stiff neck forcing them to bend their neck.

Acupressure

- B25, B31, B40, B20 (for middle back pain)
- GB20 and GV14 (upper back pain)
- B48 (to reduce stress)
- B54 (due to arthritis)
- Others: B23, B22 and B25, CV6, B18, B30, B60, B53, GV4
- Pain in ankles and feet: K3, K6, ST41, B60, B62, GB34, GB39, GB40, SP4
- Hip and pelvis pain: GB29, GB30, GB31, GB34, B28, B48
- Knee pain: B54, B57, ST36, SP10, SP8, SP6
- Upper and mid back pain: B13, B38, B18, B42, SI11, SI10
- Lower back: B23, B47, B28, B48, B54, GB30, B60, GV4

Aromatherapy

Peppermint and wintergreen oil help to cool the inflamed area. Frankincense and cypress oil reduces inflammation. Lemongrass essential oils can help to improve back spasms. Peppermint oil and lavender oil to further penetrate the area can help relax the inflamed area and help with cramps. Others that can help with pain and cramps are tarragon, coriander, camphor, grapefruit, bay laurel, niaouli, marjoram, geranium, allspice, black pepper, rosemary, ginger, anise, Canadian balsam, basil linalool, clove (bud), citriodora, fennel, geranium, ginger, niaouli, nutmeg, rosemary, jasmine. Cinnamon and eucalyptus can also help chronic pain. Along with the above, back pain can be improved with ginger, juniper, thyme, and clary sage.

CHRONIC FATIGUE

Chronic fatigue syndrome is a chronic disorder characterized by extreme fatigue, unexplained by any underlying medical condition. Symptoms include fatigue, sore throat, pain that moves from joint to joint without swelling, headaches, unrefreshing sleep, extreme exhaustion lasting more than twenty-four hours after mental or physical exercise, loss of memory or concentration, mood changes, swollen lymph glands in the armpits or neck, and unexplained muscle pain. Hormonal causes can be due to thyroid, adrenal insufficiency, DHEA, testosterone deficiency, or parasitic infections like mycoplasma incognitus, HHV-6, CMV, EBV, and Chlamydia. Diagnosis occurs after a detailed history and physical, meeting at least four symptoms previously discussed, with persistent fatigue for at least six months or more.

Additional Integrative Modalities

Supplements

- Ashwagandha (Indian ginseng 250 mg daily).
- Green superfood powder (wheatgrass, spirulina, matcha).
- Vitamin B-complex with B6, B12, helps with energy metabolism.
- Rhodiola (300 mg daily).
- Magnesium (200–300 mg daily).
- Zinc (50 mg daily for three months, then 15–25 mg daily).
- Other: Coenzyme Q10 (200–300 mg daily with meals); multivitamin with the above and malic acid (900 mg); vitamin C (500–1,000 mg three times per day); selenium (200 mcg); chromium (200 mcg) and amino acids; acetyl-L-carnitine; D-Ribose; American Ginseng or Panax ginseng (1,000–2,000 mg/day) in at least two divided doses; Guarana (Paullina cupano) 50 mg twice daily, containing no more than 40 mg of caffeine/day; NADH (10 mg on an empty stomach);

Rhodiola rosea (300 mg of a 3% rosavin extract daily); thymic protein A; vitamin E (100–200 IU per day) and licorice root.

Homeopathy

- Arnica montana can be used for fatigue with the feeling of bruised muscles.
- Kali phosphoricum is for a feeling of fatigue and mental weariness, especially if it follows an illness like the flu. Associated symptoms include anxiety; depression; nightmares; insomnia; agoraphobia; fear of crowds; loss of memory; muscle weakness and pains worse with exercise, cold, and mental effort, but improved with sleep, eating, and gentle movement.
- Gelsemium can be used for those who feel weak and have muscle aches, dizziness, trembling, twitching, bruising muscle feeling, dull heaviness of the head, and blurred vision. Symptoms worsen with cold weather and dampness with lots of anxiety. Fatigue may follow emotional grief. Symptoms improve after profuse urination.
- Phosphorus is for extreme fatigue, where the person has an unusually strong craving for carbonated drinks.
- Lacticum acidum is helpful with fatigue with pain in the bones, with aversions to exercise, and with a sensation of a plug in the throat.
- Mercurius solubilis is for fatigue after Epstein Barr virus, persistent sore throat, enlarged glands, lots of salivation, sensitive to cold and heat, memory loss, and poor recall of names.
- Physostigma venenosum is used in those with a great sense of feelings of weakness and fatigue who feel sore and stiff all over as if from a cold, with violent trembling of the body.
- Rhus toxicodendron helps fatigue that is associated with pain relieved by heat and aggravated by cold.
- Phosphoric acid is a remedy for weakness and exhaustion with prolonged diarrhea, depression, blue rings around the eyes, looking worn out, thin, pale with poor appetite while being thirsty and cold and music sensitive.
- Zincum metallicum is indicated for weakness, restlessness, depression, poor memory, hypersensitivity to noise, restless legs aggravated by alcohol.
- Calcarea carbonica is used for those with fatigue accompanied with headaches, constipation, swollen glands, anxiety, cold sensitivity, spreading easily and with multiple food allergies.

- Arsenicum album is helpful for fatigue with insomnia between the hours of midnight and 2:00 am accompanied with anxiety, depression, and cold sensitivity. Symptoms are worse from cold.
- Silica is helpful for people who have constipation and get easily sick and are thin and cold sensitive.
- China can be used for exhaustion and weakness after dehydration.
- Phosphoric acid can be used for nervous exhaustion and brain fog following intense mental activity, heaviness, and burning in limbs or spine.

Acupressure

- GB14, ST36, TW4, K27, ST36, SP4, B62, CV6, GV14
- Others: SP3, SP6, SP9, ST36, GB21 (improves circulation, decreases anxiety, headaches, irritability), P6 (for sleep, anxiety, indigestion), B23 and B47 (fatigue, confusion, and helps sleep), LU3 (fatigue, confusion, lightheadedness, head pain), Triple Warmer 5 (TW5 joint pain), GV20, and CV4

Aromatherapy

Frankincense can improve chronic fatigue syndrome to support neurological health and healing. Peppermint oil also improves focus and fatigue. Depending on the underlying root cause for fatigue and associated symptoms, the respective essential oils may help. Stimulate nervous system and muscles with lavender and rosemary. Tea tree oil strengthens the immune system, along with cinnamon, cistus, clove, myrrh, eucalyptus radiate, marjoram, rosewood, thyme linalool, and vetiver. Energizing oils like mandarin, lemon, and grapefruit can also be helpful.

FIBROMYALGIA

Fibromyalgia is a chronic condition characterized by pain in the muscles, tendons, and ligaments with multiple tender points on the body; fatigue; sleep; cognitive difficulties like "fibro fog" and inability to concentrate; and mood issues. Headaches, depression, and pain/cramping may be found. Diagnosis is made with a detailed history and physical with eighteen specific tender points and ruling out other diagnoses via a blood test.

Additional Integrative Modalities

Supplements

- Magnesium (500 mg per day).
- Fish oil (1,000 mg per day).
- Probiotic.
- Vitamin D.
- Digestive enzymes.
- Activated B vitamins.
- Supplements for sleep, detoxification, and treating chronic low-grade infections (see autoimmune section).

Supplements for mitochondrial support:

- Acetyl L carnitine (1,500 mg per day).
- Alpha lipoic acid (400–600 mg per day).
- CoQ10 (100–300 mg per day).
- Malic acid (1,200–2,400 mg per day in divided doses).
- Others: Turmeric and black pepper combo (1,000 mg per day), Ashwagandha and Rhodiola (500–1,000 mg per day), 5-HTP (50 mg one to three times per day), D-Ribose (5 g three times per day for three weeks, then two times per day), Malic acid (1,000–1,200 mg twice daily), Methylsulfonylmethane (MSM) (start with 1,000 mg three times daily, and increase the dosage until pain relief is evident, up to 10,000 mg daily; reduce the dosage if diarrhea occurs), arginine (500–600 mg/day divided between morning and bedtime), SAMe, Myers Cocktail, ascorbigen (100 mg/day), broccoli powder (400 mg/day), B1 (thiamine, 25–100 mg/day), vitamin C (3,000 mg/day) (vitamin C flush once a week), quercetin (500–1,000 mg three to four times per day), glutamine (begin with 8 g/day times 4 weeks), NAC (500–1,000 mg, NAC 650 mg/day times three months), iron and hormonal support if needed for the adrenals, thyroid, and DHEA.
- *Children:* bromelian (50–100 mg daily), fish oil (500–1,000 mg daily of EPA/DHA), magnesium (200 mg daily), zinc (10 mg daily), Calcium (200–1,000 mg daily), CoQ10 (100 mg daily).

Homeopathy

- Rhus tox can be used for pain and stiffness, which is worse with being still and improved with movement.

- Ruta grav is indicated for those with bruised feelings, which are worse with cold damp weather without definite benefit from warmth.
- Rhododendron is used for pain that is worse with storms and changes in the weather.
- Arnica is used for pain that feels bruised and tender, worse after exertion, feeling as if the bed is too hard.
- Causticum helps benefit soreness and stiffness, which worsen in dry weather, exertion, and cold and improve with warmth and rain.
- Bryonia can be used with pain that is worse with the slightest movement and warmth and improved with coolness. Person does not want to be touched.
- Kalmia latifolia is used for shooting pains in the muscle associated with numbness or cold sensations.
- Cimicifuga is used for sore bruised muscles with neck stiffness and pain, worse in the cold. Prone to hormone imbalances and depression.
- Calcarea carbonica helps those with muscle soreness, clammy hands and feet, anxiety, easily fatigued, joints and muscles feeling contracted. Symptoms improve with warmth and are aggravated by cold and dampness and with exertion.
- Ignatia helps with tight cramping muscles that can be triggered by emotional upset or stress.
- Magnesia phosphorica helps those with cramping muscles improved with warmth.
- Nux vomica can be used with tight muscles associated with cold sensitivity digestive issues, irritability, fatigue. Symptoms improve with warmth and worsen in cold weather.
- Pulsatilla is helpful for painful joints that move from joint to joint. Symptoms may be connected to hormonal imbalances or the menstrual cycle. Patient is depressed and tearful.
- Angustura vera can be used to reduce stiffness, muscle spasms, and cramps, especially in the lower back, and muscle aches that result from poor posture. Symptoms improve when the person stretches or is in contact with the cold and are aggravated by pressure and inactivity.

Acupressure

- LU1, LV3 (relaxed muscles and nerves)
- GV16, GB20, GV24.5 CV6, SP21 SP6, SP10, ST36, LI4 LI11, CV6, P6 (anxiety, heart palpitations, indigestion)
- CV17, B38 (increases sleep and relieves stress)
- CV17 (immune system and decreases depression and anxiety)

Aromatherapy

Helichrysum oil has been shown to improve healing of the nerve tissue and improve circulation. Lavender oil helps to reduce emotional stress associated with fibromyalgia. Muscle aches and pains can be relieved with eucalyptus, lavender, peppermint, nutmeg, rosemary, black pepper, cypress, clove, thyme, chamomile, and ginger, which reduce inflammation and improve circulation to the muscles. Juniper and Melissa help to break down toxins. Essential oils for stress and sleep are also key to healing fibromyalgia; these include chamomile, jasmine, lavender, and rose.

Other Recommendations

Cranial Electrotherapy Stimulation, myofacial release, floatation therapy, and magnetic therapy to help improve pain; postural therapies, Feldenkrais method, Alexander technique, prolotherapy, and laser therapy.

GOUT

Gout is a kind of arthritis due to too much uric acid in the blood leading to swelling, stiffness, burning pain in the joints, most commonly in the big toe. Other symptoms may include purplish skin, limited movement and peeling or itching, and warmth of the skin around the affected joint. Diagnosis can occur with a detailed history, exam, blood work, and imaging.

Additional Integrative Modalities

Supplements

- Celery seed extract (450 mg two to three times daily).
- Black cherry juice/extract.
- Nettles (250 mg three times daily) an antiinflammatory.
- Fish oil (1,000 mg of EPA/DHA per day).
- Proteolytic enzymes.
- Magnesium.
- Vitamin C (500 mg two to three times daily) to reduce the risk of gout.

Homeopathy

- Arnica is for deep, bruising pain. Arnica helps with gout attacks that occur after repeated trauma or physical effort. Joints are sensitive to any contact.

- Colchicum is indicated for painful joints especially at night, worse with movement and associated with irritability, weakness, nausea, and depression.
- Ledum is helpful when your joints are hot, throbging, and slightly swollen-affecting the knees or the feet. The pain improves from ice, cold water, and movement. Pain is aggravated at night and by the warmth of the bed.
- Urtica helps joints that burn and itch.
- Benzoic improves symptoms accompanied by a strong smelling urine.
- Lycopodium helps with symptoms that are worse from 4:00 to 8:00 pm. One foot feels hot, and the other foot feels cold.
- Pulsatilla helps with pains that go from joint to joint and improve with cold and gentle motion.
- Bryonia helps with pain that is worse with the slightest touch in an irritable individual. Symptoms are accompanied with painful edema and improve with rest and heat.
- Belladonna helps with joints that look red and hot, and throb where the pain comes on quickly.
- Rhododendron helps with pain in the big toe that flares before a storm and improves with warmth.
- Sulfur helps with burning sensation and itching of the skin aggravated by heat and improved by warmth.
- Arnica helps with gout attacks that occur after repeated trauma or physical effort. Joints are sensitive to any contact.
- Rhus toxicodendron helps with dark red swollen joints. Pain improves with movement and heat.
- Apis mellifica helps with reddish pink, swollen, painful joints, which improve with cold.
- Lachesis mutus help with pseudo attacks with purplish swelling, and throbbing pain accompanied with extreme sensitivity to touch.

Acupressure

- LV3, SP3, SP6, ST36, ST40

Aromatherapy

Peppermint oil serves to reduce pain, and frankincense can reduce swelling. Juniper oil helps break down toxic deposits and carries them away from the body. Add it to a hot sitz bath or a compress, dilute it in a carrier oil, and/or use in a massage (but don't rub the affected joint directly). Others that can help with the pain are basil linalool, cajeput, roman chamomile, cinnamon, cypress, fennel, fragonia, juniper, lemon, peppermint, pine, rosemary (cineole and camphor), and rosewood.

Other Recommendations

Magnet therapy can be effective in alleviating the pain of gout.

MUSCLE CRAMPS

Muscle cramps, pain, and spasms of the muscle anywhere in the body can be due to poor circulation of the legs, exercising, dehydration, magnesium or potassium deficiency, insufficient stretching, overexertion, certain medications (like statins and blood pressure medications), or malfunctioning nerves. Diagnosis to look for the root cause is determined through a detailed history, physical, blood work, and possible imaging.

Additional Integrative Modalities

Supplements

- Magnesium (250 mg twice daily).
- Potassium (300 mg daily).
- Green superfood powder (chlorella or spirulina).
- Calcium (500 mg twice daily).
- MSM (500 mg three times daily).

Homeopathy

- Cuprum helps with severe cramping that begins with twitching of the muscle, located mainly in the calves and the feet.
- Nux helps cramps, headache, constipation, nausea, loss of appetite, heartburn, fatigue, irritability, cold sensitivity. Symptoms are worse at night and in cold weather, but improve with warmth.
- Arnica helps cramping where the muscles feel fatigued, bruised, and tender, which is worse after exertion.
- Calcarea helps muscle spasm and soreness that may come on after exertion and in cold damp climates. Symptoms are associated with head sweats in those that are overweight, pale, fatigued, and cold sensitive. The person craves sweets and eggs.
- Camphora helps those with cramps in the calves and feet that feel cold.

- Veratum is useful for cramps in the calf associated with recent diarrhea and vomiting. Cramps improve with massage and are aggravated by walking.
- Chamomila helps with cramps in the thighs or legs.
- Cuprum can help prevent against cramps. Person can take it for fourteen days.
- Rhus toxicodendron is used for pain and stiffness that worsen in the morning or after immobility or in the cold. Things improve with movement and warmth.
- Magnesia phosphorica helps with cramping that improves with warmth.
- Ignatia amara helps with tight, spasmodic, cramps after being emotionally upset or stressed.
- Cimicifuga is for muscles that feel bruised and sore, which is worse in the cold. The person is prone to hormonal imbalances and depression.
- Causticum helps painful joints that become stiff and sore from overuse. Pain improves with warmth and is aggravated by cold or dry weather.
- Others: cactus grandiflorus, lachesis mutus, lacticum acidum, and viburnum opulus

Acupressure

- B57, GB34, ST36, LV3, GV26 (lower extremity)
- Leg cramps: B40, B60, B57
- Arms: LI11, TW15, P6, TW14, TW5
- Foot cramps: LV3 and LV2

Aromatherapy

Muscle aches can be relieved by peppermint oil, coconut oil, and cypress oil rubbed on sore muscles. If the muscle aches or cramps occur at night, use black pepper instead of peppermint. Frankincense and cypress oil reduce inflammation. Lemongrass essential oil can help to improve back spasms. Peppermint oil and lavender oil used to further penetrate the area can help relax inflamed area and help with cramps. Others that can be used for leg cramps are marjoram, rosemary, and hyssops.

OSTEOPOROSIS

Osteoporosis is a chronic condition that occurs when your bones gradually become brittle and weak, as the formation of new bone doesn't keep up with the removal of old bone, leading to an increased risk of fractures. As it is a "silent disease," it presents with very little symptoms until it leads to extensive vertebral damage that leads to curvature of the spin to cause a hump (kyphosis), loss of height, stooped posture, and back pain. Osteoporosis can be caused by aging, inactivity, steroid use, low vitamin D, nutritional deficiencies, emotional stress, kidney failure, chronic disease of the thyroid or adrenals, excessive alcohol, tobacco use, eating disorders, autoimmune disease, and long-term use of medications like gastric reflux drugs, cancer medications, and corticosteroids. Diagnosis is made via a bone mineral density test or other imaging as needed.

Additional Integrative Modalities

Supplements

- Magnesium (500 mg per day).
- Calcium (500–600 mg twice daily in divided doses); calcium citrate is the best absorbed; others are citrate-malate, chelate, and hydroxy apatite.
- Fish oil (4 g daily with 3,000 mg of evening primrose oil).
- Vitamin D3 (5,000 IU per day).
- Vitamin K2 (100 mcg MK7 daily).
- Others: Strontium (680 mg daily) and silicon (50–20 mg daily), B6 (25–50 mg per day), folic acid (800 mcg per day), B12 (800 mcg per day), and green tea (three to five cups per day or 250–500 mg of polyphenols per day).

Homeopathy

You may take the remedy as long your symptoms continue and stop when they improve (although you may not be able to "feel" bone density improving, symptoms of overall bone health can be observed). Work with a professional to locate the constitutional remedy. Homeopathy is most effective for prevention of osteoporosis and treatment of mild osteoporosis.

- Calcarea fluorica is best for those with malnutrition of the bones with enlarged hypermobile joints, bone spurs, depression, and increased urination at night. Symptoms improve with heat and warmth, worsen with rest and changes of weather.
- Folliculinum can be used for osteoporosis related to menopause.
- Silica is indicated with those who are nervous, cold, constantly get sick, and are thin.
- Calcarea carbonica is a remedy for those with osteoporosis who may also complain of muscle cramps, swollen joints, aching bones, fatigue,

feeling overwhelmed, and being overweight. Symptoms are aggravated in the cold and dampness. They crave sweets, eggs, and milk.
- Calcarea phosphorica is indicated for those with fractures or osteoporosis, as it helps boost bone building, and can be used for asymptomatic individuals for bone support. Osteoporosis may be associated with calcium deposits, neck and back pain with stiffness; patients feel cold drafts.
- Phosphorus is a remedy for weak bones or slow healing fractures in tall, very social, thin people, who crave ice cold drinks.
- Symphytum helps to reduce pain and heal fractures.

Acupressure

- K10, SP3, LV1 P3, ST36 (improve digestion)
- LU1 (stress)
- LI4 (pain)
- GV24.5 (hormonal balance)
- SP5 and K3 (pain in the ankles)

Aromatherapy

Essential oils like cypress, helichrysum, and fir oil can aid in bone repair. Black pepper and rosemary help to soothe aching joints and bones. Oils to help you relieve stress are also important for overall health; these include lavender, rose, and geranium.

• 21 •

Urology

We are almost to the end!!! Yay! Let's face it, a trip to the urologist can make most men quiver like babies under the covers, but lowering inflammation can keep them from quivering under the covers when they're up to bat. Did I get your attention? Good, now let's keep the fire out of the urological system!

D & D: SPECIAL CONSIDERATIONS

Optimize prostate health by eating foods like green leafy vegetables (like Brussels sprouts and other cruciferous veggies), cilantro, watercress, rosemary, dandelion leaves, basil leaves, thyme and blueberry, green tea, and lycopene-rich foods like cooked tomatoes. Optimize vitamin D, E, and omega 3. Herbs like ginger, rosemary, and turmeric have anti-inflammatory properties. Improve testosterone levels with sesame, watercress, Brazil nuts, and foods high in zinc like pumpkin seeds. Optimize urinary health by eating foods like cranberries, peaches, wheatgrass, celery, black raspberries, parsley, garlic, thyme, and oregano. Improve libido with natural aphrodisiacs like avocados, figs, and bananas; foods rich in vitamin C, zinc, magnesium, collagen, iron; and other foods like dark chocolate, watermelon, asparagus, celery, sweet potatoes, Brazil nuts, almonds, walnuts, beets, and most importantly lots of water. Tyrosine for dopamine found in seaweed, soy protein, egg whites, salmon, turkey, wild game, shrimp, and fish eggs. Also add spices like cloves, garlic, ginger, and nutmeg. It's important to avoid liquids within two hours of bedtime and to reduce medications and other substances that can lead to urinary retention, especially those with antihistamine and anticholinergic properties.

THE FOUR BIG S's: SPECIAL CONSIDERATIONS

Follow the guidelines in chapter 3. Lowering inflammation can decrease urinary retention and optimize urinary/prostatic health.

BENIGN PROSTATIC HYPERPLASIA

Benign prostatic hyperplasia (BPH) is a noncancerous enlargement of the prostate (an organ which produces the fluid that carries sperm during ejaculation). The prostate can get inflamed and enlarged, compressing the urethra and leading to problems with urination, bladder infections, and bladder stones. Benign prostatic hypertrophy refers to the addition of cell growth due to inflammation, hormonal changes (estrogen excess), zinc deficiency (that can be influenced by stress, infections, and diet) and deteriorating blood vessels that can lead to prostate problems. Symptoms include increased pressure from the bladder, sudden urge to urinate, and weak urinary flow, which results in difficulty starting urination, feeling of incomplete emptying of bladder, increasing the chances of infection and stones, dribbling after urination, urinary frequency and pain, incontinence, and even getting up to urinate more frequently during the night. BPH is diagnosed by reviewing a patient's history and other tests like digital rectal exam, transrectal ultrasound, urine tests, and lab tests (like a prostate-specific antigen test).

Additional Integrative Modalities

Supplements

- Saw palmetto (160 mg twice a day or 320 mg three times a day for four months then down to 320 mg once a day).
- Zinc (50 mg daily) is important for prostate health, and can be taken with 3 mg of copper.
- Fish oil (1,000 mg daily).
- Pumpkin seed oil (8–10 g, 320 mg daily, or 1 tbsp daily).
- Nettle root (120 mg twice daily).
- Optimize vitamin D.

- Other: Beta-sitosterol, also found in avocados (60–195 mg daily; divided doses up to 2,000–3,000 mg/day), pygeum (100–200 mg a day), flaxseed and SDG (300–600 mg/day), rye grass pollen (126 mg TID), and green tea and selenium.

Homeopathy

- Thuja occidentalis is for an enlarged prostate with frequent and urgent desire to pass urine.
- Argenticum nitricum helps those who lose their erection with penetration, have pain with intercourse, or have loss of sexual desire.
- Baryta helps those with a slow urine stream, frequency of urination, immature impotence, and persons who are thin and underweight.
- Causticum can help those who lose their urine from sneezing or coughing, sexual pleasure is lessened during orgasm; and there's a pressure feeling that starts from the bladder and goes into the prostate.
- Chimaphilla umbellate helps those with urinary retention who also feel like there is a ball in their pelvic floor, as they may experience swelling, soreness, and pressure that is worse when sitting.
- Clematis helps with hypertrophy that can cause dribbling and a weak stream.
- Ferrum picricum is indicated where a person frequently urinates at night, complains of pressure on rectum, and has sensation at the neck of the bladder.
- Iodum is indicated for those with shrunken testes, prostate gland that feels hard (may not be due to cancer), and who have a loss of potency.
- Lycopodium helps those with an enlarged prostate along with sexual dysfunction like impotence. Patients feel cold, crave sweets, and have digestive problems.
- Pulsatilla can be indicated for end of urination bladder pain; patients feel better in the fresh air and get warm easily.
- Sabal serrulata helps those with painful or difficult urination, with spasms of bladder or urethra. Can help in urinary retention, with a cold sensation of the prostate or bladder.
- Selenium can help with an enlarged prostate with symptoms of dribbling and impotence. Symptoms worse after urination and walking.
- Staphysagria helps those with chronic dribbling, urinary retention, burning sensation of the prostate, or urinary tract and impotence. These men have suppressed emotions.
- Conium maculatum is indicated for those with sclerosed hypertrophy of the prostate and position-changing vertigo.

Acupressure

- SP6 may help to reduce discomfort related with prostate enlargement.
- Bladder points along the groin (B27–B34) can help to increase circulation to the prostate and reduce inflammation.

Aromatherapy

Anti-inflammatory and antipathogenic essential oils can help to calm swelling; these include frankincense, myrrh, and rosemary. Massage oils around the genital area regularly to improve prostate health and stimulate blood flow.

CHRONIC PROSTATITIS

Chronic prostatitis (chronic pelvic pain syndrome) is a nonbacterial inflammation of the prostate that can lead to symptoms of urinary frequency, hesitancy, and persistent discomfort or pain that is present in the lower pelvic region, mainly at the base of the penis and around the anus. Other symptoms include sexual problems like difficulty getting an erection, painful ejaculation, or even pain after having sex. It is diagnosed when this pain persists for at least three months within the previous six months. Your doctor may examine your prostate, collect a urine sample, get an image of your urinary tract, and even order blood tests.

Additional Integrative Modalities

Supplements

- Zinc picolinate (60 mg daily until symptoms improve, then 30 mg daily).
- Quercetin (500 mg twice daily). Absorption can be improved if combined with equivalent doses of bromelain.
- Omega 3 fatty acids (2–4 g of EPA/DHA per day).
- Others: Rye, SAMe (600–1,200 mg per day), beta-sitosterol (60 mg two to three times daily; reduce to 30–60 mg daily for four more weeks once symptoms subside), grass pollen (Cernilton).

Homeopathy

Doses of 6C are most often used.

- Sabal is indicated when the prostate is enlarged and the area feels cold or when intercourse and/or ejaculation is painful.
- Thuja helps those with frequent urges to urinate and with a burning sensation at the neck of the bladder.
- Pulsatilla is a remedy for those with the urgent need to urinate, and it is worse with lying on the back. A thick yellow discharge may be present from the penis.

Acupressure

- P6 and ST36

Aromatherapy

Essential oils can help to reduce swelling and pain, prevent infection, increase sexual function, and improve urinary function and blood flow. Frankincense, myrrh, rosemary, and thyme can help, along with juniper, lavender, bergamot (antibacterial), chamomile, eucalyptus, lavender, cypress, myrtle (green or orange), pine, yarrow, and naiouli.

Other Recommendations

Biofeedback can be helpful.

ERECTILE DYSFUNCTION

Erectile dysfunction is when one is unable to achieve or maintain an erection. There are many degrees of erectile dysfunction, and causes can be mind- or body-related. Causes can be due to an endocrine disorder, nerve or neurological disorder, medications (like beta blockers, cancer chemotherapy medications, CNS depressants like Xanax, diuretics, antidepressants like SSRIs), cardiac conditions (high cholesterol or hypertension), lifestyle factors, emotional disorders (anxiety or depression, abuse of drugs), low levels of testosterone, stress, and heavy metal poisoning.

Additional Integrative Modalities

Supplements

- L-arginine (1,000 mg two to three times daily on an empty stomach) helps to improve blood flow and blood vessel dilation.
- L-citrulline (free form) (1,500–6,000 mg per day maximum).
- Panax ginseng (ideally Korean red ginseng) (1,800–3,000 mg/day in divided doses depending on ginsenoside content).
- Niacin (250 mg three times daily) can improve blood flow.
- Other: DHEA (25–50 mg daily) under the supervision of a doctor, as it can improve testosterone levels; Maca (an adaptogen herb) (500 mg three times daily) to improve sexual desire; potency wood (Muira puama, an herb from South America) (500 mg three times daily), Ginkgo biloba (120 mg twice daily) to improve blood flow; Cordyceps sinensis (800 mg twice daily of Cs-4 mycelium extract) can improve libido.

Homeopathy

- Agnus castus helps men whose erectile difficulties have come on recently, don't have an erection firm enough for penetration, and have a small and cold penis. The men are anxious and have memory/concentration issues.
- Selenium metallicum is indicated when the erectile dysfunction is associated with an increased desire for sex, and dribbles semen during sleep with erotic fantasies. Patients are usually tired.
- Lycopodium is a remedy for those with anticipation failure, cold and small penis, and a surge of desire. They also have digestive issues and lack of confidence.
- Staphysagria helps shy men with deep emotions who have erectile dysfunction that began after an emotional or embarrassing event.
- Arnica is indicated for erectile issues that follow a bruising injury to the penis.
- Hypericum is a remedy for erectile issues that have followed a bruised spinal cord injury.
- Conium helps those men whose erection doesn't last, whose legs feel cold and cramped. They have great surge of sexual feelings after long abstinence.
- Caladium helps those who have an erection when they are asleep, but then disappears when they wake up. The penis remains flaccid despite being sexually excited, and the person has frequent wet dreams. Men crave tobacco.

Acupressure

- B23 and B47 can reduce fatigue and improve sexual performance.
- K1, K3, CV4, B27 or B34 (treat lower back pain, sexual reproductive problems and sacral pain, impotency).
- CV6 (treat ED, seminal emission, night time urination and hernia or reproductive problems).
- SP12 (treat male infertility).
- SP13 (improve ED and abdominal discomfort).
- H7, B15, B31, K12, CV3,4,6, GV4.
- Premature ejaculation: H7, B15, B23, K12, CV3, 4, 6, and GV4.

Aromatherapy

Essential oils can increase libido. Examples include sandalwood, ylang-ylang, and rose. Others that can also help are jasmine, patchouli, anise, black pepper, cedarwood, clary sage, clove, ginger, neroli, nutmeg, peppermint, pine, rosemary (cineole and camphor), and vetiver.

INCONTINENCE

Urinary incontinence is the loss of bladder control that results in an unintentional releasing of urine. Incontinence has ranges from occasionally leaking when sneezing or coughing or having an urge to urinate that is so strong that they wet their clothes. There are several types of incontinence from stress, urge, overflow, and functional and mixed incontinence. Tests that the doctor will do include a urinalysis, bladder diary, post void residual measurements, urodynamic testing, and other imaging like a cystoscopy, cystogram, and/or a pelvic ultrasound.

Additional Integrative Modalities

Supplements

- Fish oils (3–4 g a day).
- Flaxseed oil (1 tbsp a day).
- Vitamin C (500 mg two to three times a day).
- Vitamin E (400 IU a day for anti-inflammatory support).
- Magnesium can help to reduce bladder muscle spasms.
- Bromelain (400 mg three times per day in between meals).

- Others: find herbal formulas with two or more of the following ingredients: buchu (a soothing diuretic and antiseptic for the urinary system), corn silk (which has soothing and diuretic properties), marshmallow root (which has soothing, demulcent properties) a horsetail (an astringent and mild diuretic with tissue-healing properties), cleavers (a traditional urinary tonic), and usnea (which has soothing and antiseptic properties). An herbalist can also make a formula for you. Follow the instructions on the label. Agrimony (thirty drops three times daily) can also help.

Homeopathy

- Causticum is a remedy for when the incontinence is worse with laughing or coughing.
- Gelsemium helps those with weak and trembly legs and drooping eyelids.
- Ferrum phosporicum is best for those with the inability to control bladder, frequent urge to urinate. Pain located in neck of bladder is relieved with urination.
- Nux vomica helps those who have involuntary dribbles of urine. The patient is very irritable.
- Pulsatilla helps those who leak urine when lying down, coughing, and sneezing, pass gas, or get angry. Cough may be present and is irritating and tickly at night, loosens up in the morning with yellowish green mucus.
- Sepia is a remedy for those who leak urine due to shock, laughing, sneezing, and coughing. It is accompanied by strong bearing down sensation in the pelvis.
- Natrum muriaticum can be used for stress incontinence, pain during sex, and vaginal dryness, especially with a history of grief.
- Pareira can be used for retention of urine from an enlarged prostate.
- Zincum can be used for stress incontinence, inability to urinate while standing, and prostate problems leading to urinary retention.

Acupressure

- SP6, B23, B28, B60, GV20, CV3
- CV8, CV4, GV20, and CV6

Aromatherapy

The essential oil cypress has relaxing properties and can be massaged onto the lower abdomen.

Other Recommendations

Biofeedback can improve symptoms.

INTERSTITIAL CYSTITIS

Interstitial cystitis is a chronic inflammation of the bladder characterized by the persistent need to frequently urinate, pelvic pain, and can mimic symptoms of a UTI, but there is a lack of bacterial infection. This illness results in chronic discomfort or pain in the bladder or pelvic area, usually in flares. Common symptoms include urgent need to urinate, pain with urination, frequent urination, pelvic pain, and pain with intercourse. In women, symptoms can get worse during menstruation. About half of the women spontaneously improve without any medical treatment. Conventional medicine has not been of much help to patients with this condition. Assessment includes a detailed medical history including a bladder diary, a pelvic exam, urine test, a cystoscopy (a tiny camera that shows your bladder), possible biopsy, urine cytology to rule out cancer, and possibly a potassium sensitivity test. It is usually diagnosed by exclusion.

Additional Integrative Modalities

Supplements

- Probiotics can help to reduce inflammation.
- Calcium glycerophosphate (two to three tabs or ¼ tsp two times a day or before high acid meals).
- Glucosamine and chondroitin—doses may vary—helps to reduce pain.
- Quercetin (1,000–3,000 mg daily) and grapeseed extract (10 mg daily).
- Others that can help: L-arginine (500 mg three times daily), marshmallow root, aloe vera.

Homeopathy

- Cantharis is for burning pains in the lower abdomen, nonstop urge to urinate, inability to empty bladder.
- Nux helps those with painful and frequent urges with little result.
- Apis is a remedy for sharp stinging pain in the lower abdomen; urine is scanty, hot, and occasionally bloody; symptoms worsen in heat and get better with cold, accompanied with urinary frequency.

- Belladonna is for burning sensation along the urethra, even after urination, urges persist.
- Berberis is for urine that is slimy, with fine mucus. Radiating pains are worse during rest and while passing urine.
- Causticum is best for frequent urge to pass urine, change in vaginal discharge; symptoms worsen by coughing and sneezing.
- Dulcamara is a remedy for those who experience an attack after getting cold, and after exertion in the fall.
- Sarsaparilla helps those with pain that comes on as urination stops, with urgency, and when urine passes there is pressure. Urine looks thick and milky.
- Staphysagria is indicated for an attack after sex or after catherization. The patient feels like there is constant trickling of urine. There is a constant burning sensation unrelated to urination.
- Clematis helps with stream of urine that is intermittent or slow.
- Camphora is best for pain that is worse at the start of urination; there is spasm of bladder muscles at base; symptoms are worse with cold. No urine is passed despite urgent straining.
- Arsenicum helps those with burning pains in lower abdomen, and patient feels anxious, restless, and cold.

Acupressure

- ST40, SP9, B28, B32, LV2, LV3, CV2, CV3
- Others: CV4, CV6, GV4

Aromatherapy

Essential oils that benefit urological conditions include lavender, sandalwood, peppermint, clary sage, and thyme, which are antispasmodic and antiseptic. Others include cypress, geranium, and juniper.

• 22 •

Conclusion

Extinguish the Flames and Take Back Control!

Don't let the hamster wheel own you—you are your own unique story! Your fall due to chronic illness is only the beginning of an amazing transformation—a transformation to find the better you, a healthier you, and a stronger you! Give yourself a chance to change for the better, a chance to turn your life around, and the boost you need to get yourself off the ground running! That fall was a blessing in disguise as it gave you the power and motivation to escape the wheel for good!

I'm sooo proud of you, as you already took the first, most difficult step—to acquire knowledge—the most important key that will help you to unlock unimaginable doors.

The fire that rages within your body has kept you stuck—despite that, look at all you have accomplished! It takes someone very special to have done all that you have done, competing with those who are not fighting a battle within! You are a gem—I can't say that enough.

Now imagine a life with no fire that burns within, a life full of peace, a life full of energy, a life full of unlimited possibilities—what can you accomplish, what will you do? It's already giving me goose bumps because the sky's the limit, I can't wait to watch you fly! With no other distractions and nothing to drag you down, anything you put your mind to could be yours. Your once-distant dreams can now be your reality!

Your name is not James Eczema, Amina Asthma, Thomas IBS, or Lily Hashimotos. These conditions don't have to define you. You can finally take charge of your own health! You are a blessing to this world and those around you. Let's begin that transformation, implement *The Holistic Rx*, and finally escape the hamster wheel for good! The first couple weeks are going to be hard, but once you get the hang of it, as the energy and pain improve, it will not be so bad—it's actually quite rewarding.

I am here for you! We can do this together! Take it one day at a time, one meal at a time! Slowly you will transform into who you were meant to be, the real and authentic you! Transform to a more energetic you! Transform to a pain-free you! Transform into a happier you! The ups and downs in your journey will only make you stronger! So it's time to break from the hamster wheel! You are so worth it, do this for yourself. Haven't you waited long enough? I have provided you with the information you need to set yourself free—imagine the places you could go! Look out world, here you come!!! Go get 'em—go experience *joie de vivre!*

Love unconditionally,
Madiha Saeed, MD ABIHM

Appendix

GUT AND PSYCHOLOGY SYNDROME (GAPS) DIET

The GAPS diet, by Dr. Natasha Campbell, helps to heal the digestive tract from disease. It is split up into two parts: introduction and full. Foods not allowed on GAPS are grains, sugar, processed foods, beans and legumes (except for lentils and navy beans), starchy veggies (corn, potatoes, okra, and parsnips), and soy. Dairy and other items should be avoided if there's an intolerance. The diet focuses on homemade broths, healthy fats, and veggies. See a full list of foods to include/avoid in Dr. Campbell's book, pages 159–67.

GAPS Introduction Diet

The introduction GAPS diet is designed to heal and seal the gut lining quickly to allow the body to recover. The foods are introduced gradually, structured in stages, and it's like a "boot camp" for your gut to heal. It provides foods that are gentle and healing for the gut lining, providing the beneficial microbes needed, removing food intolerances quickly, but it does require patience. The introduction diet is structured in six stages, adding new foods gradually over weeks to months, depending on your body's response. Stay on each stage for about three to five days, progressing when your body is ready (with no die-off like digestive issue or rashes). If your symptoms worsen in the next stage, return back to the previous stage for a few more days. Most importantly, listen to your body.

This diet does include some dairy, but this should be avoided if you have intolerances; like most foods, dairy can eventually be reintroduced back into the diet as tolerated (there is a step-wise approach for that introduction, starting from organic ghee, then unsalted butter, homemade yogurt, fermented kefir and cream, homemade cheese, traditional cheese, cream, and then raw milk).

Foods included in each stage:

- Start every day with glass of filtered water with fresh lemon juice.
- Stage 1: homemade stocks and soups with well-boiled veggies and meats, chopped liver, well-cooked vegetables (with fibrous stems removed and peeled), animal fats, coconut oil, sea salt, peppercorns, probiotic foods, filtered water, teas (turmeric, loose herbal like chamomile and fresh ginger root), lemon juice, and raw, organic cold pressed honey.
- Stage 2: continue with foods from previous stage and include fermented cod liver oil, fermented fish and gravlax, raw egg yolks, stews and casseroles (with boiled meats and veggies), fresh herbs, dairy if tolerated (like homemade whey, yogurt, sour cream and kefir), increased fermented juices, homemade ghee (if tolerated, start with one teaspoon per day and gradually increase).
- Stage 3: continue with previous stages and then gradually add ripened avocado, pancakes (made with squash, nut butter [optional], eggs, and a small amount of honey), almond butter, eggs, fully cooked vegetables (celeriac, asparagus, and cabbage), probiotics, fermented vegetables, and sautéed onion in animal fat.
- Stage 4: continue with previous foods, and start to simmer stocks longer, gradually add roasted and baked meats, cold pressed olive oil (start with one teaspoon per day), fresh pressed juices (on an empty stomach, start with one teaspoon a day of fresh carrot juice and then add celery, lettuce, and mint), walnut and almond flour, and nut/seed flour breads.
- Stage 5: continue with previous foods and gradually add raw vegetables and cooked apples in coconut oil and ghee, spices, fruit as a juice ingredient (avoid citrus), and pecan flour.
- Stage 6: continue with previous foods and gradually add raw fruits, honey, Brazil nuts, sweet treats, and baked goods with GAPS-approved ingredients.

Full GAPS Diet

Now you're an expert on how your body responds to food in its own individual way. This is unique and very valuable knowledge, which can serve you well for the rest of your life. So keep a diary through the introduction phase, where you record the whole process of food introduction and the individual symptoms and reactions.

- Start day with a glass of still mineral or filtered water with a slice of lemon or teaspoon of apple cider vinegar (warm or cold) or glass of freshly pressed fruit/vegetable juice.
- Our body is detoxifying from 4:00 am to 10:00 am; eating fresh fruit, drinking water and freshly pressed juices, and having probiotic foods will assist in this process, so have breakfast at around 10:00 am.

Digestive Health and Detoxification

Remember to continue juicing and bathing (in Epsom salt alternating with bicarbonate of soda, sea salt, seaweed powder, and cider vinegar) as it is an excellent way to detox and reduce toxic load as discussed in chapter 2, along with having natural chelators (like juice, seaweed, coriander and other herbs, fermented foods, etc.).

Supplements

GAPS children and adults should have a group of essential supplements: essential therapeutic-strength probiotic, essential fatty acid, cod liver oil, digestive enzymes, and vitamin and mineral supplements.

Essential fatty acid

a. A seed/nut blend of omega 3 and 6 (ratio 2:1). Start with a small amount (depending on age of child)—start with a few drops building up to 1–3 tbsp a day.
    - For children under age eighteen months: 1–2 tsp.
    - Adults: build up to 4–5 tbsp a day.

b. Fish oil (high EPA/DHA).
    - Adults: start with a small dosage and build up to 3 to 4 teaspoons a day.
    - Children under two: gradually increase to 1 teaspoon per day.
    - Children over two: start small and gradually increase to 1 to 3 teaspoons daily.

Cod liver oil

- (ratio of A:D is 10:1)
- Adults: Start with 2–2.5 mL (about ½ tsp/day) and gradually increase to 1 tsp daily.
- Lactating or pregnant women: gradually increase to 1.5–2 tsp per day.
- Children: Start half that dose and gradually increase to ½ tsp.
- For babies and very small children: Rub cod liver oil onto their skin (diaper area), gradually increase to ⅓ tsp.

Digestive Enzymes

- Betaine HCl with added pepsin (200–300 mg of betaine, 100 mg pepsin)
- Child: eighteen months to twenty-four months: 1 pinch
- Two to three years: 2 to 3 pinches
- Four to six years: half a capsule
- Six to ten years: half to a full capsule
- Greater than ten and adults: at least one capsule at the beginning of each meal

Other ways to increase acidity and optimize digestion: cabbage juice and stock with your meals.

GAPS Feeding Schedule

For those children and families who are prone to disease, when ready to introduce foods, do so according to the GAPS introduction schedule (minding sensitivities).

Week 1: Start with homemade meat stock with the fat, and freshly pressed vegetable juice mixed with warm water between meals (start with carrot juice then add cabbage, celery, and lettuce).

Week 2: Continue with previous foods, add probiotic gradually, homemade sauerkraut juice, soups with pureed nonstarchy vegetables. If yogurt is well tolerated, you are gradually increasing its daily amount, introduce sour cream, fermented with yogurt culture.

Week 3: Continue with previous foods; add boiled meats (starting with chicken); introduce ripe avocado, starting with a teaspoon added to the vegetable puree, gradually increasing the amount. Increase amount of yogurt and sour cream to 1–2 tsp with meals.

Weeks 4 and 5: Continue with previous foods; add raw egg yolks to vegetable puree (do a sensitivity test first); add cooked apples; increase amount of butter, coconut oil, or ghee.

Weeks 6 and 7: Carry on with previous foods, increase the amount of homemade yogurt or sour cream to 3 tsp with every meal. Gradually increase raw egg yolks to two a day, adding to your baby's soup or cups of meat stock. Increase the meat intake, particularly gelatinous meats around the joints and bones (well cooked in water).

Weeks 8 and 9: Continue with previous foods. Add pancakes made with nut butter and eggs. Increase the amount of freshly pressed juices, add some yogurt to the juice. Try to add some fresh apple to the juice mixture. Add raw vegetables starting with lettuce and peeled cucumbers (blended in a food processor and added to soup or vegetable puree). After these two vegetables are well tolerated, gradually add other raw vegetables, finely blended.

Week 10 and onward: Carry on with previous foods, add scrambled egg with raw butter or animal fat, with avocados and raw or cooked vegetables. Try some ripe raw apples (without the skin), ripe banana with all fruit given between meals. Introduce gradually your homemade cottage cheese (made from homemade yogurt) starting with a tiny amount and gradually increasing.

When on full GAPS diet, you can start adding small amounts of natural salt to the food.

RESOURCES

Madiha Saeed, MD
HolisticMom, MD
@HolisticMomMD
www.holisticmommd.com

Books

General

Boosting Your Immunity for Dummies by Kellyann Petrucci and Wendy Warner, MD
The Supplement Handbook by Mark Moyad, MD, MPH
The Doctor's Book of Natural Health Remedies by Peg Moline
Effortless Healing by Joseph Mercola, MD

Autoimmune disease

The Autoimmune Solution and *The Thyroid Connection* by Amy Myers, MD
Hashimoto's Thyroiditis: Lifestyle Interventions for Finding and Treating the Root Cause and *Hashimoto's Protocol* by Izabella Wentz, PharmD
The Paleo Approach by Sarah Ballantyne, PhD

Cardiology

The Paleo Cardiologist by Dr. John Wolfson, DO

Dental Health

Cure Tooth Decay by Ramiel Nagel
How to Stop Cavities by Judene Benoit, DDS

Dermatology

Feed Your Face by Dr. Jessica Wu, MD

Ear, Nose, and Throat

The Allergy Book by Dr. Robert Sears, MD, and William Sears, MD
The Allergy Solution by Leo Galland, MD, and Jonathan Galland, JD

Endocrinology

Dr. Mark Hyman's books
Smart Fat by Steven Masley, MD, and Jonny Bowden, PhD, CNS
The Obesity Code by Jason Fung, MD
The Adrenal Thyroid Revolution by Aviva Romm, MD

Gastroenterology

Digestive Wellness by Elizabeth Lipski, PhD
Gutbliss by Robynne Chutkan, MD
Eat Dirt by Dr. Josh Axe
The Microbiome Solution by Robynne Chutkan, MD

Gynecology

The Hormone Reset Diet by Sara Gottfried, MD

Neurology

Grain Brain by David Perlmutter, MD
Sugar Crush by Richard Jacoby and Raquel Baldelomar

Oncology

Radical Remission by Kelly Turner, PhD
The Anti-Cancer Diet by David Khayat, MD

Ophthalmology

The Eye Care Revolution by Robert Abel Jr., MD

Pediatrics

Super Nutrition for Babies by Katherine Erlich, MD
The Dirt Cure by Maya Shetreat Klein, MD

Psychiatry

Healing ADD by Daniel Amen, MD
A Mind of Your Own by Kelly Brogan, MD

Rheumatology

Healthy Joints for Life by Richard Diana, MD
No Grain, No Pain by Dr. Peter Osborne
Holistic Pain Relief by Heather Tick, MD
The FibroManual by Ginevra Liptan, MD
Fibro Fix by Dr. David Brady

Laboratories

23 and Me: www.23andme.com
Commonwealth Laboratories: www.hydrogenbreathtesting.com
Cyrex Laboratories: www.cyrexlabs.com
DiagnosTechs: www.diagnostechs.com/
Doctor's Data: www.doctorsdata.com
Genova Diagnostics: www.gdx.net
IGeneX: www.igenex.com/
Immuno Laboratories: www.immunolabs.com/patients/
Immunosciences Lab: www.immunoscienceslab.com
iSpot Lyme: http://ispotlyme.com
Laboratory Corporation of America: www.labcorp.com/
Quest Diagnostics: www.questdiagnostics.com/
RealTime Laboratories: www.realtimelab.com

Other Resources

http://www.localharvest.org: locate a local and seasonal CSA.
http://www.realmilk.com/wherel.html: find local fresh milk.
http://www.ewg.org: this source provides a "Clean 15/Dirty Dozen" produce list, information guide to safe skin care, house cleaning products, and other sources to empower people to live healthier lives in a healthier environment.

An Organization You Might Consider Supporting

Documenting Hope: www.documentinghope.com: dedicated to healing chronic disease in children

Integrative Entities

Academy of Integrative Health & Medicine: www.aihm.org
Institute for Functional Medicine: www.functionalmedicine.org

CONSTITUTIONAL HOMEOPATHIC REMEDIES

For chronic illnesses, adding a constitutional homeopathic remedy can optimize health and well-being. Based on the person's symptoms and personality, choose a constitutional remedy to help bring a person back into balance. Choose the remedy that best matches you and take 30C or 12C/15C once a week. Some acute remedies may be used as chronic remedies.

Types

Depending on your symptoms, choose a category below, then find the medicine within that category that best fits you.

- *Psoric:* Presents with skin, mucous membrane, and serous manifestations. Symptoms tend to follow an oscillatory pattern returning to baseline symptoms. A tendency toward parasites and lack of good reaction.
- *Sycotic:* Slows progressive development of symptoms. Tendency to grow benign tumors, chronic catarrh of mucus membranes, general inhibition of tissues infiltration, sensitivity to cold and humidity, patients may have general depressive and obsessive tendency.
- *Tuberculinics:* Patients have loss of appetite, hypersensitivity and nervous instability, easily tired, hypersensitivity to cold, variability to symptoms and demineralization.

Psoric

Sulfur: This homeopathic targets metabolism, the circulatory system, and has detoxifying action. Person feels burning pain or heat with itching. Symptoms are aggravated by heat (especially the heat of the bed) and at 11:00 am, improved with dry weather or movement. Associated symptoms are discharge, cravings for sweets, spices and alcohol, the need for fresh air, diarrhea that wakes the patient in the morning, redness of the orifices, localized general sweating, and the light sleep. This person is generally overweight or thin, and when in good health the individual is optimistic and very active, but in sickness they become irritable.

Psorinum: This homeopathic targets those that have irritated skin and mucous membranes, along with allergies and reactional depressive tendencies. This homeopathic works on the nervous system and works well with those who experience overall weakness/fatigue and weight loss. Their symptoms are worse in the cold winter or with any contact with wool that can lead to itching; improvement in symptoms occur with heat (except in bed), or when eating. Accompanied symptoms maybe bad discharge, extreme cold sensitivity, feeling exceptionally well, compulsive snacking during migraines, and intense itching (worse with the heat of the bed or showering). The person looks thin, pale, dirty, and is pessimistic, and anxious.

Lycopodium: This homeopathic targets the liver, digestive tract, nervous system, kidneys, genital tract, skin, mucous membranes, metabolism, and issues with cholesterol or uric acid. Persons feel fatigued, bloated at the belt level, have itching that is improved by cold, have sensations of one foot being cold while the other is hot, and are quickly satiated after eating. There is redness after meals, and the patients crave sweet and have food intolerances to oysters and onions. These patients have dermatological and digestive disorders and have general symptoms like fatigue. Symptoms are present predominantly on the right side. Symptoms are made worse with heat and contraindication and aggravated between 4:00 and 8:00 pm and improved with hot foods and fresh air. They have underdeveloped musculature and may present with facial tics, lack self-esteem, are proud, like being in charge, seek affection, and are very emotional.

Arsenicum album: Can be used in those whose symptoms have come on by allergy, toxic food poisoning, and severe infections. It targets the heart, blood vessels; nervous system; skin; digestive, respiratory, and urogenital systems. Patients have necrosing irritations of the mucous membranes in the digestive, respiratory, and urogenital systems with intense burning, extreme cold sensitivity, extreme weakness, thirst during a fever, and have corrosive discharge. Patients are cold-sensitive, meticulous, anemic, and fatigued with the reactional anxiety. Symptoms are worsened with cold between the times of 1:00 to 3:00 am and improved with heat.

Nux vomica: Is helpful for those whose symptoms were triggered by burnout or business worries, sedentary lifestyle, or excessive intake of drugs, alcohol, or stimulants. This homeopathic targets the nervous and digestive systems. Patients have hypersensitivity to light, noise, odors, cold; experience spasms, hyperreflectivity, false urges, sensation of incomplete bowel movement, coated tongue, sleepiness after meals; and are hypersensitive, impatient, and irritated. They can present with reactional depression. They crave alcohol and stimulants. Symptoms are worse after meals, with alcohol, stimulants, cold, air drafts, and upon waking up; they improve with heat and with shortened sleep.

Arsenicum iodatum: This homeopathic targets those symptoms associated with mucous membranes like watery, nasal discharge that feels as if it is burning or blocking nasal passages; skin is lichen-like, the patient complains of enlarged lymph nodes; and symptoms related to vascular sclerosis or arrhythmia. These individuals are weak, thin, anxious, impatient, do not sweat during a fever, and are prone to chronic respiratory infections. Symptoms are aggravated with extreme temperatures and when they are hungry, and they are improved with eating and exposure to cold air.

Calcarea carbonica: Is best for those whose problems are related to metabolism, bone, or lymphoid tissues. Patients are fatigued, have localized sweating, have discharge with an odor, experience spasms, have a hard time digesting foods and are slow, fearful, and overweight. They crave eggs, sweets, and those foods that they can't digest well. Their symptoms are worse with the full moon, cold, and dampness and are improved by dry weather.

Sycotic

Thuja occidentalis: Patient's symptoms begin after a long period of internal or external stress (i.e., vaccines, pollution, repeated stress, recurrent infections and their treatments, long lasting or over current chemotherapy). Symptoms are related to skin, lymphatic tissue, nervous system, or their urogenital tract. Symptoms may include neuralgia, cellulitis, a rumbling stomach, yellow or greenish discharge, odorous sweat, benign tumors, and depressive and obsessive ideas/tendencies. Symptoms are worse around 3:00 am and 3:00 pm, aggravated by cold and damp weather or vaccines.

Medorrhinum: Patient's symptoms were triggered by gonorrhea, antibiotics, steroids, or multiple vaccines. This homeopathic can be used when they have symptoms related to mucous membranes, like yellowish white thick irritating discharge, triggering a rash, skin issues especially where the skin merges with the mucous membranes, joints (swollen stiffness and/or sclerosed), and symptoms related to the nervous system. Other symptoms include burning localized pain on the palms, soles; or along the spinal cord, generalized itching aggravated by undressing. Patients crave alcohol, have a constant fear of getting sick, and can be depressed. Symptoms are worse during the daytime, when they think about their ailments, or in cold weather. They notice an improvement next to the water or seaside, in warm/damp weather, during sunsets, when they lay on their abdomen or in knee chest position and with constant movement.

Natrum sulphuricum: Is a helpful homeopathic if the patient's symptoms had been brought on by a result of a concussion, damp weather, or an intake of medications (specifically related to quinine). Symptoms include digestive symptoms like diarrhea or bloating, respiratory symptoms like irritation of mucous membranes with congestion, rheumatological complaints of general stiffness, dermatological issues like dry, flaky skin or cellulitis, general symptoms of depression, anxiety, or obsessions and generalized bruising. The individual is slow to process information, fatigued, irritable upon waking, overweight, and has dirty looking skin with lots of skin growths and warts. Their symptoms are improved with dry weather, after diarrhea or a soft stool, and are made worse by damp weather that could either be hot or cold.

Nitricum acidum: This homeopathic can be used after your symptoms are triggered by burnout or late nights. Symptoms that may be related to skin include induration, yellowish warts with cracks, mucous membrane symptoms accompanied with ulcerations and bleeding, oozing, cracking polyps, benign tumors, anal fissure, stinging pain, headaches, anxiety about health, and possible depressive tendencies. Their symptoms are aggravated by the cold, noise, slightest touch, and at night and are improved with slow movement and heat.

Dulcamara: Patient's symptoms may have been triggered by exposure to damp or rainy weather or subsequently after sweating or being wet. Symptoms include greenish-yellow diarrhea after getting a cold, plugged nose in the rainy or foggy weather, always feeling a need to clear the throat, enlarged lymph nodes, sensitivity to cold weather, and stiffness in the joints aggravated by dampness and improved with movement. Skin may have large warts on the back of the hands or back and feels wet and itchy accompanied with oozing rashes that feel worse by cold water and touch. Symptoms are worse with lying down at night and with damp weather and improved with movement, dry weather, heat (beside the cough), and by breathing in hot air (especially rhinitis). Patients are always thirsty.

Psoric/Sycotic

Sepia: Sepia can be used when symptoms are triggered by recurrent worries, events that occur in a woman's genital lifetime, and hormonal changes. Organs that may be affected are the circulatory system, mucous membranes, and skin with irritation and suppuration. Symptoms may include pelvic heaviness, constipation, emptiness in the epigastric, lump in the rectum, hot flashes, depressive tendencies, migraines, indigestion, menstrual herpes, lack of stamina, and being indifferent. Their symptoms are aggravated by anything that increases venous stasis, contraindication or consolation and improved by whatever improves the blood flow. They crave acid foods and vinegar and experience aversions to sight or smell of foods. These individuals have brown facial spots, dry cracked lips, brown hair, and are thin women.

Silicea: This medication can be used when symptoms are triggered by malnutrition, nutritional disorders, vaccine reactions, chronic ENT and digestive problems, repeated intake of antibiotics, and intellectual burnout. These patients have general lack of stamina, are thin, cold sensitive, have perfuse sweating, white spots on nails, decreased intellectual capacities, suppuration of chronic infections, neck and feet sweat, general hyperesthesia, and experience thorn- or splinter-like pain. They crave cold foods and experience aversions for meat. Their symptoms are worse with the new moon, inadequate vaccine shots, dampness, and in cold. Thir symptoms are improved by hot wraps, dry weather, and heat. These individuals are frail with bright eyes and frontal bone hypertrophy. They may possess cervical adenopathies and are nervous, agitated, and angry. This homeopathic can be used with the hypersensitive child.

Others: Calcarea carbonica and graphites.

Tuberculinics

Natrum muriaticum: This homeopathic is used when your symptoms are triggered by sadness, grief, emotional shock, sentimental disappointment, allergy, or loss of vital fluids. Symptoms may include tingling, burning or stinging pain of the mucous membranes, hyperventilation, fatigue, cold sensitivity, their tongue is like a geographic map, have abnormal cravings for salt, thirst and appetite disorders. These patients have oily skin, cracked upper lips, depression; they give up easily, are introverts, have problems in memory, are easily distracted, have sleep disorders, and have a thin upper body. Their symptoms worsen around 10:00 am, at the seaside, with consolation, and with sun exposure.

Sulphur: Patients will benefit from this homeopathic if they have symptoms related to their skin, mucous membranes, serous membrane, lymph nodes or have general metabolism concerns. The symptoms they experience may be exhaustion at the peak of 11:00 am; sensation of local burning pain in the nose, the anus after a stool, or feet; palpitations occur with the slightest effort; irritating discharge; cold extremities; and they crave acidic foods like lemon. Symptoms are worse with the slightest effort and with heat. Sulfur can be used in thin children and teenagers.

Tuberculinum: This homeopathic can be used with those that have symptoms triggered by bad personal hygiene and diet, debilitating disease, inadequate vaccines, and recurrent viral or bacterial aggression. Organs that may be affected are the nervous system, skin, lymphatic tissue, mucous membranes, and overall general health. Symptoms include cold sensitivity, weight loss, sweating triggered by the slightest effort, emotional instability, are thin, nervousness, hypersensitivity to cold, easily exhausted with venous congestion. Symptoms are worse with the slightest effort, and they improve by being outside in the fresh air.

HAPPY HEALTHY TUMMIES: FAST AND EASY RECIPES (THAT HEAL TOO . . . SHHHH)

Eating healthy can be delicious and fast! Remember to follow the list to optimize health and lower inflammation: 1. Veggies; 2. Clean Protein; and 3. Healthy Fat. Stay hydrated with water and bone broth. Following are some hits in my house. I like to keep it simple, turning one base recipe into whatever my heart desires! It's so much fun!!!! If you have food sensitivities, I have laid out tips at the end of this section on how you can adjust the recipe.

Breakfast

Vanilla Chia Pudding

Ingredients:

- ¾ cup nondairy milk of choice
- 1 tsp vanilla extract
- 3–4 tbsp chia seeds
- Stevia or honey to taste

Directions:

1. Mix together ingredients in a ceramic dish or mason jar.
2. Refrigerate for at least six hours.
3. Enjoy!

Can top with berries or dairy-free dark chocolate chips.

Nut/Seed Porridge

Ingredients:

- ½ cup sunflower seeds
- ½ cup pecans
- ½ cup walnuts
- 5 dates
- 1 can coconut milk
- Stevia to taste
- 2 cups nondairy milk of choice
- Coconut flakes (optional)

Directions:

1. Finely chop nuts and seeds along with coconut milk in a food processer.
2. Add dates to mixture and blend.
3. Transfer mixture to a ceramic skillet on mild heat.
4. Add nondairy milk of choice and bring to a boil.
5. Add coconut flakes for garnish.

No-Grain Cereal

Ingredients:

- ½ cup raw sunflower seeds
- ½ cup flax seeds
- ½ cup pumpkin seeds
- ½ cup unsweetened coconut flakes
- ½ cup cashew pieces
- ½ cup slivered almonds
- 2 tbsp coconut oil
- Stevia, cinnamon, and vanilla

Directions:

1. Mix all the ingredients together in a bowl.
2. Add stevia, cinnamon, and vanilla to taste.
3. Bake at 325°F until golden.

This recipe is great for kids with dairy and egg allergies, and can be tailored for nut allergies by simply taking out the nuts. For a quick breakfast or meal: my kids love this cereal with almond milk or coconut cream or topped on top of homemade raw yogurt with fresh berries (and dark chocolate chips if they are being extra good). The cereal also can be mixed with dried apples and cinnamon or blueberries, cherries, or other berries.

Green "Hulk" Smoothie

Ingredients:

- Base: water or nondairy milk of choice
- 1 cup low-glycemic fruits
- 2–3 cups greens
- ½ avocado
- Stevia to taste
- ½ cucumber
- Ice
- Protein: hemp, egg white, pea protein powder, or gelatin
- Additional: glutamine powder

Directions:

Blend and enjoy.

Blueberry Waffles

Ingredients:

- 1½ cups almond flour
- 4 large eggs
- ¼ tsp baking soda
- ¼ tsp salt
- 2 ripe bananas, mashed
- ½ cup blueberries
- Coconut oil spray

Directions:

1. Plug in/preheat your waffle iron.
2. While that heats up, mix everything together.
3. Once the waffle iron is warm, spray on coconut oil to the waffle iron plate.
4. Pour the waffle batter onto the plate.
5. Close the waffle iron and allow it to thoroughly cook.
6. Once done (usually when the light turns on), take off the plate and enjoy! My kids love it with a drizzle of honey and/or butter.

This is my FAVORITE recipe, because it is SOOOO easy and delicious! Best yet, I can change it regularly to what my family is in the mood for, as I have made jelly cakes and blueberry muffins with this same recipe!!

Turmeric Eggs

Ingredients:

- One onion, sliced thin
- 3 tomatoes chopped
- 1 tbsp ghee
- ¼ tsp salt
- ¼ tsp turmeric
- ¼ tsp black powder
- ¼ tsp paprika
- 5–6 eggs
- Cilantro as garnish

Directions:

1. Sauté onions and tomatoes in ghee until soft.
2. Add in spices, adjust as needed.
3. Add in eggs, but don't touch them until they start to cook. Cover.
4. When they look like they are almost done cooking, stir.
5. Enjoy.

Lunch/Dinner

Mushroom Burger

Ingredients:

- 2 lbs grass-fed ground beef
- Salt and pepper to taste
- 3 portobello mushrooms or red peppers, diced
- Half an onion, diced
- ½ tsp garlic
- Fresh cilantro

Directions:

1. Mix together.
2. Form into patties.
3. Brown on a skillet with ghee.

My kids love lettuce-wrapped burgers! Serve with sweet potato fries (may not be appropriate for someone following a yeast-free diet plan).

Thai Soup with Healing Bone Broth

Bone Broth Ingredients

- 2 lbs (or more) bones from a healthy source
- Kosher salt and freshly ground black pepper, to taste
- 2 cloves garlic, minced
- 1 onion, diced
- 6 cups water to yield four cups of broth
- A large stockpot to cook the broth in
- Strainer to remove the pieces

Thai Soup Ingredients

- 2 tbsp unsalted butter
- 1 lb medium shrimp, peeled and deveined
- 1 can mushrooms
- 1 tbsp ginger
- ¼ tsp paprika
- 2 (12-ounce) cans unsweetened coconut milk
- Juice of 1 lime
- 2 tbsp chopped fresh cilantro leaves

Bone Broth Directions:

1. Place the bones in a large stock pot.
2. Pour water over the bones.
3. Add onion and garlic.
4. Boil for three to eight hours (or more if tolerated).
5. Remove bones with fine metal strainer.

Thai Soup Directions:

1. Melt butter (or oil of choice) in a large stockpot over medium high heat.
2. Add onions in butter until soft.
3. Add shrimp, salt, ginger, and pepper, to taste. Cook until pink.

4. Add garlic, onion, mushrooms, and bell pepper to the stockpot.
5. Gradually stir coconut milk and bone stock, mix until incorporated.
6. Bring to a boil; reduce heat to simmer until soup starts to thicken.
7. Stir in shrimp, lime juice, and cilantro.
8. Enjoy! Feel the healthy powder!

Broccoli Slaw

Ingredients:

- One package broccoli slaw
- ½ cup all natural mayo or olive oil
- ¼ tsp pepper
- 1 tsp honey

Directions:

Mix all the ingredients together.

Basic Cauliflower Rice

Ingredients:

- One package frozen cooked diced cauliflower rice, thawed
- Salt
- Pepper
- Oil of your choice

Directions:

1. Heat oil in pan.
2. Add in cauliflower rice.
3. Add spices to taste and sauté as normal.

This "rice" can be made into all rice dishes. Simply replace the rice for this, and spice and sautee as you would do for those dishes.

Sesame French Cut Green Beans

Ingredients:

- 1 lb green beans
- 1 tsp coconut amines
- ¼ tsp salt
- ¼ tsp garlic
- 2 tsp ghee
- ¼ tsp black pepper
- ¼ tsp Italian seasoning
- ¼ tsp sesame seeds or roasted almonds

Directions:

Mix together and cook in skillet until done.

Mom's Famous Fried Chicken

Ingredients:

- Juice of 1 lemon
- ¼ tsp crushed red pepper
- ¼ tsp cumin
- 1 tsp garlic
- ½ tsp salt
- 4 tbsp chickpea flour and extra for dry coating
- 2 eggs
- ¼ tsp baking powder
- 2 lbs chicken thighs cut in half

Directions:

1. Mix ingredients together (except the baking powder, which is to be added one-half hour before cooking) and leave for two hours.
2. Coat with dry chickpea flour.
3. Fry in oil.

Use the same method for coating fish and shrimp. Great treat!

Stuffed Paratha (Flatbread)

Ingredients:

- ½ cup almond flour
- ½ cup tapioca
- 1 cup canned full fat coconut milk
- One cup already prepared ground beef
- Butter or coconut oil for frying
- Spices to taste (garlic, onion powder, salt, pepper, turmeric, etc.)

Directions:

1. Mix almond flour, tapioca, and coconut milk together into a thin batter.
2. In the fry pan, add a teaspoon of butter/coconut oil.
3. Add a small ladle of mixture to the pan.
4. Thin out like a pancake.
5. When one side starts to firm up, add in two tablespoons ground beef.
6. Add another layer of batter to cover all the ground beef.
7. Flip.
8. Allow both sides to cook on low heat. Enjoy!

The stuffing in this recipe can vary according to your preferences, and can be turned into desserts if filled with apples and cinnamon or other fruits.

Grape Leaf Wrapped Salmon

Ingredients:

- 10 grape leaves, jarred or fresh
- 1 tbsp chopped dill
- 1 tsp garlic and ginger paste
- ½ tsp salt
- 1 tsp paprika
- ½ tsp chili pepper (optional)
- 5 salmon fillets (4 ounce)

Directions:

1. Preheat oven to 400°F.
2. Wash grape leaves, if using all natural jarred; or if using fresh boil for five to six minutes until it softens.
3. Mix rest of the ingredients together.
4. Lay two grape leaves out.
5. Add two teaspoons of the mixture to the middle of the grape leaves.
6. Lay salmon on top of the leaves and spices.
7. Fold and roll the fish until it is completely covered by the leaves.
8. Bake for fifteen to twenty minutes depending on the thickness of the steaks.
9. Serve hot on top of cauliflower dill rice! My mouth is watering!

Yellow Anti-inflammatory Chicken

Ingredients:

- 2 lbs chicken cut up into 1-inch pieces
- 1 tsp turmeric
- ½ teaspoon salt
- ¼ tsp black pepper
- Juice of one lemon
- ¼ tsp cumin
- 1 tsp garlic paste
- 1 tsp ginger paste
- 1 small diced tomato (optional)
- ¼ cup oil

Directions:

1. Heat oil in a skillet.
2. Mix ginger, garlic for one minute and add rest (except the tomato) on high heat.
3. Five to six minutes before the chicken looks done, add the tomatoes.
4. Then cover till water evaporates.
5. Yum!

DESSERT

Chewy Coconut Cookie

Ingredients:

- 1⅓ cup almond flour
- 2 tbsp finely shredded coconut, unsweetened
- ¼ cup coconut oil
- ⅓ cup maple syrup or honey
- ½ tsp baking soda
- ⅛ tsp salt

Directions:

1. Mix all ingredients in a bowl. This is a crumbly mixture, but does stick together.
2. Roll into balls.
3. Line on a cookie sheet.
4. Slightly flatten/form the batter to form a cookie.
5. Bake them at 325°F for fifteen to twenty minutes. Make sure you watch them and take out when golden brown.
6. Don't touch until cool.

Can use base recipe and make a lemon cookie (with lemon zest and lemon extract), with chocolate chips or just nuts.

Chocolate Swirl Cake

Ingredients:

- ½ cup almond flour
- 3 eggs
- 2 tbsp honey
- Squeeze of lemon
- ½ tsp baking soda
- ¼ tbsp nondairy milk
- Unsweetened raw cacao powder (for chocolate swirl)

Directions:

1. Mix ingredients together except the cacao powder.
2. Poor into oiled cake pan.
3. Leave a couple tablespoons of batter in the bowl and mix in the cacao powder.
4. Add a couple spots of cacao powder batter to the cake horizontally.
5. Use the end of a spoon to gently make a swirl.
6. Bake at 350°F for fifteen minutes or until cake is done (knife comes out clean in center).

Use this as the base of all your cakes, add apples (with cinnamon swirl), lemon, orange, nuts, chocolate chips or anything to change up the cake.

Apple Cinnamon Cake

Ingredients:

- ½ cup honey
- ½ cup grass-fed butter
- 3 eggs
- 1 tsp baking soda
- 1 tsp salt
- 1½ cups almond flour
- 2 apples, diced
- ½ tsp cinnamon

Directions:

1. Mix all ingredients together.
2. Pour into baking sheet lined with unbleached parchment paper.
3. Bake at 350°F for twenty minutes or until knife comes out clean.

Healing Brownies

Ingredients:

- ⅔ cup honey
- 1 cup nut flour
- 3 eggs
- ½ cup cocoa unsweetened, raw
- ½ cup butter
- ¼ tsp baking soda
- ¼ tsp salt (if butter is unsalted)
- ½ cup walnuts or pecans

Directions:

1. Mix together and bake at 350°F until knife comes out clean.
2. Add puréed/whole raspberries or strawberries and shredded coconut flakes for garnish.

Creamy Coconut with Fruit

Ingredients:

- One can coconut milk
- ½ cup blueberries or strawberries
- Nuts or seeds to top
- Stevia to taste

Directions:

Mix together and enjoy!

Chocolate Chip Cookies

Ingredients:

- 3 cups almond flour
- ½ cup nut butter
- ½ cup honey or maple syrup
- 1 tbsp salt
- 1 tbsp baking soda
- 3 eggs
- Dairy-free dark chocolate chips

Directions:

1. Mix ingredients together.
2. Roll into balls.
3. Place on greased cookie sheet.
4. Bake at 350°F for ten to fifteen minutes or until golden.

Can add walnuts, figs, raisins, or any other add-in to make a new cookie! If in a rush, I add two extra eggs and put it all in a pan for cookie bars! Adding raisins and cinnamon and using almond butter makes delicious raisin cookies!

Lemon Poppy Muffins

Ingredients:

- ½ cups almond flour
- 1 tsp baking soda
- 3 tbsn coconut flour
- ¼ tsp salt
- ⅓ cup coconut milk
- ⅓ cup honey or maple syrup
- 2 lemons
- Zest from 2 lemons
- 3 eggs
- 2 tbsp coconut oil
- 2 tbsp poppy seeds

Directions:

1. Mix together.
2. Place in lined minimuffin bakeware.
3. Bake at 350°F for fifteen minutes or until knife comes out clean.

Drinks

- Filtered water (try adding wedges of orange, cucumber, mint to the water to help add extra flavors)
- Carbonated water
- Green tea
- Soups with bone broth

Lemonade

Ingredients:

- Water
- Lemon
- Stevia

Directions:

Mix to taste and drink.

Dairy-free nut milks

Ingredients:

- 1 cup almonds, cashews, hazelnuts, or pecans
- 2 cups water
- 1 date
- Pinch of sea salt
- Vanilla
- cheese cloth

Directions:

1. Place nuts in a large bowl; cover with cold water.
2. Stand, covered for four hours or overnight.
3. Rinse the nuts under cold water and drain.
4. In a blender, blend all ingredients.
5. Strain milk through a cheesecloth.
6. Squeeze all remaining milk from almond pulp.

For Allergies/Sensitivities

Nut flours can be switched easily. I have had patients switch nut flours for seed flours (use raw sunflower or pumpkin seeds) with success. Nut flours and coconut flour cannot easily be swapped. Milks can be swapped.

For egg allergy, flax "egg" can be used in those recipes calling for just one or two flax eggs.

Ingredients (equivalent to one egg)

- 1 tsp ground flax or chia seeds
- 3 tbsp water

Directions

1. Stir together until well combined.
2. Place in the refrigerator for fifteen minutes.
3. Use in place of eggs.

I hope you enjoyed these recipes (is your mouth watering, like mine is?)! Stay connected on social media and my website (HolisticMom, MD, www.holis ticmommd.com) as we continue to share easy tips and recipes that you can incorporate in your busy lifestyle to help gain optimal health and happiness!

SELECTED CONTRAINDICATIONS/ CAUTIONS/INTERACTIONS/SIDE EFFECTS

- *Ashwagandha:* Caution in pregnancy (has been reported to have abortifacient properties), don't use in congestion, can exacerbate barbiturates effects, can lead to GI distress in children.
- *Astragalus:* Not recommended in severe congestion, overactive immune system or extreme tension, fever, inflammation, severe dryness, hot skin lesions, or onset of the cold/flu symptoms.
- *Black Cohosh:* Avoid in pregnancy, heart conditions; and it can lead to digestive distress like nausea, vomiting, or irritating the nervous system (headaches and low blood pressure) if used in excess. It can be used in estrogen-dependent tumors, fibrocystic disease, pancreatitis, gallbladder disease, endometriosis, and uterine bleeding.
- *Chamomile:* Avoid use in those who have a sensitivity to ragweed, or who may be severely allergic to chamomile. Avoid therapeutic doses

during pregnancy. It may lead to contact dermatitis (Roman more than German).

- *Dandelion:* Few cases may report digestive symptoms like nausea, heartburn, diarrhea, abdominal discomfort (an allergic reaction), and fresh latex of plant.
- *Ginger:* Avoid in cases of peptic ulcers, hyperacidity; avoid excessive amounts in herpes, eczema, and acne.
- *Lavender:* Avoid large doses in pregnancy.
- *Licorice:* Avoid in cases of edema, nausea, vomiting, and rapid heart beat, pregnancy, if taking steroid or digoxin. Prolonged use may lead to sodium retention, depletion of potassium, headaches, and vertigo. Don't take for longer than six weeks.
- *Milk thistle:* Can lead to digestive complaints like bloating or diarrhea.
- *St. John's wort:* Don't combine with other antidepressant medications, protease inhibitors, or organ antirejection drugs. Not recommended for children under two, during pregnancy or nursing. May cause photosensitivity, nausea, or dizziness.
- *Valerian:* Large doses can cause fatigue, nausea, headaches, depression, or a stimulating effect. Avoid in pregnancy. Don't give to children under three. Avoid in cases of low sugar or blood pressure.
- *Vitamin A:* Cautioned in pregnant women.
- *B12:* Should be avoided with Leber's disease.
- *Vitamin C:* Do not take vitamin C when you are going to have lab tests.
- *Vitamin D:* Caution, if you have hyperparathyroidism; Hodgkin's or non-Hodgkin's lymphoma; granulomatous disease, like sarcoidosis and tuberculosis; kidney stone; kidney disease; or liver disease.
- *Coenzyme Q10:* May reduce effectiveness of blood thinning medications. Doses up to 2,400 mg per day have been well tolerated. Some note heartburn, digestive upset, and headaches with doses more than 600 mg per day.
- *Glucosamine and chondroitin:* Caution if severely allergic to shellfish. Chondroitin is made from bovine cartilage, so vegetarians, be cautioned.
- *Alpha lipoic acid:* Doses up to 2,400 mg per day have not been shown to have any serious adverse effects.
- *Choline:* No drug interactions; do not exceed the upper limit of 3,500 mg per day.
- *SAMe:* Don't take it if taking an antidepressant medication and levodopa as it may lead to serotonin syndrome.

MEDICAL DISCLAIMER: Information here is provided for informational purposes only. Please see a medical professional before applying any recommendations.

Notes

INTRODUCTION

1. "Multiple Chronic Conditions," Centers for Disease Control and Prevention. January 20, 2016. Accessed January 9, 2017. http://www.cdc.gov/chronicdisease/about/multiple-chronic.htm.

CHAPTER 1. UNDERSTANDING THE SILENT FIRE WITHIN: THE ROLE OF INFLAMMATION IN CHRONIC ILLNESS

1. Husain, Awal Al, and Ian N. Bruce. "Risk Factors for Coronary Heart Disease in Connective Tissue Diseases." *Therapeutic Advances in Musculoskeletal Disease,* June 2010. Accessed January 9, 2017. https://www.ncbi.nlm.nih.gov/pmc/articles/PMC3382674/.

2. Centers for Disease Control and Prevention. Accessed January 5, 2017. http://www.cdc.gov/nccdphp/overview.htm.

3. Centers for Disease Control and Prevention. November 14, 2016. Accessed January 9, 2017. http://www.cdc.gov/chronicdisease/.

4. Anderson, Gerard. *Chronic Conditions: Making the Case for Ongoing Care*. Baltimore, MD: Johns Hopkins University, November 2007. http://www.fightchronicdisease.com/news/pfcd/pr12102007.cfm.

5. "One in Three Kids Will Develop Diabetes." WebMD. Accessed January 9, 2017. http://www.webmd.com/diabetes/news/20030616/one-in-three-kids-will-develop-diabetes#1.

6. Egger, G. "In Search of a Germ Theory Equivalent for Chronic Disease." *Preventing Chronic Disease*, May 2012. doi:10.5888/pcd9.110301.

7. Kruger, Monika, Philipp Schledorn, Wieland Schrodl, Hans-Wolfgang Hoppe, Walburga Lutz, and Awad A. Shehata. "Detection of Glyphosate Residue in Animals and Humans." *Environmental & Analytical Toxicology*, 2014. Accessed January 9, 2017.

https://www.omicsonline.org/open-access/detection-of-glyphosate-residues-in-animals-and-humans-2161-0525.1000210.pdf.

8. Woodyard, Catherine. "Exploring the Therapeutic Effects of Yoga and Its Ability to Increase Quality of Life." *International Journal of Yoga,* 2011. Accessed January 9, 2017. http://www.ncbi.nlm.nih.gov/pmc/articles/PMC3193654/.

9. "Inflammation, Pain, and Chronic Disease: An Integrative Approach to Treatment and Prevention." National Center for Biotechnology Information. Accessed January 9, 2017. http://www.ncbi.nlm.nih.gov/m/pubmed/16320856/.

10. Kiecolt-Glaser, Janice K. "Stress, Food, and Inflammation: Psychoneuroimmunology and Nutrition at the Cutting Edge." *Psychosomatic Medicine.* May 2010. Accessed January 9, 2017. http://www.ncbi.nlm.nih.gov/pmc/articles/PMC2868080/.

11. Coleab, Steven W., John P. Capitanio, Katie Chun, Jesusa M. G. Arevaloa, and Jeffrey Maab And. "Steven W. Cole." *Proceedings of the National Academy of Sciences.* Accessed January 9, 2017. http://www.pnas.org/content/early/2015/11/18/1514249112.abstract?sid=90997c16-880d-4069-8968-67c6122e1554.

12. Woodyard, Catherine. "Exploring the Therapeutic Effects of Yoga and Its Ability to Increase Quality of Life." *International Journal of Yoga,* 2011. Accessed January 9, 2017. http://www.ncbi.nlm.nih.gov/pmc/articles/PMC3193654/.

CHAPTER 2. DIGESTIVE HEALTH AND DETOXIFICATION

Notes: Digestion

1. "Inflammation: Maintaining the Mucosal Barrier in Intestinal Inflammation." Nature Reviews. *Gastroenterology & Hepatology.* Accessed January 9, 2017. http://www.ncbi.nlm.nih.gov/pubmed/26701373.

2. Hadhazy, Adam. "Think Twice: How the Gut's 'Second Brain' Influences Mood and Well-Being." *Scientific American.* February 11, 2010. Accessed January 9, 2017. https://www.scientificamerican.com/article/gut-second-brain/.

3. "NIH Human Microbiome Project Defines Normal Bacterial Makeup of the Body." National Institutes of Health News Reviews. June 13, 2012. Accessed January 9, 2017. https://www.nih.gov/news-events/news-releases/nih-human-microbiome-project-defines-normal-bacterial-makeup-body.

4. "The Anxiolytic Effect of Bifidobacterium Longum NCC3001 Involves Vagal Pathways for Gut-brain Communication." *Neurogastroenterology and Motility: The Official Journal of the European Gastrointestinal Motility Society.* Accessed January 9, 2017. http://www.ncbi.nlm.nih.gov/pubmed/21988661.

5. Martín, Rebeca, Sylvie Miquel, Jonathan Ulmer, Noura Kechaou, Philippe Langella, and Luis G. Bermúdez-Humarán. "Role of Commensal and Probiotic Bacteria in Human Health: A Focus on Inflammatory Bowel Disease." *Microbial Cell Factories* 12, no. 1 (2013): 71. doi:10.1186/1475-2859-12-71.

6. http://www.facebook.com/drjoshaxe. "Probiotics Benefits, Foods and Supplements." Dr. Axe. December 22, 2016. Accessed January 9, 2017. http://draxe.com/probiotics-benefits-foods-supplements.

7. Le Chatelier, E., et al. "Richness of human gut microbiome correlates with/ metabolic markers." *Nature*. August 29, 2013; 500 (7464): 541–46.

8. http://advances.sciencemag.org/content/1/3/e1500183.

9. "[Role of Intestinal Flora in Health and Disease]." *Nutricion Hospitalaria*. Accessed January 9, 2017. http://www.ncbi.nlm.nih.gov/pubmed/17679289.

10. Aagaard, K. M. "Author Response to Comment on 'The Placenta Harbors a Unique Microbiome.'" *Science Translational Medicine* 6, no. 254 (September 2014). doi:10.1126/scitranslmed.3010007.

11. "Your Changing Microbiome." *Your Changing Microbiome*. Accessed January 9, 2017. http://learn.genetics.utah.edu/content/microbiome/changing/.

12. "The Role of Intestinal Microbiota and the Immune System." *European Review for Medical and Pharmacological Sciences*. Accessed January 9, 2017. http://www.ncbi.nlm.nih.gov/pubmed/23426535.

13. "Leaky Gut." Nursing Standard (Royal College of Nursing [Great Britain]: 1987). Accessed January 9, 2017. http://www.ncbi.nlm.nih.gov/pubmed/27317075.

14. Arrieta, M. C., L. Bistritz, and J. B. Meddings. "Alterations in Intestinal Permeability." *Gut*. October 2006. Accessed January 5, 2017. http://www.ncbi.nlm.nih.gov/pmc/articles/PMC1856434/.

15. Bischoff, Stephan C., Giovanni Barbara, Wim Buurman, Theo Ockhuizen, Jörg-Dieter Schulzke, Matteo Serino, Herbert Tilg, Alastair Watson, and Jerry M. Wells. "Intestinal Permeability—A New Target for Disease Prevention and Therapy." *BMC Gastroenterology*. 2014. Accessed January 9, 2017. http://www.ncbi.nlm.nih.gov/pmc/articles/PMC4253991/.

16. Ibid.

17. "[Physiological Patterns of Intestinal Microbiota. The Role of Dysbacteriosis in Obesity, Insulin Resistance, Diabetes and Metabolic Syndrome]." *Orvosi Hetilap*. Accessed January 9, 2017. http://www.ncbi.nlm.nih.gov/pubmed/26708682.

18. "Regulation of Intestinal Epithelial Permeability by Tight Junctions." *Cellular and Molecular Life Sciences: CMLS*. Accessed January 9, 2017. http://www.ncbi.nlm.nih.gov/pubmed/22782113.

19. "Maternal Immune Activation and Abnormal Brain Development across CNS Disorders." *Nature Reviews. Neurology*. Accessed January 9, 2017. http://www.ncbi.nlm.nih.gov/pubmed/25311587.

20. "Maternal Inflammation Promotes Fetal Microglial Activation and Increased Cholinergic Expression in the Fetal Basal Forebrain: Role of Interleukin-6." *Pediatric Research*. Accessed January 9, 2017. http://www.ncbi.nlm.nih.gov/pubmed/23877071.

21. Wang, Wen Le. "Zonula Occludin Toxin, a Microtubule Binding Protein." *World Journal of Gastroenterology* 6, no. 3 (2000): 330. doi:10.3748/wjg.v6.i3.330.

22. Fasano, A. "Zonulin and Its Regulation of Intestinal Barrier Function: The Biological Door to Inflammation, Autoimmunity, and Cancer." *Physiological Reviews* 91, no. 1 (January 2011): 151–75. doi:10.1152/physrev.00003.2008.

23. Fasano, Alessio. "Intestinal Permeability and Its Regulation by Zonulin: Diagnostic and Therapeutic Implications." *Clinical Gastroenterology and Hepatology* 10, no. 10 (October 2012): 1096–100. doi:10.1016/j.cgh.2012.08.012.

24. "Children and Toxic Chemicals." Mount Sinai Hospital. Accessed January 9, 2017. http://www.mountsinai.org/patient-care/service-areas/children/areas-of-care/childrens-environmental-health-center/childrens-disease-and-the-environment/children-and-toxic-chemicals.

25. Dethlefsen, L., and D. A. Relman. "Incomplete Recovery and Individualized Responses of the Human Distal Gut Microbiota to Repeated Antibiotic Perturbation." *Proceedings of the National Academy of Sciences* 108, no. Supplement_1 (September 2010): 4554–561. doi:10.1073/pnas.1000087107.

26. "Exercise, Intestinal Barrier Dysfunction and Probiotic Supplementation." *Medicine and Sport Science.* Accessed January 5, 2017. http://www.ncbi.nlm.nih.gov/pubmed/23075554.

27. Campbell, Andrew W. "Autoimmunity and the Gut." Autoimmune Diseases. Accessed January 9, 2017. https://www.ncbi.nlm.nih.gov/pmc/articles/PMC4036413/.

28. Arrieta, M. C., L. Bistritz, and J. B. Meddings. "Alterations in Intestinal Permeability." *Gut.* October 2006. Accessed January 9, 2017. https://www.ncbi.nlm.nih.gov/pmc/articles/PMC1856434/.

29. Bardella, Maria Teresa, Luca Elli, Sara De Matteis, Irene Floriani, Valter Torri, and Luca Piodi. "Autoimmune Disorders in Patients Affected by Celiac Sprue and Inflammatory Bowel Disease." *Annals of Medicine* 41, no. 2 (January 2009): 139–43. doi:10.1080/07853890802378817.

30. Camilleri, M., K. Madsen, R. Spiller, B. G. Van Meerveld, and G. N. Verne. "Intestinal Barrier Function in Health and Gastrointestinal Disease." *Neurogastroenterology & Motility* 24, no. 6 (May 2012): 503–12. doi:10.1111/j.1365-2982.2012.01921.x.

31. Fresko, I. "Intestinal Permeability in Behcet's Syndrome." *Annals of the Rheumatic Diseases* 60, no. 1 (January 2001): 65–66. doi:10.1136/ard.60.1.65.

32. Nouri, Mehrnaz, Anders Bredberg, Björn Weström, and Shahram Lavasani. "Intestinal Barrier Dysfunction Develops at the Onset of Experimental Autoimmune Encephalomyelitis, and Can Be Induced by Adoptive Transfer of Auto-Reactive T Cells." *PLoS ONE* 9, no. 9 (September 2014). doi:10.1371/journal.pone.0106335.

33. "Rheumatoid Arthritis-Celiac Disease Relationship: Joints Get That Gut Feeling." Autoimmunity Reviews. Accessed January 9, 2017. https://www.ncbi.nlm.nih.gov/pubmed/26190704.

34. PA, Jose, D, Raj. "Gut Microbiota in Hypertension." *Curr Opin Nehrol Hyperten* 2015; September 24 (5): 403–9. doi: 10.1097/MNH.0000000000000149. https://www.ncbi.nlm.nih.gov/pubmed/26125644.

35. Bischoff, Stephan C., Giovanni Barbara, Wim Buurman, Theo Ockhuizen, Jörg-Dieter Schulzke, Matteo Serino, Herbert Tilg, Alastair Watson, and Jerry M. Wells. "Intestinal Permeability—A New Target for Disease Prevention and Therapy." *BMC Gastroenterology.* 2014. Accessed January 9, 2017. https://www.ncbi.nlm.nih.gov/pmc/articles/PMC4253991/.

36. Pike, Michael G., Robert J. Heddle, Peter Boulton, Malcolm W. Turner, and David J. Atherton. "Increased Intestinal Permeability in Atopic Eczema." *Journal of Investigative Dermatology* 86, no. 2 (February 1986): 101–4. doi:10.1111/1523-1747.ep12284035.

37. Bischoff, Stephan C., Giovanni Barbara, Wim Buurman, Theo Ockhuizen, Jörg-Dieter Schulzke, Matteo Serino, Herbert Tilg, Alastair Watson, and Jerry M. Wells. "Intestinal Permeability—A New Target for Disease Prevention and Therapy." *BMC Gastroenterology*. 2014. Accessed January 9, 2017. https://www.ncbi.nlm.nih.gov/pmc/articles/PMC4253991/.

38. "Gut Microbiota and Obesity." Cellular and Molecular Life Sciences: CMLS. Accessed January 9, 2017. http://www.ncbi.nlm.nih.gov/pbmed/26459447/.

39. Li, Xia, and Mark A. Atkinson. "The Role for Gut Permeability in the Pathogenesis of Type 1 Diabetes—A Solid or Leaky Concept?" *Pediatric Diabetes* 16, no. 7 (August 2015): 485–92. doi:10.1111/pedi.12305.

40. Vaarala, O., M. A. Atkinson, and J. Neu. "The 'Perfect Storm' for Type 1 Diabetes: The Complex Interplay between Intestinal Microbiota, Gut Permeability, and Mucosal Immunity." *Diabetes* 57, no. 10 (September 2008): 2555–562. doi:10.2337/db08-0331.

41. Gomes, J. M. G., J. A. Costa, and R. C. Alfenas. "Could the Beneficial Effects of Dietary Calcium on Obesity and Diabetes Control Be Mediated by Changes in Intestinal Microbiota and Integrity?" *British Journal of Nutrition* 114, no. 11 (September 2015): 1756–765. doi:10.1017/s0007114515003608.

42. Merga, Yvette, Barry J. Campbell, and Jonathan M. Rhodes. "Mucosal Barrier, Bacteria and Inflammatory Bowel Disease: Possibilities for Therapy." *Digestive Diseases* 32, no. 4 (2014): 475–83. doi:10.1159/000358156.

43. Prager, Matthias, Janine Buettner, and Carsten Buening. "Genes Involved in the Regulation of Intestinal Permeability and Their Role in Ulcerative Colitis." *Journal of Digestive Diseases* 16, no. 12 (December 2015): 713–22. doi:10.1111/1751-2980.12296.

44. "New and Emerging Treatment Options for Irritable Bowel Syndrome." *Gastroenterology & Hepatology*. Accessed January 9, 2017. https://www.ncbi.nlm.nih.gov/pubmed/26491416.

45. Camilleri, M., K. Madsen, R. Spiller, B. G. Van Meerveld, and G. N. Verne. "Intestinal Barrier Function in Health and Gastrointestinal Disease." *Neurogastroenterology & Motility* 24, no. 6 (May 2012): 503–12. doi:10.1111/j.1365-2982.2012.01921.x.

46. Bischoff, Stephan C., Giovanni Barbara, Wim Buurman, Theo Ockhuizen, Jörg-Dieter Schulzke, Matteo Serino, Herbert Tilg, Alastair Watson, and Jerry M. Wells. "Intestinal Permeability—A New Target for Disease Prevention and Therapy." *BMC Gastroenterology*. 2014. Accessed January 9, 2017. https://www.ncbi.nlm.nih.gov/pmc/articles/PMC4253991/.

47. "Role of Gut Microbiota in Liver Disease." *Journal of Clinical Gastroenterology*. Accessed January 9, 2017. https://www.ncbi.nlm.nih.gov/pubmed/26447960.

48. Nature.com. Accessed January 9, 2017. http://www.nature.com/pr/journal/v39/n6/full/pr19962558a.html.

49. Mosci, Paolo, Elena Gabrielli, Eugenio Luciano, Stefano Perito, Antonio Cassone, Eva Pericolini, and Anna Vecchiarelli. "Involvement of IL-17A in Preventing the Development of Deep-seated Candidiasis from Oropharyngeal Infection." *Microbes and Infection* 16, no. 8 (August 2014): 678–89. doi:10.1016/j.micinf.2014.06.007.

50. Zhang, D., L. Zhang, F. Yue, Y. Zheng, and R. Russell. "Serum Zonulin Is Elevated in Women with Polycystic Ovary Syndrome and Correlates with Insulin

Resistance and Severity of Anovulation." *European Journal of Endocrinology* 172, no. 1 (October 2014): 29–36. doi:10.1530/eje-14-0589.

51. "Leaky Intestine and Impaired Microbiome in an Amyotrophic Lateral Sclerosis Mouse Model." *Physiological Reports*. Accessed January 9, 2017. https://www.ncbi.nlm.nih.gov/pubmed/25847918.

52. Bekkering, Pjotr, Ismael Jafri, Frans J. Van Overveld, and Ger T. Rijkers. "The Intricate Association between Gut Microbiota and Development of Type 1, Type 2 and Type 3 Diabetes." *Expert Review of Clinical Immunology* 9, no. 11 (November 2013): 1031–41. doi:10.1586/1744666x.2013.848793.

53. Roos, N. M. De, C. G. T. Giezenaar, J. M. P. Rovers, B. J. M. Witteman, M. G. Smits, and S. Van Hemert. "The Effects of the Multispecies Probiotic Mixture Ecologic®Barrier on Migraine: Results of an Open-Label Pilot Study." *Beneficial Microbes* 6, no. 5 (October 2015): 641–46. doi:10.3920/bm2015.0003.

54. Forsyth, Christopher B., Kathleen M. Shannon, Jeffrey H. Kordower, Robin M. Voigt, Maliha Shaikh, Jean A. Jaglin, Jacob D. Estes, Hemraj B. Dodiya, and Ali Keshavarzian. "Increased Intestinal Permeability Correlates with Sigmoid Mucosa Alpha-Synuclein Staining and Endotoxin Exposure Markers in Early Parkinson's Disease." *PLoS ONE* 6, no. 12 (December 2011). doi:10.1371/journal.pone.0028032.

55. Bischoff, Stephan C., Giovanni Barbara, Wim Buurman, Theo Ockhuizen, Jörg-Dieter Schulzke, Matteo Serino, Herbert Tilg, Alastair Watson, and Jerry M. Wells. "Intestinal Permeability—A New Target for Disease Prevention and Therapy." *BMC Gastroenterology*. 2014. Accessed January 9, 2017. https://www.ncbi.nlm.nih.gov/pmc/articles/PMC4253991/.

56. Leclercq, Sophie, Sébastien Matamoros, Patrice D. Cani, Audrey M. Neyrinck, François Jamar, Peter Stärkel, Karen Windey, Valentina Tremaroli, Fredrik Bäckhed, Kristin Verbeke, Philippe De Timary, and Nathalie M. Delzenne. "Intestinal Permeability, Gut-Bacterial Dysbiosis, and Behavioral Markers of Alcohol-Dependence Severity." Proceedings of the National Academy of Sciences of the United States of America. October 21, 2014. Accessed January 9, 2017. https://www.ncbi.nlm.nih.gov/pmc/articles/PMC4210345/.

57. Kelly, John R., Paul J. Kennedy, John F. Cryan, Timothy G. Dinan, Gerard Clarke, and Niall P. Hyland. "Breaking Down the Barriers: The Gut Microbiome, Intestinal Permeability and Stress-Related Psychiatric Disorders." *Frontiers in Cellular Neuroscience* 9 (October 2015). doi:10.3389/fncel.2015.00392.

58. Vojdani, Aristo. "Immune Reactivity against Food Proteomes." *Journal of Food Processing & Technology* 6, no. 7 (2015). doi:10.4172/2157-7110.s1.019.

59. Bischoff, Stephan C., Giovanni Barbara, Wim Buurman, Theo Ockhuizen, Jörg-Dieter Schulzke, Matteo Serino, Herbert Tilg, Alastair Watson, and Jerry M. Wells. "Intestinal Permeability—A New Target for Disease Prevention and Therapy." *BMC Gastroenterology*. 2014. Accessed January 9, 2017. https://www.ncbi.nlm.nih.gov/pmc/articles/PMC4253991/.

60. Maes, Michael, Ivana Mihaylova, and Jean-Claude Leunis. "Increased Serum IgA and IgM against LPS of Enterobacteria in Chronic Fatigue Syndrome (CFS): Indication for the Involvement of Gram-Negative Enterobacteria in the Etiology of CFS

and for the Presence of an Increased Gut–Intestinal Permeability." *Journal of Affective Disorders* 99, no. 1–3 (April 2007): 237–40. doi:10.1016/j.jad.2006.08.021.

61. Goebel, A., S. Buhner, R. Schedel, H. Lochs, and G. Sprotte. "Altered Intestinal Permeability in Patients with Primary Fibromyalgia and in Patients with Complex Regional Pain Syndrome." *Rheumatology* 47, no. 8 (April 2008): 1223–227. doi:10.1093/rheumatology/ken140.

62. "The Gut Microbiome and the Brain." *Journal of Medicinal Food*. Accessed January 9, 2017. https://www.ncbi.nlm.nih.gov/pubmed/25402818.

63. Julio-Pieper, M., J. A. Bravo, E. Aliaga, and M. Gotteland. "Review Article: Intestinal Barrier Dysfunction and Central Nervous System Disorders—A Controversial Association." *Alimentary Pharmacology & Therapeutics* 40, no. 10 (September 2014): 1187–1201. doi:10.1111/apt.12950.

64. Bischoff, Stephan C., Giovanni Barbara, Wim Buurman, Theo Ockhuizen, Jörg-Dieter Schulzke, Matteo Serino, Herbert Tilg, Alastair Watson, and Jerry M. Wells. "Intestinal Permeability—A New Target for Disease Prevention and Therapy." *BMC Gastroenterology*. 2014. Accessed January 9, 2017. https://www.ncbi.nlm.nih.gov/pmc/articles/PMC4253991/.

65. Bouchaud, Gregory, Paxcal Gourbeyre, Tiphaine Bihouée, Phillippe Aubert, David Lair, Marie-Aude Cheminant, Sandra Denery-Papini, Michel Neunlist, Antoine Magnan, and Marie Bodinier. "Consecutive Food and Respiratory Allergies Amplify Systemic and Gut but Not Lung Outcomes in Mice." *Journal of Agricultural and Food Chemistry* 63, no. 28 (July 2015): 6475-483. Doi:10.1021/acs.jafe.5b02338.

66. "Small Intestinal Transit, Absorption, and Permeability in Patients with AIDS with and without Diarrhoea." *Gut*. Accessed January 9, 2017. https://www.ncbi.nlm.nih.gov/pubmed/10369707.

67. Ludvigsson, Jonas F., Johan Reutfors, Urban Ösby, Anders Ekbom, and Scott M. Montgomery. "Coeliac Disease and Risk of Mood Disorders—A General Population-Based Cohort Study." *Journal of Affective Disorders* 99, no. 1–3 (April 2007): 117–26. doi:10.1016/j.jad.2006.08.032.

68. Ludvigsson, Jonas F., Urban Osby, Anders Ekbom, and Scott M. Montgomery. "Coeliac Disease and Risk of Schizophrenia and Other Psychosis: A General Population Cohort Study." *Scandinavian Journal of Gastroenterology* 42, no. 2 (January 2007): 179–85. doi:10.1080/00365520600863472.

69. Millward, C., M. Ferriter, S. Calver, and G. Connell-Jones. "Gluten- and Casein-free Diets for Autistic Spectrum Disorder." *Cochrane Database of Systematic Reviews*, April 2004. doi:10.1002/14651858.cd003498.pub2.

70. "Cognitive Impairment and Celiac Disease." *Archives of Neurology*. Accessed January 9, 2017. https://www.ncbi.nlm.nih.gov/pubmed/17030661.

71. Ludvigsson, Jonas F. "Small-Intestinal Histopathology and Mortality Risk in Celiac Disease." *JAMA* 302, no. 11 (September 2009): 1171. doi:10.1001/jama.2009.1320.

72. Punzi, John S., Martha Lamont, Diana Haynes, and Robert L. Epstein. "USDA Pesticide Data Program: Pesticide Residues on Fresh and Processed Fruit and Vegetables, Grains, Meats, Milk, and Drinking Water." *Outlooks on Pest Management* 16, no. 3 (June 2005): 131–37. doi:10.1564/16jun12.

73. Bernardo, D., J. A. Garrote, L. Fernandez-Salazar, S. Riestra, and E. Arranz. "Is Gliadin Really Safe for Non-Coeliac Individuals? Production of Interleukin 15 in Biopsy Culture from Non-Coeliac Individuals Challenged with Gliadin Peptides." *Gut* 56, no. 6 (June 2007): 889–90. doi:10.1136/gut.2006.118265.

74. "Food and Nutrition Sciences—SCIRP." Food and Nutrition Sciences—SCIRP. Accessed January 9, 2017. http://www.scirp.org/journal/fns/.

75. Punder, Karin De, and Leo Pruimboom. "The Dietary Intake of Wheat and Other Cereal Grains and Their Role in Inflammation." *Nutrients*. March 2013. Accessed January 9, 2017. http://www.ncbi.nlm.nih.gov/pmc/articles/PMC3705319/.

76. "Evidence That Intermittent, Excessive Sugar Intake Causes Endogenous Opioid Dependence." *Obesity Research*. Accessed January 9, 2017. http://www.ncbi.nlm.nih.gov/pubmed/12055324/.

77. Neuroreport, November 16, 2001; 12(16): 3549–52. Sugar stimulates the brain reward centers via the neurotransmitter dopamine like other addictive drugs.

78. "Added Sugar Intake and Cardiovascular Diseases Mortality among US Adults—Journals—NCBI." National Center for Biotechnology Information. Accessed January 9, 2017. https://www.ncbi.nlm.nih.gov/labs/articles/24493081/.

79. Swithers, Susan E. "Artificial Sweeteners Produce the Counterintuitive Effect of Inducing Metabolic Derangements." *Trends in Endocrinology & Metabolism* 24, no. 9 (September 2013): 431–41. doi:10.1016/j.tem.2013.05.005.

80. Schiffman, Susan S., and Kristina I. Rother. "Sucralose, A Synthetic Organochlorine Sweetener: Overview of Biological Issues." *Journal of Toxicology and Environmental Health, Part B* 16, no. 7 (October 2013): 399–451. doi:10.1080/10937404.2013.842523.

81. Abou-Donia, Mohamed B., Eman M. El-Masry, Ali A. Abdel-Rahman, Roger E. Mclendon, and Susan S. Schiffman. "Splenda Alters Gut Microflora and Increases Intestinal P-Glycoprotein and Cytochrome P-450 in Male Rats." *Journal of Toxicology and Environmental Health, Part A* 71, no. 21 (September 2008): 1415–29. doi:10.1080/15287390802328630.

82. Nettleton, J. A., P. L. Lutsey, Y. Wang, J. A. Lima, E. D. Michos, and D. R. Jacobs. "Diet Soda Intake and Risk of Incident Metabolic Syndrome and Type 2 Diabetes in the Multi-Ethnic Study of Atherosclerosis (MESA)." *Diabetes Care* 32, no. 4 (January 2009): 688–94. doi:10.2337/dc08-1799.

83. Suez, Jotham, Tal Korem, David Zeevi, Gili Zilberman-Schapira, Christoph A. Thaiss, Ori Maza, David Israeli, Niv Zmora, Shlomit Gilad, Adina Weinberger, Yael Kuperman, Alon Harmelin, Ilana Kolodkin-Gal, Hagit Shapiro, Zamir Halpern, Eran Segal, and Eran Elinav. "Artificial Sweeteners Induce Glucose Intolerance by Altering the Gut Microbiota." *Obstetrical & Gynecological Survey* 70, no. 1 (January 2015): 31–32. doi:10.1097/01.ogx.0000460711.58331.94.

84. Purohit, Vishnudutt, J. Christian Bode, Christiane Bode, David A. Brenner, Mashkoor A. Choudhry, Frank Hamilton, Y. James Kang, Ali Keshavarzian, Radhakrishna Rao, R. Balfour Sartor, Christine Swanson, and Jerrold R. Turner. "Alcohol, Intestinal Bacterial Growth, Intestinal Permeability to Endotoxin, and Medical Consequences: Summary of a Symposium." Alcohol (Fayetteville, NY). August 2008. Accessed January 9, 2017. https://www.ncbi.nlm.nih.gov/pmc/articles/PMC2614138/.

85. Azzouz, Abdelmonaim, Beatriz Jurado-Sánchez, Badredine Souhail, and Evaristo Ballesteros. "Simultaneous Determination of 20 Pharmacologically Active Substances in Cow's Milk, Goat's Milk, and Human Breast Milk by Gas Chromatography–Mass Spectrometry." *Journal of Agricultural and Food Chemistry* 59, no. 9 (May 2011): 5125–32. doi:10.1021/jf200364w.

86. Harkinson, Josh. "You're Drinking the Wrong Kind of Milk." Mother Jones. Accessed January 9, 2017. http://www.motherjones.com/environment/2014/03/a1-milk-a2-milk-america.

87. "How Glyphosate Worsens Modern Diseases." Mercola.com. Accessed January 9, 2017. http://articles.mercola.com/sites/articles/archive/2013/05/14/glyphosate.aspx.

88. Amit Dutta. "The Microbiome for Gastroenterologists." *Gastroenterology & Endoscopy News*. 2015; 66: 4.

89. Prudden, John F., and Leslie L. Balassa. "The Biological Activity of Bovine Cartilage Preparations." *Seminars in Arthritis and Rheumatism* 3, no. 4 (June 1974): 287–321. doi:10.1016/0049-0172(74)90003-1.

90. Samonina, G., L. Lyapina, G. Kopylova, V. Pastorova, Z. Bakaeva, N. Jeliaznik, S. Zuykova, and I. Ashmarin. "Protection of Gastric Mucosal Integrity by Gelatin and Simple Proline-Containing Peptides." *Pathophysiology* 7, no. 1 (April 2000): 69–73. doi:10.1016/s0928-4680(00)00045-6.

91. Hertzler, Steven R., and Shannon M. Clancy. "Kefir Improves Lactose Digestion and Tolerance in Adults with Lactose Maldigestion." *Journal of the American Dietetic Association* 103, no. 5 (May 2003): 582–87. doi:10.1053/jada.2003.50111.

92. Mandel, David R., Katy Eichas, and Judith Holmes. "Bacillus Coagulans: A Viable Adjunct Therapy for Relieving Symptoms of Rheumatoid Arthritis according to a Randomized, Controlled Trial." *BMC Complementary and Alternative Medicine* 10, no. 1 (January 2010). doi:10.1186/1472-6882-10-1.

93. Abedon, Stephen T., Sarah J. Kuhl, Bob G. Blasdel, and Elizabeth Martin Kutter. "Phage Treatment of Human Infections." *Bacteriophage* 1, no. 2 (March 2011): 66–85. doi:10.4161/bact.1.2.15845.

94. Guslandi, Mario, Patrizia Giollo, and Pier Alberto Testoni. "A Pilot Trial of Saccharomyces Boulardii in Ulcerative Colitis." *European Journal of Gastroenterology & Hepatology* 15, no. 6 (June 2003): 697–98. doi:10.1097/00042737-200306000-00017.

95. Castagliuolo, I., L. Valenick, M. Riegler, Jt Lamont, and C. Pothoulakis. "Saccharomyces Boulardii Protease Inhibits Clostridium Difficile Toxin a and B-induced Effects in Human Colonic Mucosa." *Gastroenterology* 114 (April 1998). doi:10.1016/s0016-5085(98)83862-6.

96. Buts, Jean-Paul, Nadine De Keyser, and Laurence De Raedemaeker. "Saccharomyces Boulardii Enhances Rat Intestinal Enzyme Expression by Endoluminal Release of Polyamines." *Pediatric Research* 36, no. 4 (October 1994): 522–27. doi:10.1203/00006450-199410000-00019.

97. Sanchez, Marina, Christian Darimont, Vicky Drapeau, Shahram Emady-Azar, Lionel Philippe, Corinne Ammon-Zuffrey, Jean Doré, and Angelo Tremblay. "Effect of Lactobacillus Rhamnosus CGMCC1.3724 Supplementation on Weight Loss and Maintenance in Obese Men and Women." *Canadian Journal of Diabetes* 37 (April 2013). doi:10.1016/j.jcjd.2013.03.270.

98. "Recent Developments in Prebiotics to Selectively Impact Beneficial Microbes and Promote Intestinal Health." Current Opinion in Biotechnology. Accessed January 9, 2017. http://www.ncbi.nlm.nih.gov/pubmed/25448231.

99. "Glutamine and Intestinal Barrier Function." Amino Acids. Accessed January 9, 2017. http://www.ncbi.nlm.nih.gov/pubmed/24965526.

100. Hulst, R. R. W. J. Van Der, M. F. Von Meyenfeldt, N. E. P. Deutz, P. B. Soeters, R. J. M. Brummer, B. K. Von Kreel, and J. W. Arends. "Glutamine and the Preservation of Gut Integrity." *The Lancet* 341, no. 8857 (May 1993): 1363–65. doi:10.1016/0140-6736(93)90939-e.

101. Catanzaro, Daniela, Serena Rancan, Genny Orso, Stefano Dall'Acqua, Paola Brun, Maria Cecilia Giron, Maria Carrara, Ignazio Castagliuolo, Eugenio Ragazzi, Laura Caparrotta, and Monica Montopoli. "Boswellia Serrata Preserves Intestinal Epithelial Barrier from Oxidative and Inflammatory Damage." *Plos One* 10, no. 5 (May 2015). doi:10.1371/journal.pone.0125375.

102. Katz, Uriel, Yehuda Shoenfeld, Varda Zakin, Yaniv Sherer, and Shaul Sukenik. "Scientific Evidence of the Therapeutic Effects of Dead Sea Treatments: A Systematic Review." *Seminars in Arthritis and Rheumatism* 42, no. 2 (October 2012): 186–200. doi:10.1016/j.semarthrit.2012.02.006.

103. Wegienka, G., C. C. Johnson, S. Havstad, D. R. Ownby, C. Nicholas, and E. M. Zoratti. "Lifetime Dog and Cat Exposure and Dog- and Cat-Specific Sensitization at Age 18 Years." *Clinical & Experimental Allergy* 41, no. 7 (June 2011): 979–86. doi:10.1111/j.1365-2222.2011.03747.x.

Notes: Nutrition

1. Shoelson, Steven E., Jongsoon Lee, and Allison B. Goldfine. "Inflammation and Insulin Resistance." *Journal of Clinical Investigation.* July 3, 2006. Accessed January 9, 2017. http://www.ncbi.nlm.nih.gov/pmc/articles/PMC1483173/.

2. "Acute Psychological Stress Results in the Rapid Development of Insulin Resistance." *The Journal of Endocrinology.* Accessed January 9, 2017. http://www.ncbi.nlm.nih.gov/pubmed/23444388.

3. Paolisso, G. "Hypertension, Diabetes Mellitus, and Insulin Resistance: The Role of Intracellular Magnesium." *American Journal of Hypertension* 10, no. 3 (March 1997): 346–55. doi:10.1016/s0895-7061(96)00342-1.

4. "Prediabetes." Centers for Disease Control and Prevention. December 28, 2016. Accessed January 9, 2017. http://www.cdc.gov/diabetes/basics/prediabetes.html.

5. "Metabolic and Physiologic Effects from Consuming a Hunter-gatherer (Paleolithic)-type Diet in Type 2 Diabetes." *European Journal of Clinical Nutrition.* Accessed January 9, 2017. https://www.ncbi.nlm.nih.gov/pubmed/25828624.

6. Alcock, Joe, Carlo C. Maley, and C. Athena Aktipis. "Is Eating Behavior Manipulated by the Gastrointestinal Microbiota? Evolutionary Pressures and Potential Mechanisms." *BioEssays* 36, no. 10 (August 2014): 940–49. doi:10.1002/bies.201400071.

7. "Adults Meeting Fruit and Vegetable Intake Recommendations—United States, 2013." Centers for Disease Control and Prevention. July 10, 2015. Accessed January 9, 2017. http://www.cdc.gov/mmwr/preview/mmwrhtml/mm6426a1.htm.

8. "Fruit and Vegetable Consumption and Its Relation to Markers of Inflammation and Oxidative Stress in Adolescents." *Journal of the American Dietetic Association.* Accessed January 9, 2017. http://www.ncbi.nlm.nih.gov/pubmed/19248856.

9. "2,4,5-trimethoxybenzaldehyde, a Bitter Principle in Plants, Suppresses Adipogenesis through the Regulation of ERK1." *Journal of Agricultural and Food Chemistry.* Accessed January 9, 2017. http://www.ncbi.nlm.nih.gov/pubmed/25222709.

10. "Insulin Release: The Receptor Hypothesis." Diabetologia. Accessed January 9, 2017. http://www.ncbi.nlm.nih.gov/pubmed/24700279.

11. "Oral Dose of Citrus Peel Extracts Promotes Wound Repair in Diabetic Rats." *Pakistan Journal of Biological Sciences: PJBS.* Accessed January 9, 2017. http://www.ncbi.nlm.nih.gov/pubmed/24506007.

12. Choi, In Hwa, Jeong Sook Noh, Ji-Sook Han, Hyun Ju Kim, Eung-Soo Han, and Yeong Ok Song. "Kimchi, a Fermented Vegetable, Improves Serum Lipid Profiles in Healthy Young Adults: Randomized Clinical Trial." *Journal of Medicinal Food* 16, no. 3 (March 2013): 223–29. doi:10.1089/jmf.2012.2563.

13. Sun, P., J. Q. Wang, and H. T. Zhang. "Effects of Bacillus Subtilis Natto on Performance and Immune Function of Preweaning Calves." *Journal of Dairy Science* 93, no. 12 (December 2010): 5851–55. doi:10.3168/jds.2010-3263.

14. Lindequist, Ulrike, Timo H. J. Niedermeyer, and Wolf-Dieter Jülich. "The Pharmacological Potential of Mushrooms." *Evidence-Based Complementary and Alternative Medicine* 2, no. 3 (2005): 285–99. doi:10.1093/ecam/neh107.

15. "Increased Lean Red Meat Intake Does Not Elevate Markers of Oxidative Stress and Inflammation in Humans." *The Journal of Nutrition.* Accessed January 9, 2017. https://www.ncbi.nlm.nih.gov/pubmed/17237312.

16. Simopoulos, Artemis P. "Omega-3 Fatty Acids in Inflammation and Autoimmune Diseases." *Journal of the American College of Nutrition* 21, no. 6 (December 2002): 495–505. doi:10.1080/07315724.2002.10719248.

17. Mutungi, Gisella, David Waters, Joseph Ratliff, Michael Puglisi, Richard M. Clark, Jeff S. Volek, and Maria Luz Fernandez. "Eggs Distinctly Modulate Plasma Carotenoid and Lipoprotein Subclasses in Adult Men Following a Carbohydrate-restricted Diet." *The Journal of Nutritional Biochemistry* 21, no. 4 (April 2010): 261–67. doi:10.1016/j.jnutbio.2008.12.011.

18. Duckett, S. K., J. P. S. Neel, J. P. Fontenot, and W. M. Clapham. "Effects of Winter Stocker Growth Rate and Finishing System On: III. Tissue Proximate, Fatty Acid, Vitamin, and Cholesterol Content." *Journal of Animal Science* 87, no. 9 (June 2009): 2961–70. doi:10.2527/jas.2009-1850.

19. "Prediabetes." Centers for Disease Control and Prevention. December 28, 2016. Accessed January 9, 2017. http://www.cdc.gov/diabetes/basics/prediabetes.html.

20. "Red Meat from Animals Offered a Grass Diet Increases Plasma and Platelet N-3 PUFA in Healthy Consumers." *The British Journal of Nutrition.* Accessed January 9, 2017. http://www.ncbi.nlm.nih.gov/pubmed/20807460.

21. "Human Health Benefits of Vaccenic Acid." *Applied Physiology, Nutrition, and Metabolism = Physiologie Appliquee, Nutrition Et Metabolisme*. Accessed January 9, 2017. http://www.ncbi.nlm.nih.gov/pubmed/19935865.

22. Margioris, Andrew N. "Fatty Acids and Postprandial Inflammation." *Current Opinion in Clinical Nutrition and Metabolic Care* 12, no. 2 (March 2009): 129–37. doi:10.1097/mco.0b013e3283232a11.

23. Gardner, Christopher D., Alexandre Kiazand, Sofiya Alhassan, Soowon Kim, Randall S. Stafford, Raymond R. Balise, Helena C. Kraemer, and Abby C. King. "Comparison of the Atkins, Zone, Ornish, and LEARN Diets for Change in Weight and Related Risk Factors Among Overweight Premenopausal Women. The A to Z Weight Loss Study: A Randomized Trial." *Obstetrical & Gynecological Survey* 62, no. 7 (July 2007): 454–56. doi:10.1097/01.ogx.0000269084.43998.38.

24. "Association of Dietary, Circulating, and Supplement Fatty Acids with Coronary Risk: A Systematic Review and Meta-analysis." Association of Dietary, Circulating, and Supplement Fatty Acids with Coronary Risk A Systematic Review and Meta-analysis A Systematic Review and Meta-analysis | Annals of Internal Medicine | American College of Physicians. March 18, 2014. Accessed January 9, 2017. http://annals.org/aim/article/1846638/association-dietary-circulating-supplement-fatty-acids-coronary-risk-systematic-review.

25. Hämäläinen, E., H. Adlercreutz, P. Puska, and P. Pietinen. "Diet and Serum Sex Hormones in Healthy Men." *Journal of Steroid Biochemistry* 20, no. 1 (January 1984): 459–64. doi:10.1016/0022-4731(84)90254-1.

26. Hession, M., C. Rolland, U. Kulkarni, A. Wise, and J. Broom. "Systematic Review of Randomized Controlled Trials of Low-carbohydrate vs. Low-fat/low-calorie Diets in the Management of Obesity and Its Comorbidities." *Obesity Reviews* 10, no. 1 (January 2009): 36–50. doi:10.1111/j.1467-789x.2008.00518.x.

27. Lawrence, G. D. "Dietary Fats and Health: Dietary Recommendations in the Context of Scientific Evidence." *Advances in Nutrition: An International Review Journal* 4, no. 3 (May 2013): 294–302. doi:10.3945/an.113.003657.

28. Volk, Brittanie M., Laura J. Kunces, Daniel J. Freidenreich, Brian R. Kupchak, Catherine Saenz, Juan C. Artistizabal, Maria Luz Fernandez, Richard S. Bruno, Carl M. Maresh, William J. Kraemer, Stephen D. Phinney, and Jeff S. Volek. "Effects of Step-Wise Increases in Dietary Carbohydrate on Circulating Saturated Fatty Acids and Palmitoleic Acid in Adults with Metabolic Syndrome." *PLoS ONE* 9, no. 11 (November 2014). doi:10.1371/journal.pone.0113605.

29. Ameer, Fatima, Lisa Scandiuzzi, Shahida Hasnain, Hubert Kalbacher, and Nousheen Zaidi. "De Novo Lipogenesis in Health and Disease." *Metabolism* 63, no. 7 (July 2014): 895–902. doi:10.1016/j.metabol.2014.04.003.

30. Nickols-Richardson, Sharon M., Mary Dean Coleman, Joanne J. Volpe, and Kathy W. Hosig. "Perceived Hunger Is Lower and Weight Loss Is Greater in Overweight Premenopausal Women Consuming a Low-Carbohydrate/High-Protein vs High-Carbohydrate/Low-Fat Diet." *Journal of the American Dietetic Association* 105, no. 9 (September 2005): 1433–37. doi:10.1016/j.jada.2005.06.025.

31. "Flaxseed Oil." University of Maryland Medical Center. Accessed January 9, 2017. http://umm.edu/health/medical/altmed/supplement/flaxseed-oil.

32. Ogbolu, D. O., A. A. Oni, O. A. Daini, and A. P. Oloko. "In Vitro Antimicrobial Properties of Coconut Oil on Candida Species in Ibadan, Nigeria." *Journal of Medicinal Food* 10, no. 2 (June 2007): 384–87. doi:10.1089/jmf.2006.1209.

33. Bergsson, G., J. Arnfinnsson, O. Steingrimsson, and H. Thormar. "In Vitro Killing of Candida Albicans by Fatty Acids and Monoglycerides." *Antimicrobial Agents and Chemotherapy* 45, no. 11 (November 2001): 3209–12. doi:10.1128/aac.45.11.3209-3212.2001.

34. "The Serum LDL/HDL Cholesterol Ratio Is Influenced More Favorably by Exchanging Saturated with Unsaturated Fat Than by Reducing Saturated Fat in the Diet of Women." *The Journal of Nutrition*. Accessed January 9, 2017. https://www.ncbi.nlm.nih.gov/pubmed/12514271.

35. Lindeberg, Staffan, Mats Eliasson, Bernt Lindahl, and Bo Ahrén. "Low Serum Insulin in Traditional Pacific Islanders—The Kitava Study." *Metabolism* 48, no. 10 (October 1999): 1216–19. doi:10.1016/s0026-0495(99)90258-5.

36. "Dietary Intake and the Risk of Coronary Heart Disease among the Coconut-Consuming Minangkabau in West Sumatra, Indonesia." *Asia Pacific Journal of Clinical Nutrition*. Accessed January 9, 2017. https://www.ncbi.nlm.nih.gov/pubmed/15563444.

37. Boon, Chee-Meng, Mei-Han Ng, Yuen-May Choo, and Shiueh-Lian Mok. "Super, Red Palm and Palm Oleins Improve the Blood Pressure, Heart Size, Aortic Media Thickness and Lipid Profile in Spontaneously Hypertensive Rats." *PLoS ONE* 8, no. 2 (February 2013). doi:10.1371/journal.pone.0055908.

38. Fattore, E., C. Bosetti, F. Brighenti, C. Agostoni, and G. Fattore. "Palm Oil and Blood Lipid-Related Markers of Cardiovascular Disease: A Systematic Review and Meta-analysis of Dietary Intervention Trials." *American Journal of Clinical Nutrition* 99, no. 6 (April 2014): 1331–50. doi:10.3945/ajcn.113.081190.

39. "Palm Oil and the Heart: A Review." *World Journal of Cardiology*. Accessed January 9, 2017. https://www.ncbi.nlm.nih.gov/pubmed/25810814.

40. Covas, María-Isabel. "The Effect of Polyphenols in Olive Oil on Heart Disease Risk Factors." *Annals of Internal Medicine* 145, no. 5 (September 2006): 333. doi:10.7326/0003-4819-145-5-200609050-00006.

41. Elnagar, Ahmed, Paul Sylvester, and Khalid El Sayed. "(−)-Oleocanthal as a C-Met Inhibitor for the Control of Metastatic Breast and Prostate Cancers." *Planta Medica* 77, no. 10 (February 2011): 1013–19. doi:10.1055/s-0030-1270724.

42. Teres, S., G. Barcelo-Coblijn, M. Benet, R. Alvarez, R. Bressani, J. E. Halver, and P. V. Escriba. "Oleic Acid Content Is Responsible for the Reduction in Blood Pressure Induced by Olive Oil." *Proceedings of the National Academy of Sciences* 105, no. 37 (September 2008): 13811–16. doi:10.1073/pnas.0807500105.

43. Roos, Baukje De, Xuguang Zhang, Guillermo Rodriguez Gutierrez, Sharon Wood, Garry J. Rucklidge, Martin D. Reid, Gary J. Duncan, Louise L. Cantlay, Garry G. Duthie, and Niamh O'Kennedy. "Anti-platelet Effects of Olive Oil Extract: In Vitro Functional and Proteomic Studies." *European Journal of Nutrition* 50, no. 7 (January 2011): 553–62. doi:10.1007/s00394-010-0162-3.

44. "Nutrition and Atherosclerosis." *Archives of Medical Research*. Accessed January 9, 2017. https://www.ncbi.nlm.nih.gov/pubmed/26031780.

45. Romero, Concepción, Eduardo Medina, Julio Vargas, Manuel Brenes, and Antonio De Castro. "In Vitro Activity of Olive Oil Polyphenols against Helicobacter Pylori." *Journal of Agricultural and Food Chemistry* 55, no. 3 (February 2007): 680–86. doi:10.1021/jf0630217.

46. D'Imperio, Marco, Marco Gobbino, Antonio Picanza, Simona Costanzo, Anna Della Corte, and Luisa Mannina. "Influence of Harvest Method and Period on Olive Oil Composition: An NMR and Statistical Study." *Journal of Agricultural and Food Chemistry* 58, no. 20 (October 2010): 11043–51. doi:10.1021/jf1026982.

47. Givens, D. I. "Milk in the Diet: Good or Bad for Vascular Disease?" *Proceedings of the Nutrition Society* 71, no. 01 (October 2011): 98–104. doi:10.1017/s0029665111003223.

48. Watson, Stephen John, Gerald Bishop, Jack Cecil Drummond, Albert Edward Gillam, and Isidor Morris Heilbron. "The Relation of the Colour and Vitamin A Content of Butter to the Nature of the Ration Fed." *Biochemical Journal* 28, no. 3 (1934): 1076–85. doi:10.1042/bj0281076.

49. Organicvalley.coop. Accessed January 9, 2017. https://www.organicvalley.coop/products/butter/pasture-butter/pasture-butter-cultured-1-lb-4-quarters/.

50. Grosso, G., J. Yang, S. Marventano, A. Micek, F. Galvano, and S. N. Kales. "Nut Consumption on All-Cause, Cardiovascular, and Cancer Mortality Risk: A Systematic Review and Meta-analysis of Epidemiologic Studies." *American Journal of Clinical Nutrition* 101, no. 4 (February 2015): 783–93. doi:10.3945/ajcn.114.099515.

51. Hshieh, T. T., A. B. Petrone, J. M. Gaziano, and L. Djousse. "Nut Consumption and Risk of Mortality in the Physicians' Health Study." *American Journal of Clinical Nutrition* 101, no. 2 (December 2014): 407–12. doi:10.3945/ajcn.114.099846.

52. Jenkins, David J. A., Julia M. W. Wong, Cyril W. C. Kendall, Amin Esfahani, Vivian W. Y. Ng, Tracy C. K. Leong, Dorothea A. Faulkner, Ed Vidgen, Gregory Paul, Ratna Mukherjea, Elaine S. Krul, and William Singer. "Effect of a 6-month Vegan Low-carbohydrate ('Eco-Atkins') Diet on Cardiovascular Risk Factors and Body Weight in Hyperlipidaemic Adults: A Randomised Controlled Trial." *BMJ Open* 4, no. 2 (February 2014). doi:10.1136/bmjopen-2013-003505.

53. Dhiman, T. R., S. H. Nam, A. L. Ure. "Factors Affecting Conjugated Linoleic Acid Content in Milk and Meat." *Crit Rev Food Sci Nutr.* 2005;45(6):463–82. https://www.ncbi.nlm.nih.gov/pubmed/16183568.

54. Jiang, Rui. "Nut and Peanut Butter Consumption and Risk of Type 2 Diabetes in Women." *Jama* 288, no. 20 (November 2002): 2554. doi:10.1001/jama.288.20.2554.

55. "Cognition: The New Frontier for Nuts and Berries." *The American Journal of Clinical Nutrition.* Accessed January 9, 2017. http://www.ncbi.nlm.nih.gov/pubmed/24871475.

56. Guasch-Ferré, Marta, Mònica Bulló, Miguel Ángel Martínez-González, Emilio Ros, Dolores Corella, Ramon Estruch, Montserrat Fitó, Fernando Arós, Julia Wärnberg, Miquel Fiol, José Lapetra, Ernest Vinyoles, Rosa Maria Lamuela-Raventós, Lluís Serra-Majem, Xavier Pintó, Valentina Ruiz-Gutiérrez, Josep Basora, and Jordi Salas-Salvadó. "Frequency of Nut Consumption and Mortality Risk in the PREDIMED Nutrition Intervention Trial." *BMC Medicine* 11, no. 1 (July 2013). doi:10.1186/1741-7015-11-164.

57. "Evidence for Anti-cancer Properties of Blueberries: A Mini-Review." Anticancer Agents in Medicinal Chemistry. Accessed January 9, 2017. http://www.ncbi.nlm.nih.gov/pubmed/23387969.

58. "Punicic Acid Is an Omega-5 Fatty Acid Capable of Inhibiting Breast Cancer Proliferation." *International Journal of Oncology*. Accessed January 9, 2017. http://www.ncbi.nlm.nih.gov/pubmed/20043077.

59. "Antiproliferative Effects of Pomegranate Extract in MCF-7 Breast Cancer Cells Are Associated with Reduced DNA Repair Gene Expression and Induction of Double Strand Breaks." *Molecular Carcinogenesis*. Accessed January 9, 2017. http://www.ncbi.nlm.nih.gov/pubmed/23359482.

60. Shukla, Meenakshi, Kalpana Gupta, Zafar Rasheed, Khursheed A. Khan, and Tariq M. Haqqi. "Bioavailable Constituents/Metabolites of Pomegranate (*Punica Granatum* L) Preferentially Inhibit COX2 Activity *ex Vivo* and IL-1beta-induced PGE2 Production in Human

61. "Clinical Investigation of the Acute Effects of Pomegranate Juice on Blood Pressure and Endothelial Function in Hypertensive Individuals." ARYA Atherosclerosis. Accessed January 9, 2017. http://www.ncbi.nlm.nih.gov/pubmed/24575134.

62. "Total Antioxidant Content of Alternatives to Refined Sugar." *Journal of the American Dietetic Association*. Accessed January 9, 2017. http://www.ncbi.nlm.nih.gov/pubmed/19103324.

63. "Neurological Effects of Honey: Current and Future Prospects." Evidence-based Complementary and Alternative Medicine: ECAM. Accessed January 9, 2017. http://www.ncbi.nlm.nih.gov/pubmed/24876885.

64. "Antioxidant Activity, Inhibition of Nitric Oxide Overproduction, and in Vitro Antiproliferative Effect of Maple Sap and Syrup from Acer Saccharum." *Journal of Medicinal Food*. Accessed January 9, 2017. http://www.ncbi.nlm.nih.gov/pubmed/20132041; "Canadian Forest Service Publications." Government of Canada, Natural Resources Canada, Canadian Forest Service. January 9, 2017. Accessed January 9, 2017. http://cfs.nrcan.gc.ca/publications?id=28297.

65. "Effects of Maple (Acer) Plant Part Extracts on Proliferation, Apoptosis and Cell Cycle Arrest of Human Tumorigenic and Non-tumorigenic Colon Cells." Phytotherapy Research: PTR. Accessed January 9, 2017. http://www.ncbi.nlm.nih.gov/pubmed/22147441; "Maple Polyphenols, Ginnalins A-C, Induce S- and G2/M-cell Cycle Arrest in Colon and Breast Cancer Cells Mediated by Decreasing Cyclins A and D1 Levels." *Food Chemistry*. Accessed January 9, 2017. http://www.ncbi.nlm.nih.gov/pubmed/23122108.

66. Yamamoto, T., K. Uemura, K. Moriyama, K. Mitamura, A. Taga. "Inhibitory Effect of Maple Syrup on the Cell Growth and Invasion of Human Colorectal Cancer Cells. *Oncol Rep*. April 2015; 33(4):1579–84. doi: 10.3892/or.2015.3777. Epub February 2, 2015. https://www.ncbi.nlm.nih.gov/pubmed/25647359.

67. "Polyphenolic Extract from Maple Syrup Potentiates Antibiotic Susceptibility and Reduces Biofilm Formation of Pathogenic Bacteria." *Applied and Environmental Microbiology*. Accessed January 9, 2017. http://www.ncbi.nlm.nih.gov/pubmed/25819960; "The Beneficial Effect of the Sap of Acer Mono in an Animal with Low-Calcium

Diet-Induced Osteoporosis-like Symptoms." The British Journal of Nutrition. Accessed January 9, 2017. http://www.ncbi.nlm.nih.gov/pubmed/18377679.

68. "Comparison of the Enhancement of Plasma Glucose Levels in Type 2 Diabetes Otsuka Long-Evans Tokushima Fatty Rats by Oral Administration of Sucrose or Maple Syrup." *Journal of Oleo Science*. Accessed January 9, 2017. http://www.ncbi.nlm.nih.gov/pubmed/24005018; "Changes in Plasma Glucose in Otsuka Long-Evans Tokushima Fatty Rats after Oral Administration of Maple Syrup." *Journal of Oleo Science*. Accessed January 9, 2017. http://www.ncbi.nlm.nih.gov/pubmed/25757438.

69. "Total Antioxidant Content of Alternatives to Refined Sugar." *Journal of the American Dietetic Association*. Accessed January 9, 2017. http://www.ncbi.nlm.nih.gov/pubmed/19103324.

70. "Organic Foods vs Supermarket Foods: Element Levels." Organic Foods vs Supermarket Foods: Element Levels. Accessed January 9, 2017. https://journeytoforever.org/farm_library/bobsmith.html.

71. Castro-Quezada, Itandehui, Almudena Sánchez-Villegas, Ramón Estruch, Jordi Salas-Salvadó, Dolores Corella, Helmut Schröder, Jacqueline Álvarez-Pérez, María Dolores Ruiz-López, Reyes Artacho, Emilio Ros, Mónica Bulló, María-Isabel Covas, Valentina Ruiz-Gutiérrez, Miguel Ruiz-Canela, Pilar Buil-Cosiales, Enrique Gómez-Gracia, José Lapetra, Xavier Pintó, Fernando Arós, Miquel Fiol, Rosa María Lamuela-Raventós, Miguel Ángel Martínez-González, and Lluís Serra-Majem. "A High Dietary Glycemic Index Increases Total Mortality in a Mediterranean Population at High Cardiovascular Risk." *PLoS ONE* 9, no. 9 (September 2014). doi:10.1371/journal.pone.0107968.

72. Samsel, Anthony, and Stephanie Seneff. "Glyphosate, Pathways to Modern Diseases II: Celiac Sprue and Gluten Intolerance." *Interdisciplinary Toxicology*. December 2013. Accessed January 9, 2017. http://www.ncbi.nlm.nih.gov/pmc/articles/PMC3945755/.

73. Punder, Karin De, and Leo Pruimboom. "The Dietary Intake of Wheat and Other Cereal Grains and Their Role in Inflammation." *Nutrients*. March 2013. Accessed January 9, 2017. http://www.ncbi.nlm.nih.gov/pmc/articles/PMC3705319/.

74. Santarelli, Raphaëlle, Fabrice Pierre, and Denis Corpet. "Processed Meat and Colorectal Cancer: A Review of Epidemiologic and Experimental Evidence." *Nutrition and Cancer* 60, no. 2 (March 2008): 131–44. doi:10.1080/01635580701684872.

75. "Home Use of Vegetable Oils, Markers of Systemic Inflammation, and Endothelial Dysfunction among Women." *The American Journal of Clinical Nutrition*. Accessed January 9, 2017. https://www.ncbi.nlm.nih.gov/pubmed/18842776.

76. Lerner, Aaron, and Torsten Matthias. "Changes in Intestinal Tight Junction Permeability Associated with Industrial Food Additives Explain the Rising Incidence of Autoimmune Disease." *Autoimmunity Reviews* 14, no. 6 (June 2015): 479–89. doi:10.1016/j.autrev.2015.01.009.

77. Cressey, Daniel. "Widely Used Herbicide Linked to Cancer." *Nature* (March 2015). doi:10.1038/nature.2015.17181.

78. "Trans Fat Leads to Weight Gain Even on Same Total Calories, Animal Study Shows." Wake Forest Baptist Health - Winston-Salem, North Carolina - Wake Forest Baptist, North Carolina. June 19, 2006. Accessed January 9, 2017. http://www.wakehealth.edu/News-Releases/2006/Trans_Fat_Leads_To_Weight_Gain_Even_on_Same_Total_Calories,_Animal_Study_Shows.htm.

79. "Shining the Spotlight on Trans Fats." *The Nutrition Source*. May 26, 2015. Accessed January 9, 2017. https://www.hsph.harvard.edu/nutritionsource/transfats/.

80. "A Real Killer: Trans Fat Causes Colon Cancer." *NaturalNews*. Accessed January 9, 2017. http://www.naturalnews.com/025960_fat_trans_colon.html.

81. Chajès, Véronique, Anne C. M. Thiébaut, Maxime Rotival, Estelle Gauthier, Virginie Maillard, Marie-Christine Boutron-Ruault, Virginie Joulin, Gilbert M. Lenoir, and Françoise Clavel-Chapelon. "Association between Serum Trans-monounsaturated Fatty Acids and Breast Cancer Risk in the E3N-EPIC Study." *American Journal of Epidemiology*. June 2008. Accessed January 9, 2017. https://www.ncbi.nlm.nih.gov/pmc/articles/PMC2679982/.

82. Ramsden, C. E., D. Zamora, B. Leelarthaepin, S. F. Majchrzak-Hong, K. R. Faurot, C. M. Suchindran, A. Ringel, J. M. Davis, and J. R. Hibbeln. "Use of Dietary Linoleic Acid for Secondary Prevention of Coronary Heart Disease and Death: Evaluation of Recovered Data from the Sydney Diet Heart Study and Updated Meta-analysis." *Bmj* 346, no. 3 (February 2013). doi:10.1136/bmj.e8707.

83. Patterson, E., R. Wall, G. F. Fitzgerald, R. P. Ross, and C. Stanton. "Health Implications of High Dietary Omega-6 Polyunsaturated Fatty Acids." *Journal of Nutrition and Metabolism* 2012 (2012): 1–16. doi:10.1155/2012/539426.

84. Simopoulos, A. P. "Importance of the Ratio of Omega-6/Omega-3 Essential Fatty Acids: Evolutionary Aspects." *World Review of Nutrition and Dietetics Omega-6/Omega-3 Essential Fatty Acid Ratio: The Scientific Evidence*, 2003, 1–22. doi:10.1159/000073788.

85. Ludwig, David S., and Walter C. Willett. "Three Daily Servings of Reduced-Fat Milk." *JAMA Pediatrics* 167, no. 9 (September 2013): 788. doi:10.1001/jamapediatrics.2013.2408.

86. Hertzler, Steven R., and Shannon M. Clancy. "Kefir Improves Lactose Digestion and Tolerance in Adults with Lactose Maldigestion." *Journal of the American Dietetic Association* 103, no. 5 (May 2003): 582–87. doi:10.1053/jada.2003.50111.

87. "Eat Wild—Super Natural." Eat Wild—Super Natural. Accessed January 9, 2017. http://www.eatwild.com/articles/superhealthy.html.

88. "Diets Containing High Amylose vs Amylopectin Starch: Effects on Metabolic Variables in Human Subjects." *The American Journal of Clinical Nutrition*. Accessed January 9, 2017. https://www.ncbi.nlm.nih.gov/pubmed/2644803.

89. Trinidad, Trinidad P., Anacleta S. Loyola, Aida C. Mallillin, Divinagracia H. Valdez, Faridah C. Askali, Joan C. Castillo, Rosario L. Resaba, and Dina B. Masa. "The Cholesterol-Lowering Effect of Coconut Flakes in Humans with Moderately Raised Serum Cholesterol." *Journal of Medicinal Food*. August 2004, 7(2): 136–40. https://doi.org/10.1089/1096620041224148.

90. Koehler, Peter, Georg Hartmann, Herbert Wieser, and Michael Rychlik. "Changes of Folates, Dietary Fiber, and Proteins in Wheat As Affected by Germination." *Journal of Agricultural and Food Chemistry* 55, no. 12 (June 2007): 4678–83. doi:10.1021/jf0633037.

91. Cortés-Giraldo, Isabel, Julio Girón-Calle, Manuel Alaiz, Javier Vioque, and Cristina Megías. "Hemagglutinating Activity of Polyphenols Extracts from Six Grain Legumes." *Food and Chemical Toxicology* 50, no. 6 (June 2012): 1951–54. doi:10.1016/j.fct.2012.03.071.

92. Sandberg, Ann-Sofie. "Bioavailability of Minerals in Legumes." *British Journal of Nutrition* 88, no. S3 (December 2002): 281. doi:10.1079/bjn/2002718.

93. "Genetics of Dietary Habits and Obesity—A Twin Study." *Danish Medical Bulletin.* Accessed January 9, 2017. https://www.ncbi.nlm.nih.gov/pubmed/20816022.

94. "The Implication of Vitamin D and Autoimmunity: A Comprehensive Review." *Clinical Reviews in Allergy & Immunology*. Accessed January 9, 2017. http://www.ncbi.nlm.nih.gov/pubmed/23359064.

95. Geiger, Helmut, and Christoph Wanner. "Magnesium in Disease." *Clinical Kidney Journal.* February 2012. Accessed January 9, 2017. http://www.ncbi.nlm.nih.gov/pmc/articles/PMC4455821/.

96. "Suboptimal Magnesium Status in the United States: Are the Health Consequences Underestimated?" *Nutrition Reviews*. Accessed January 9, 2017. http://www.ncbi.nlm.nih.gov/pubmed/22364157.

97. "The Multifaceted and Widespread Pathology of Magnesium Deficiency." Medical Hypotheses. Accessed January 9, 2017. http://www.ncbi.nlm.nih.gov/pubmed/11425281.

98. Efstratiadis, G., M. Sarigianni, and I. Gougourelas. "Hypomagnesemia and Cardiovascular System." *Hippokratia*. 2006. Accessed January 9, 2017. https://www.ncbi.nlm.nih.gov/pmc/articles/PMC2464251/.

99. Surette, M. E., J. Whelan, K. S. Broughton, and J. E. Kinsella. "Evidence for Mechanisms of the Hypotriglyceridemic Effect of N − 3 Polyunsaturated Fatty Acids." *Biochimica Et Biophysica Acta (BBA—Lipids and Lipid Metabolism)* 1126, no. 2 (June 1992): 199–205. doi:10.1016/0005-2760(92)90291-3.

100. "Omega-3 Fatty Acids." University of Maryland Medical Center. Accessed January 9, 2017. http://umm.edu/health/medical/altmed/supplement/omega3-fatty-acids.

101. *Nutr Cancer* (2010) 62:284–96; *Cancer Prev Res*. (2011) 2062-71; *Cancer* (2011); 117: 3774–80.

Notes: Detoxification

1. Meyer, Joel N., K. Leung, C. Maxwell, John P. Rooney, Ataman Sendoel, Michael O. Hengartner, Glen E. Kisby, and Amanda S. Bess. "Mitochondria as a Target of Environmental Toxicant." *Toxicol.Sci.* April 2013. doi: 10.1093/toxsci/kft102. http://toxsci.oxfordjournals.org/content/early/2013/05/22/toxsci.kft102.full.

2. Bitto, Alessandra, Gabriele Pizzino, Natasha Irrera, Federica Galfo, and Francesco Squadrito. "Epigenetic Modifications Due to Heavy Metals Exposure in Children Living in Polluted Areas." *Current Genomics*. December 2014. Accessed January 9, 2017. http://www.ncbi.nlm.nih.gov/pmc/articles/PMC4311390/.

3. Rice, Kevin M., Ernest M. Walker, Miaozong Wu, Chris Gillette, and Eric R. Blough. "Environmental Mercury and Its Toxic Effects." *Journal of Preventive Medicine and Public Health*. March 2014. Accessed January 9, 2017. http://www.ncbi.nlm.nih.gov/pmc/articles/PMC3988285/.

4. Hong, Young-Seoub, Ki-Hoon Song, and Jin-Yong Chung. "Health Effects of Chronic Arsenic Exposure." *Journal of Preventive Medicine and Public Health*. September 2014. Accessed January 9, 2017. http://www.ncbi.nlm.nih.gov/pmc/articles/PMC4186552/.

5. "Health Risk of Exposure to Bisphenol A (BPA)." *Roczniki Panstwowego Zakladu Higieny*. Accessed January 9, 2017. http://www.ncbi.nlm.nih.gov/pubmed/25813067.

6. "Toxic Effects of the Easily Avoidable Phthalates and Parabens." *Alternative Medicine Review: A Journal of Clinical Therapeutic*. Accessed January 9, 2017. http://www.ncbi.nlm.nih.gov/pubmed/21155623.

7. "Bactericidal Effects of Triclosan in Soap Both in Vitro and in Vivo." *The Journal of Antimicrobial Chemotherapy*. Accessed January 9, 2017. http://www.ncbi.nlm.nih.gov/pubmed/26374612.

8. http://www.accessdata.fda.gov/scripts/cdrh/cfdocs/cfcfr/cfrsearch.cfmfr=355.10, http://www.fluoridealert.org/wp-content/uploads/fda-2005a.pdf.

9. "Prevalence and Severity of Dental Fluorosis in the United States, 1999–2004." Centers for Disease Control and Prevention. November 8, 2010. Accessed January 9, 2017. http://www.cdc.gov/nchs/data/databriefs/db53.htm.

10. Grandjean, Phillippe, Philip J. Landrigan. "Neurobehavioral Effects of Developmental Toxicity." *The Lancet*. February 2014. http://dx.doi.org/10.1016/S1474-4422(13)70278-3. http://www.thelancet.com/journals/laneur/article/PIIS1474-4422(13)70278-3/abstract.

11. "Systemic versus Topical Fluoride." Caries Research. Accessed January 9, 2017. http://www.ncbi.nlm.nih.gov/pubmed/15153698.

12. "Blue-green Algae." Memorial Sloan Kettering Cancer Center. Accessed January 9, 2017. https://www.mskcc.org/cancer-care/integrative-medicine/herbs/blue-green-algae.

13. Morita, Kunimasa, Masahiro Ogata, and Takashi Hasegawa. "Chlorophyll Derived from Chlorella Inhibits Dioxin Absorption from the Gastrointestinal Tract and Accelerates Dioxin Excretion in Rats." *Environmental Health Perspectives* 109, no. 3 (March 2001): 289. doi:10.2307/3434698.

14. Soltani, M., A.-R. Khosravi, F. Asadi, and H. Shokri. "Evaluation of Protective Efficacy of Spirulina Platensis in Balb/C Mice with Candidiasis." *Journal De Mycologie Médicale / Journal of Medical Mycology* 22, no. 4 (December 2012): 329–34. doi:10.1016/j.mycmed.2012.10.001.

15. "Spirulina." University of Maryland Medical Center. Accessed January 9, 2017. http://umm.edu/health/medical/altmed/supplement/spirulina.

16. "The Average Woman Puts 515 Synthetic Chemicals on Her Body Every Day without Knowing." *The Huffington Post*. Accessed January 9, 2017. http://www.huffingtonpost.com/entry/synthetic-chemicals-skincare_us_56d8ad09e4b0000de403d995.

CHAPTER 3. THE BIG FOUR Ss: STRESS, SLEEP, SOCIAL HEALTH, AND SPIRITUALITY

Notes: Stress

1. "Linking Stress to Inflammation." Anesthesiology Clinics. Accessed January 9, 2017. http://www.ncbi.nlm.nih.gov/pubmed/16927932.

2. Kivimaki, M., D. A. Lawlor, A. Singh-Manoux, G. D. Batty, J. E. Ferrie, M. J. Shipley, H. Nabi, S. Sabia, M. G. Marmot, and M. Jokela. "Common Mental Disorder and Obesity: Insight from Four Repeat Measures over 19 Years: Prospective Whitehall II Cohort Study." *Bmj* 339, no. 2 (October 6, 2009). doi:10.1136/bmj.b3765.

3. Eriksson, A.-K., A. Ekbom, F. Granath, A. Hilding, S. Efendic, and C.-G. Stenson. "Psychological Distress and Risk of Pre-diabetes and Type2 Diabetes in a Prospective Study of Swedish Middle-aged Men and Women." *Diabetic Medicine* 25, no. 7 (July 2008): 834–42. doi:10.1111/j.1464-5491.2008.02463.x.

4. Vogelzangs, Nicole, Aartjan T. F. Beekman, Yuri Milaneschi, Stefania Bandinelli, Luigi Ferrucci, and Brenda W. J. H. Penninx. "Urinary Cortisol and Six-Year Risk of All-Cause and Cardiovascular Mortality." *The Journal of Clinical Endocrinology & Metabolism* 95, no. 11 (November 2010): 4959–64. doi:10.1210/jc.2010-0192.

5. Johansson, L., X. Guo, M. Waern, S. Ostling, D. Gustafson, C. Bengtsson, and I. Skoog. "Midlife Psychological Stress and Risk of Dementia: A 35-Year Longitudinal Population Study." *Brain* 133, no. 8 (May 2010): 2217–24. doi:10.1093/brain/awq116.

6. Kuper, Hannah, Ling Yang, Tores Theorell, and Elisabete Weiderpass. "Job Strain and Risk of Breast Cancer." *Epidemiology* 18, no. 6 (November 2007): 764–68. doi:10.1097/ede.0b013e318142c534.

7. Rai, Dheeraj, Kyriaki Kosidou, Michael Lundberg, Ricardo Araya, Glyn Lewis, and Cecilia Magnusson. "Psychological Distress and Risk of Long-Term Disability: Population-based Longitudinal Study." *Journal of Epidemiology and Community Health* 66, no. 7 (March 2011): 586–92. doi:10.1136/jech.2010.119644.

8. Aboa-Éboulé, Corine, Chantal Brisson, Elizabeth Maunsell, Benoît Mâsse, Renée Bourbonnais, Michel Vézina, Alain Milot, Pierre Théroux, and Gilles R. Dagenais. "Job Strain and Risk of Acute Recurrent Coronary Heart Disease Events." *JAMA* 298, no. 14 (October 2007): 1652. doi:10.1001/jama.298.14.1652.

9. "Acute Psychological Stress Results in the Rapid Development of Insulin Resistance." *The Journal of Endocrinology*. Accessed January 9, 2017. http://www.ncbi.nlm.nih.gov/pubmed/23444388.

10. "Psychosocial Stress Is Positively Associated with Body Mass Index Gain over 5 Years: Evidence from the Longitudinal AusDiab Study." Obesity (Silver Spring, MD). Accessed January 9, 2017. http://www.ncbi.nlm.nih.gov/pubmed/23512679.

11. Wellen, Kathryn E., and Gökhan S. Hotamisligil. "Inflammation, Stress, and Diabetes." *Journal of Clinical Investigation*. May 2, 2005. Accessed January 9, 2017. http://www.ncbi.nlm.nih.gov/pmc/articles/PMC1087185.

12. Alcock, Joe, Carlo C. Maley, and C. Athena Aktipis. "Is Eating Behavior Manipulated by the Gastrointestinal Microbiota? Evolutionary Pressures and Potential Mechanisms." *BioEssays* 36, no. 10 (August 2014): 940–49. doi:10.1002/bies.201400071.

13. Kelly, John R., Paul J. Kennedy, John F. Cryan, Timothy G. Dinan, Gerard Clarke, and Niall P. Hyland. "Breaking Down the Barriers: The Gut Microbiome, Intestinal Permeability and Stress-Related Psychiatric Disorders." *Frontiers in Cellular Neuroscience* 9 (October 2015). doi:10.3389/fncel.2015.00392.

14. Bested, Alison C., Alan C. Logan, and Eva M. Selhub. "Intestinal Microbiota, Probiotics and Mental Health: From Metchnikoff to Modern Advances: Part II—Contemporary Contextual Research." *Gut Pathogens* 5, no. 1 (2013): 3. doi:10.1186/1757-4749-5-3.

15. "Why Being Mindful Matters." Taking Charge of Your Health & Wellbeing. Accessed January 9, 2017.

16. Bercik, P., A. J. Park, D. Sinclair, A. Khoshdel, J. Lu, X. Huang, Y. Deng, P. A. Blennerhassett, M. Fahnestock, D. Moine, B. Berger, J. D. Huizinga, W. Kunze, P. G. Mclean, G. E. Bergonzelli, S. M. Collins, and E. F. Verdu. "The Anxiolytic Effect of Bifidobacterium Longum NCC3001 Involves Vagal Pathways for Gut-Brain Communication." *Neurogastroenterology & Motility* 23, no. 12 (October 2011): 1132–39. doi:10.1111/j.1365-2982.2011.01796.x.

17. "Ingestion of Lactobacillus Strain Regulates Emotional Behavior and Central GABA Receptor Expression in a Mouse via the Vagus Nerve." Proceedings of the National Academy of Sciences of the United States of America. Accessed January 9, 2017. http://www.ncbi.nlm.nih.gov/pubmed/21876150.

18. Schmidt, K., P. Cowen, C. J. Harmer, G. Tzortzis, and P. W. J. Burnet. "P.1.e.003 Prebiotic Intake Reduces the Waking Cortisol Response and Alters Emotional Bias in Healthy Volunteers." *European Neuropsychopharmacology* 24 (October 2014). doi:10.1016/s0924-977x(14)70294-9.

19. Campos-Rodríguez, Rafael, Marycarmen Godínez-Victoria, Edgar Abarca-Rojano, Judith Pacheco-Yépez, Humberto Reyna-Garfias, Reyna Elizabeth Barbosa-Cabrera, and Maria Elisa Drago-Serrano. "Stress Modulates Intestinal Secretory Immunoglobulin A." *Frontiers in Integrative Neuroscience*. 2013. Accessed January 9, 2017. http://www.ncbi.nlm.nih.gov/pmc/articles/PMC3845795/.

20. Vanuytsel, Tim, Sander Van Wanrooy, Hanne Vanheel, Christophe Vanormelingen, Sofie Verschueren, Els Houben, Shadea Salim Rasoel, Joran Tóth, Lieselot Holvoet, Ricard Farré, Lukas Van Oudenhove, Guy Boeckxstaens, Kristin Verbeke, and Jan Tack. "Psychological Stress and Corticotropin-Releasing Hormone Increase Intestinal Permeability in Humans by a Mast Cell-Dependent Mechanism." *Gut* 63, no. 8 (October 2013): 1293–99. doi:10.1136/gutjnl-2013-305690.

21. Vanuytsel, Tim, Sander Van Wanrooy, Hanne Vanheel, Christophe Vanormelingen, Sofie Verschueren, Els Houben, Shadea Salim Rasoel, Joran Tóth, Lieselot Holvoet, Ricard Farré, Lukas Van Oudenhove, Guy Boeckxstaens, Kristin Verbeke, and Jan Tack. "Psychological Stress and Corticotropin-Releasing Hormone Increase Intestinal Permeability in Humans by a Mast Cell-Dependent Mechanism." *Gut* 63, no. 8 (October 2013): 1293–99. doi:10.1136/gutjnl-2013-305690.

22. Hanson, Rick. "Relaxed and Contented: Activating the Parasympathetic Wave of Your Nervous System," Accessed January 9, 2017. http://www.wisebrain.org/ParasympatheticNS.pdf.

23. "Restoring the Balance of the Autonomic Nervous System as an Innovative Approach to the Treatment of Rheumatoid Arthritis." Molecular Medicine (Cambridge, MA). Accessed January 9, 2017. https://www.ncbi.nlm.nih.gov/pubmed/21607292.

24. "The Anti-inflammatory Effect of Exercise." *Journal of Applied Physiology* (Bethesda, MD: 1985). Accessed January 9, 2017. http://www.ncbi.nlm.nih.gov/pubmed/15772055.

25. Vina, J., F. Sanchis-Gomar, V. Martinez-Bello, and MC Gomez-Cabrera. "Exercise Acts as a Drug; The Pharmacological Benefits of Exercise." *British Journal of Pharmacology*. September 2012. Accessed January 9, 2017. http://www.ncbi.nlm.nih.gov/pmc/articles/PMC3448908/.

26. Khazaei, Majid. "Chronic Low-Grade Inflammation after Exercise: Controversies." *Iranian Journal of Basic Medical Sciences*. 2012. Accessed January 9, 2017. http://www.ncbi.nlm.nih.gov/pmc/articles/PMC3586919/.

27. Puri, Harsharnjit S. "Rasayana: Ayurvedic Herbs for Longevity and Rejuvenation: Volume 2 of Traditional Herbal Medicines for Modern Times." *The Journal of Alternative and Complementary Medicine* 9, no. 2 (April 2003): 331–32. doi:10.1089/107555303360623446.

Notes: Sleep

1. Mullington, Janet M., Norah S. Simpson, Hans K. Meier-Ewert, and Monika Haack. "Sleep Loss and Inflammation." *Best Practice & Research. Clinical Endocrinology & Metabolism*. October 2010. Accessed January 9, 2017. http://www.ncbi.nlm.nih.gov/pmc/articles/PMC3548567/.

2. Jackson, Melinda L., Ewa M. Sztendur, Neil T. Diamond, Julie E. Byles, and Dorothy Bruck. "Sleep Difficulties and the Development of Depression and Anxiety: A Longitudinal Study of Young Australian Women." *Archives of Women's Mental Health* 17, no. 3 (March 2014): 189–98. doi:10.1007/s00737-014-0417-8.

3. "News & Events." Sleep Deprivation Doubles Risks of Obesity in Both Children and Adults. Accessed January 9, 2017. http://www2.warwick.ac.uk/newsandevents/pressreleases/ne100000021440/.

4. Patel, S. R., A. Malhotra, D. P. White, D. J. Gottlieb, and F. B. Hu. "Association between Reduced Sleep and Weight Gain in Women." *American Journal of Epidemiology* 164, no. 10 (September 2006): 947–54. doi:10.1093/aje/kwj280.

5. "Sleep Your Way to a Slimmer Body." *New Scientist*. Accessed January 9, 2017. https://www.newscientist.com/article/mg19025535-600-sleep-your-way-to-a-slimmer-body/

6. Känel, Roland Von, José S. Loredo, Sonia Ancoli-Israel, Paul J. Mills, Loki Natarajan, and Joel E. Dimsdale. "Association between Polysomnographic Measures of Disrupted Sleep and Prothrombotic Factors." *Chest* 131, no. 3 (March 2007): 733–39. doi:10.1378/chest.06-2006.

7. "Sleep Deprivation: Treatments—National Library of Medicine—PubMed Health." National Center for Biotechnology Information. Accessed January 9, 2017. http://www.ncbi.nlm.nih.gov/pubmedhealth/PMHT0023523/.

Notes: Social Health

1. "Oxytocin Revisited: Its Role in Cardiovascular Regulation.—PubMed—NCBI." National Center for Biotechnology Information. Accessed January 9, 2017. http://www.ncbi.nlm.nih.gov/m/pubmed/21981277/.

2. Kearns, Ade, Elise Whitley, Carol Tannahill, and Anne Ellaway. "Loneliness, Social Relations and Health and Wellbeing in Deprived Communities." *Psychology, Health & Medicine*. 2015. Accessed January 9, 2017. http://www.ncbi.nlm.nih.gov/pmc/articles/PMC4697361/.

3. "Psychological Distress and Salivary Secretory Immunity." *Brain, Behavior, and Immunity*. Accessed January 9, 2017. http://www.ncbi.nlm.nih.gov/pubmed/26318411.

Notes: Spirituality

1. "Short-term Meditation Increases Blood Flow in Anterior Cingulate Cortex and Insula.—PubMed—NCBI." National Center for Biotechnology Information. Accessed January 9, 2017. http://www.ncbi.nlm.nih.gov/m/pubmed/25767459/.

2. "Decrease in Blood Pressure and Improved Psychological Aspects through Meditation Training in Hypertensive Older Adults: A Randomized Control Study.—PubMed—NCBI." National Center for Biotechnology Information. Accessed January 9, 2017. http://www.ncbi.nlm.nih.gov/m/pubmed/25407688/.

3. "NCCIH." National Institutes of Health. May 24, 2016. Accessed January 9, 2017. https://nccih.nih.gov/health/meditation/overview.htm.

4. "Regulation of Gene Expression by Yoga, Meditation and Related Practices: A Review of Recent Studies.—PubMed—NCBI." National Center for Biotechnology Information. Accessed January 9, 2017. http://www.ncbi.nlm.nih.gov/m/pubmed/23380323/.

5. "Mindfulness Meditation and the Immune System: A Systematic Review of Randomized Controlled Trials.—PubMed—NCBI." National Center for Biotechnology Information. Accessed January 9, 2017. http://www.ncbi.nlm.nih.gov/m/pubmed/26799456/.

6. Publications, Harvard Health. "In Praise of Gratitude." *Harvard Health*. Accessed January 9, 2017. http://www.health.harvard.edu/newsletter_article/in-praise-of-gratitude.

7. "The Role of Gratitude in Spiritual Well-being in Asymptomatic Heart Failure Patients.—PubMed—NCBI." National Center for Biotechnology Information. Accessed January 9, 2017. http://www.ncbi.nlm.nih.gov/m/pubmed/26203459/.

8. "Forever Young(er): Potential Age-defying Effects of Long-term Meditation on Gray Matter Atrophy." *Frontiers*. Accessed January 9, 2017. http://journal.frontiersin.org/article/10.3389/fpsyg.2014.01551/full.

9. Breweral, Judson A., Patrick D. Worhunskya, Jeremy R. Grayb, Yi-Yuan Tangc, and And Jochen Weberd. "Judson A. Brewer." Proceedings of the National Academy of Sciences. Accessed January 9, 2017. http://www.pnas.org/content/108/50/20254.short.

10. MPH, Madhav Goyal MD. "Meditation for Psychological Stress and Well-being." Meditation for Psychological Stress and Well-being | Complementary and Alternative Medicine | JAMA Internal Medicine | The JAMA Network. March 1, 2014. Accessed January 9, 2017. http://archinte.jamanetwork.com/article.aspx?articleid=1809754.

11. Zeidan, Fadel, Katherine T. Martucci, Robert A. Kraft, John G. McHaffie, and Robert C. Coghill. "Neural Correlates of Mindfulness Meditation-Related Anxiety Relief." Social Cognitive and Affective Neuroscience | Oxford Academic. May 21, 2013. Accessed January 9, 2017. http://scan.oxfordjournals.org/content/9/6/751.short.

12. "Sign In: Registered Users." SAGE Journals: Your Gateway to World-Class Journal Research. Accessed January 9, 2017. http://pss.sagepub.com/content/24/5/776.

Bibliography

Abaci, Peter. *Take Charge of Your Chronic Pain: The Latest Research, Cutting-edge Tools, and Alternative Treatments for Feeling Better.* Guilford, CT: GPP Life, 2010.

Abel, Robert. *The Eye Care Revolution: Prevent and Reverse Common Vision Problems.* New York, NY: Kensington Books, 2014.

Amen, Daniel G. *Healing ADD: The Breakthrough Program That Allows You to See and Heal the Six Types of Attention Deficit Disorder.* New York: G.P. Putnam's Sons, 2001.

Andrews, Synthia, and Bobbi Dempsey. *Acupressure & Reflexology for Dummies.* Hoboken, NJ: Wiley, 2007.

Axe, Josh. *Eat Dirt: Why Leaky Gut May Be the Root Cause of Your Health Problems and 5 Surprising Steps to Cure It.* New York: Harper Wave, an Imprint of HarperCollinsPublishers, 2016.

Balch, James F., Mark Stengler, and Robin Young-Balch. *Prescription for Natural Cures: A Self-care Guide for Treating Health Problems with Natural Remedies Including Diet, Nutrition, Supplements, and Other Holistic Methods.* Hoboken, NJ: Wiley, 2011.

Ballantyne, Sarah. *The Paleo Approach: Reverse Autoimmune Disease and Heal Your Body.* Las Vegas: Victory Belt Publishing, 2013.

Bauer, Brent A., Philip T. Hagen, and Martha Millman. *Mayo Clinic Book of Alternative Medicine & Home Remedies.* New York: Time Home Entertainment, 2013.

Bock, Kenneth, Cameron Stauth, and Korri Fink. *Healing the New Childhood Epidemics: Autism, ADHD, Asthma, and Allergies: The Groundbreaking Program for the 4-A Disorders.* New York: Ballantine Books, 2007.

Bollinger, Ty M. *The Truth about Cancer: What You Need to Know about Cancer's History, Treatment, and Prevention.* Carlsbad, CA: Hay House, 2016.

Brady, David M. *The Fibro Fix: Get to the Root of Your Fibromyalgia and Start Reversing Your Chronic Pain and Fatigue in 21 Days.* Emmaus, PA: Rodale Books, 2016.

Brogan, Kelly, and Kristin Loberg. *A Mind of Your Own: The Truth about Depression and How Women Can Heal Their Bodies to Reclaim Their Lives: Featuring a 30-day Plan for Transformation.* New York: Harper Wave, 2016.

Campbell, Thomas M. *The Campbell Plan: The Simple Way to Lose Weight and Reverse Illness, Using the China Study's Whole-Food, Plant-Based Diet.* Emmaus, PA: Rodale Books, 2015.

Campbell-McBride, Natasha. *Gut and Psychology Syndrome: Natural Treatment for Autism, Dyspraxia, A.D.D., Dyslexia, A.D.H.D., Depression, Schizophrenia.* Cambridge, UK: Medinform Pub., 2010.

Challa, Shekhar. *Probiotics for Dummies.* Hoboken, NJ: Wiley, 2012.

Chutkan, Robynne. *Gutbliss: A 10-Day Plan to Ban Bloat, Flush Toxins, and Dump Your Digestive Baggage.* New York: Avery, A Member of Penguin Group (USA), 2013.

Chutkan, Robynne. *The Microbiome Solution: A Radical New Way to Heal Your Body from the Inside Out.* New York: Avery, an Imprint of Penguin Random House, 2015.

Curtis, Susan, Pat Thomas, and Fran Johnson. *Essential Oils: All-Natural Remedies and Recipes for Your Mind, Body, and Home.* New York: DK Publishing, 2016.

Dalet, Roger. *The Encyclopedia of Healing Points: The Home Guide to Acupoint Treatment.* Rochester, VT: Healing Arts Press, 2010.

Diana, Richard. *Healthy Joints for Life: An Orthopedic Surgeon's Proven Plan to Reduce Pain and Inflammation, Avoid Surgery, and Get Moving Again.* Don Mills, Ontario: Harlequin, 2013.

Ditchek, Stuart H., Russell H. Greenfield, and Lynn Murray Willeford. *Healthy Child, Whole Child: Integrating the Best of Conventional and Alternative Medicine to Keep Your Kids Healthy.* New York: William Morrow, 2009.

Dog, Tieraona Low. *Fortify Your Life: Your Guide to Vitamins, Minerals, and More.* Washington, DC: National Geographic, 2016.

Fung, Jason. *The Obesity Code: Unlocking the Secrets of Weight Loss.* Vancouver: Greystone Books, 2016.

Gaynor, Mitchell L. *The Gene Therapy Plan: Taking Control of Your Genetic Destiny with Diet and Lifestyle.* New York: Viking, 2015.

Genzlinger, Kelly, Kathy Erlich, and David Brownstein. *Super Nutrition for Babies: The Right Way to Feed Your Baby for Optimal Health.* Beverly, MA: Fair Winds Press, 2012.

Goodman, Dennis. *Magnificent Magnesium: Your Essential Key to a Healthy Heart and More.* Garden City Park, NY: Square One Publishers, 2014.

Gottfried, Sara. *The Hormone Reset Diet: Heal Your Metabolism to Lose up to 15 Pounds in 21 Days.* New York: HarperOne, an Imprint of HarperCollinsPublishers, 2015.

Greenblatt, James. *Answers to Anorexia: A Breakthrough Nutritional Treatment That Is Saving Lives.* North Branch, MN: Sunrise River Press, 2010.

Hayfield, Robin. *Homeopathy: A Practical Guide: Simple Remedies for Natural Health.* England: Anness Publishing, 2013.

Herbert, Martha R., and Karen Weintraub. *The Autism Revolution: Whole-Body Strategies for Making Life All It Can Be.* New York: Ballantine Books, 2012.

Hyman, Mark. *Eat Fat, Get Thin: Why the Fat We Eat Is the Key to Sustained Weight Loss and Vibrant Health.* New York: Little, Brown and Company, 2016.

Hyman, Mark. *The Blood Sugar Solution 10-Day Detox Diet: Activate Your Body's Natural Ability to Burn Fat and Lose Weight Fast.* New York: Little, Brown and Company, 2014.

Hyman, Mark. *The Blood Sugar Solution: The Ultrahealthy Program for Losing Weight, Preventing Disease, and Feeling Great Now!* New York: Little, Brown and, 2012.

Jacoby, Richard, and Raquel Baldelomar. *Sugar Crush: How to Reduce Inflammation, Reverse Nerve Damage, and Reclaim Good Health.* New York: HarperWave, 2015.

Johnson, Rebecca L., and Steven Foster. *National Geographic Guide to Medicinal Herbs: The World's Most Effective Healing Plants.* Washington, DC: National Geographic, 2010.

Jouanny, Jacques. *Homeopathic Therapeutics: Possibilities in Chronic Pathology.* France: Editions Boiron, 1994.

Kahn, Joel. *The Whole Heart Solution: Halt Heart Disease Now with the Best Alternative and Traditional Medicine.* New York: Reader's Digest Association, 2013.

Kang, Shimi K. *The Dolphin Way: A Parent's Guide to Raising Healthy, Happy, and Motivated Kids—without Turning into a Tiger.* New York: Jeremy P. Tarcher, Penguin, 2014.

Kellman, Raphael. *The Microbiome Diet: The Scientifically Proven Way to Restore Your Gut Health and Achieve Permanent Weight Loss.* Boston: Da Capo Press, 2014.

Kemper, Kathi. *Mental Health, Naturally: The Family Guide to Holistic Care for a Healthy Mind and Body.* Elk Grove Village, IL: American Academy of Pediatrics, 2010.

Khayat, David, Nathalie Hutter-Lardeau, and France Carp. *The Anticancer Diet: Reduce Cancer Risk through the Foods You Eat.* New York: W.W. Norton & Company, 2015.

Kolster, Bernard C., and Astrid Waskowiak. *The Reflexology Atlas.* Rochester, VT: Healing Arts Press, 2005.

Kubiena, Gertrude, B. Sommer, and Dorothee Bergfeld. *Practice Handbook of Acupuncture.* Edinburgh: Churchill Livingstone/Elsevier, 2010.

Lancer, Harold, and Diane Reverand. *Younger: The Breakthrough Anti-aging Method for Radiant Skin and Total Rejuvenation.* New York: Grand Central Life & Style, 2014.

Lipman, Frank. *10 Reasons You Feel Old and Get Fat—And How You Can Stay Young, Slim, and Happy!* Carlsbad, CA: Hay House, 2016.

Lipski, Elizabeth. *Digestive Wellness: Strengthen the Immune System and Prevent Disease through Healthy Digestion.* Chicago: Contemporary, 2010.

Liptan, Ginevra. *The Fibromanual: A Complete Fibromyalgia Treatment Guide for You and Your Doctor.* New York: Ballantine Books, 2016.

Lockie, Andrew. *The Family Guide to Homeopathy: Symptoms and Natural Solutions.* New York: Simon & Schuster, 1993.

Maccaro, Janet C. *Natural Health Remedies: Your A-Z Blueprint for Vibrant Health.* Lake Mary, FL: Siloam, 2015.

Mars, Brigitte, and Chrystle Fiedler. *The Home Reference to Holistic Health & Healing: Easy-to-use Natural Remedies, Herbs, Flower Essences, Essential Oils, Supplements, and Therapeutic Practices for Health, Happiness, and Well-being.* Beverly, MA: Fair Winds Press, 2015.

Mars, Brigitte, and Chrystle Fiedler. *The Home Reference to Holistic Health & Healing: Easy-to-Use Natural Remedies, Herbs, Flower Essences, Essential Oils, Supplements, and Therapeutic Practices for Health, Happiness, and Well-being.* Beverly, MA: Fair Winds Press, 2015.

Masley, Steven, and Jonny Bowden. *Smart Fat: Eat More Fat, Lose More Weight, Get Healthy Now.* New York: HarperOne, an Imprint of HarperCollins Publishers, 2016.

McCarthy, Jenny, and Jerry Kartzinel. *Healing and Preventing Autism: A Complete Guide.* New York: Dutton, 2009.

Mercola, Joseph. *Effortless Healing: 9 Simple Ways to Sidestep Illness, Shed Excess Weight, and Help Your Body Fix Itself.* New York: Harmony Books, 2015.

Moline, Peg. *The Doctor's Book of Natural Health Remedies: Unlock the Power of Alternative Healing and Find Your Path Back to Health.* New York: Galvanized Brands, 2014.

Moyad, Mark A., and Janet Lee. *The Supplement Handbook: A Trusted Expert's Guide to What Works & What's Worthless for More than 100 Conditions.* Emmaus, PA: Rodale, 2014.

Murray, Michael T., and Joseph E. Pizzorno. *The Encyclopedia of Natural Medicine.* New York: Atria Books, 2012.

Myers, Amy. *The Autoimmune Solution: Prevent and Reverse the Full Spectrum of Inflammatory Symptoms and Diseases.* San Francisco: HarperOne, an Imprint of HarperCollinsPublsihers, 2015.

Myers, Amy. *The Thyroid Connection: Why You Feel Tired, Brain-Fogged, and Overweight—And How to Get Your Life Back.* New York: Little, Brown and Company, 2016.

Nagel, Ramiel. *Cure Tooth Decay: Heal & Prevent Cavities with Nutrition.* Los Gatos, CA: Golden Child Pub., 2009.

Null, Gary. *Reboot Your Brain: A Natural Approach to Fighting Memory Loss, Dementia, Alzheimer's, Brain Aging, and More.* New York: Gary Null Publishing, an Imprint of Skyhorse Publishing, 2013.

Perlmutter, David, and Kristin Loberg. *Brain Maker: The Power of Gut Microbes to Heal and Protect Your Brain—For Life.* New York: Little, Brown and Company, 2015.

Phelan, Thomas W. *Tantrums!: Managing Meltdowns in Public and Private.* Glen Ellyn, IL: ParentMagic, 2014.

Purchon, Nerys, Lora Cantele, and Tracy Bordian. *The Complete Aromatherapy & Essential Oils Handbook for Everyday Wellness.* Toronto, Ontario: Robert Rose, 2014.

Rhéaume-Bleue, Kate. *Vitamin K2 and the Calcium Paradox: How a Little-Known Vitamin Could Save Your Life.* Toronto: HarperCollins Canada, 2013.

Ring, Melinda. *The Natural Menopause Solution: Expert Advice for Melting Stubborn Midlife Pounds, Reducing Hot Flashes, and Getting Relief from Menopause Symptoms.* Emmaus, PA: Rodale, 2012.

Romm, Aviva. *Adrenal Thyroid Revolution: A Proven 4-Week Program to Rescue Your Metabolism, Hormones, Mind & Mood.* New York: HarperCollins, 2017.

Scott, Elizabeth Anne. *8 Keys to Stress Management: Simple and Effective Strategies to Transform Your Experience of Stress.* New York: W.W. Norton & Company, 2013.

Sears, Robert W., and William Sears. *The Allergy Book: Solving Your Family's Nasal Allergies, Asthma, Food Sensitivities, and Related Health and Behavioral Problems.* New York: Little, Brown & Company, 2015.

Shannon, Scott M., and Noah Gallagher. Shannon. *Mental Health for the Whole Child: Moving Young Clients from Disease & Disorder to Balance & Wellness*. New York: W.W. Norton & Company, 2013.

Shannon, Scott M., and Emily Heckman. *Parenting the Whole Child: A Holistic Child Psychiatrist Offers Practical Wisdom on Behavior, Brain Health, Nutrition, Exercise, Family Life, Peer Relationships, School Life, Trauma, Medication, and More*. New York: W.W. Norton & Company, 2013.

Shepherd, Sue, and P. R. Gibson. *The Complete Low-FODMAP Diet: A Revolutionary Plan for Managing IBS and Other Digestive Disorders*. New York: Experiment, 2013.

Shetreat-Klein, Maya, and Rachel Holtzman. *The Dirt Cure: Growing Healthy Kids with Food Straight from Soil*. New York, NY: Atria Books, 2016.

Sierpina, Victor S. *1000 Cures for 200 Ailments: Integrated Alternative and Conventional Treatments for the Most Common Illnesses*. New York: Collins, 2007.

Skowron, Jared. *100 Natural Remedies for Your Child: The Complete Guide to Safe, Effective Treatments for Childhood's Most Common Ailments, from Allergies to Weight Loss*. Emmaus, PA: Rodale Books, 2011.

Snyder, R. Bradley. *The 5 Simple Truths of Raising Kids: How to Deal with Modern Problems Facing Your Tweens and Teens*. New York: Demos Health, 2013.

Sollars, David. *The Complete Idiot's Guide to Acupuncture and Acupressure*. New York: Alpha Books, 2000.

Sood, Amit. *The Mayo Clinic Guide to Stress-Free Living*. Cambridge, MA: Da Capo Press/Lifelong Books, 2013.

Stengler, Mark, James F. Balch, Robin Young-Balch, and James F. Balch. *Prescription for Natural Cures: A Self-care Guide for Treating Health Problems with Natural Remedies Including Diet, Nutrition, Supplements, and Other Holistic Methods*. Nashville, TN: Turner Publishing Company, 2016.

Sunderland, Margot. *The Science of Parenting*. New York: Penguin Random House, 2016.

Teeguarden, Iona. *A Complete Guide to Acupressure—Jin Shin Do*. Tokyo: Japan Publications, 1996.

Teitelbaum, Jacob. *The Fatigue and Fibromyalgia Solution: The Essential Guide to Overcoming Chronic Fatigue and Fibromyalgia, Made Easy!* New York: Avery, a Member of Penguin Group (USA), 2013.

Teitelbaum, Jacob, and Bill Gottlieb. *Real Cause, Real Cure: The 9 Root Causes of the Most Common Health Problems and How to Solve Them*. Emmaus, PA: Rodale, 2011.

Teta, Jillian Sarno, and Jeannette Bessinger. *Natural Solutions for Digestive Health: Relief from the Most Common Problems Including: Acid Reflux, IBS, Gas, Constipation, Diarrhea, Crohn's Disease, Ulcers, Children's Digestive Issues, and More*. New York: Sterling Publishing, 2014.

Thompson, Rob. *The Sugar Blockers Diet Eat Great, Lose Weight: Eat Great, Lose Weight: A Doctor's 7-Step Plan to Lose Weight, Lower Blood Sugar, and Beat Diabetes—While Eating the Carbs You Love*. Emmaus, PA: Rodale, 2012.

Tick, Heather. *Holistic Pain Relief: Dr. Tick's Breakthrough Strategies to Manage and Eliminate Pain*. Novato, CA: New World Library, 2013.

Turner, Kelly A. *Radical Remission: Surviving Cancer against All Odds*. New York: HarperOne, 2014.

Wahls, Terry L., and Eve Adamson. *The Wahls Protocol: How I Beat Progressive MS Using Paleo Principles and Functional Medicine*. New York: Avery, a Member of Penguin Group (USA), 2014.

Warner, Wendy, and Kellyann Petrucci. *Boosting Your Immunity for Dummies*. Hoboken, NJ: John Wiley & Sons, 2013.

Weil, Andrew. *Spontaneous Happiness*. New York: Little, Brown and, 2011.

Wentz, Izabella. *Hashimoto's Protocol: A 90 Day Plan for Reversing Thyroid Symptoms and Getting Your Life Back*. New York: HarperCollins, 2017.

Wentz, Izabella, and Marta Nowosadzka. *Hashimoto's Thyroiditis: Lifestyle Interventions for Finding and Treating the Root Cause*. Lexington, KY: Wentz, LLC, 2013.

Wolfson, Jack. *The Paleo Cardiologist: The Natural Way to Heart Health*. New York: Morgan James Publishing, 2015.

Wu, Jessica. *Feed Your Face: Younger, Smoother Skin and a Beautiful Body in 28 Delicious Days*. New York: St. Martin's Press, 2011.

Your Guide to Reflexology: Relieve Pain, Reduce Stress, and Bring Balance to Your Life. Avon, MA: Adams Media, 2016.

Index

About the Author

Madiha M. Saeed, MD, ABIHM, is a board-certified integrative holistic family physician practicing in Illinois. She completed her residency in family medicine at St. Joseph Regional Medical Center, South Bend, Indiana. She received the Resident Teacher Award from the Society of Teachers of Family Medicine in 2010. She is a diplomate of the American Board of Integrative Holistic Medicine and holds a diploma in homeopathy from the Center for Education and Development of Clinical Homeopathy. Dr. Saeed has had numerous articles published in *Holistic Primary Care* magazine. She was featured in the Academy of Integrative Health and Medicine member spotlight titled "Walking the Talk: One Member Brings Holism Everywhere She Goes." She is the Director of Education for Documenting Hope, a national organization dedicated to healing chronic disease in children. She speaks and lectures nationally, igniting the world with her passion to educate and heal.